ACTS OF DEFIANCE

ACTS
OF DEFIANCE

———

Jack Ashley

REINHARDT BOOKS

IN ASSOCIATION WITH

VIKING

REINHARDT BOOKS
in association with Viking

Published by the Penguin Group
Penguin Books Ltd, 27 Wrights Lane, London w8 5tz, England
Penguin Books USA Inc., 375 Hudson Street, New York, New York 10014, USA
Penguin Books Australia Ltd, Ringwood, Victoria, Australia
Penguin Books Canada Ltd, 10 Alcorn Avenue, Toronto, Ontario, Canada m4v 3b2
Penguin Books (NZ) Ltd, 182–190 Wairau Road, Auckland 10, New Zealand

Penguin Books Ltd, Registered Offices: Harmondsworth, Middlesex, England

First published 1992
1 3 5 7 9 10 8 6 4 2

Typeset by DatIX International Limited, Bungay, Suffolk
Set in $10\frac{1}{2}$/13 pt Lasercomp Ehrhardt
Printed in England by Clays Ltd, St Ives plc

A CIP catalogue record for this book is available from the British Library

isbn 1–871–06131–8

TO PAULINE

AND MY FAMILY

CONTENTS

ILLUSTRATIONS

PREFACE

At a reception to mark my twenty-five years in Parliament, Neil Kinnock said, 'When I see "Mr and Mrs Jack Ashley, Companion of Honour", I know that Companion is in the plural.' That pithy and perceptive comment gave substance to a shadow. For throughout those years Pauline, while never seeking publicity for herself, played an outstanding role in our partnership.

She kept herself in the background partly because in the early years we were both uncertain as to whether I could remain as a totally deaf Member of Parliament. If I were to show reliance on her it could be misinterpreted as inability to do the job. It was also partly because, as the MP, I was the spokesman, and research work, however distinguished, is rarely acknowledged in public speeches and debates.

Pauline's work was of the highest quality and it fertilized all my Parliamentary activity including the campaigns. When I have written in the following pages that I tabled Parliamentary Questions, they were usually drafted by Pauline, as were many of my letters and speeches. Nor was it solely research that occupied her, because she often initiated ideas. It is no coincidence that much of my Parliamentary work concerned feminist issues such as the law on rape and battered wives. We also shared an anger against injustice which meant that we worked in harmony on subjects about which we both felt deeply.

With her clarity of mind and powers of concentration, Pauline would undoubtedly have made a success of any career she had chosen. I was fortunate that she chose to work for me; and I know she enjoyed and was fascinated by the issues that perpetually came our way.

It has been a remarkable contribution from the person without whom this book could not have been written and to whom it is dedicated.

ACKNOWLEDGEMENTS

I am grateful most of all to my wife Pauline, who corrected errors, remedied omissions and, like all good wives, generally pressed me to do better. My daughters and their partners gave me similar loving criticism from a more objective viewpoint. I am grateful to them.

Joe Haines cast his perceptive journalist's eye over my words and warmly encouraged me. He frowned on clichés and snapped at obfuscation.

Two good friends, Norman Howard and Maureen Chartres, read early drafts and made many valuable suggestions. My editor, Caroline Muir, sharpened my final scripts with precision and good humour, while my secretary Sue Hopper typed and retyped my words as quickly as I could write them. The House of Commons Library staff were, as always, extremely helpful.

My thanks to them all.

Jack Ashley was made a Peer
in June 1992

I

Childhood in Widnes

Widnes, where I was born in 1922, was an unlikely place for a happy childhood. A small industrial town squatting on the banks of the River Mersey, it was a citadel of the chemical industry, reeking with smoke and fumes. At the beginning of the century, as the factories were built, rows of small terraced houses went up alongside them. So there was no escape from the pungent smells which varied only with the wind. Yet, like everyone else, I assumed in my childhood that they were part of the natural order of things.

The main road through Widnes is now called Ashley Way, an honour which gives me disproportionate pleasure. Widnes is where my roots are and where I have always felt at home. As a child, I was acutely conscious of the industrial environment. In bed I often listened to the Liverpool–London express trains thundering over the Mersey Bridge a quarter of a mile from my home. The sound of their whistles fading in the distance, especially at night, trailed a melancholy note in contrast to the lively crack of shunted wagon-buffers in nearby factories. Every morning at 7.30, factory hooters, urgent and demanding, shrieked their strident instructions; when they signalled the working day's end at 5 p.m. they seemed oddly resigned.

Despite some pleasant localities, Widnes was mainly a poor, working-class town. Men who were employed in the 1920s and 1930s worked long, dirty hours. Those out of work were bored and often demoralized, dividing their time between dole queues and the street corners. But hardship creates its own comradeship, and the town's grace was its fine community spirit.

Number 34 Wellington Street, where I was born and reared, was a decrepit terraced house with a parlour, two bedrooms, kitchen and tiny scullery. It had no bathroom, and the lavatory was at the far end of the back yard. This was inadequate accommodation for one family, let alone for the two who lived there. My parents, two sisters and myself shared with my aunt's family of the same size. We had the parlour and front bedroom, while they lived in the kitchen and the other bedroom; both families cooked meals in the scullery and shared the lavatory. I was never conscious of feeling overcrowded when I was very young, though my parents must have felt it, with three children and only two rooms. My father was a labourer, and later a night-watchman, at ICI. He died of pneumonia when he was thirty-five. I was five years old at the time. A quiet and devout Catholic, he went regularly to early morning Mass even when seriously ill. Everyone seemed to have a high regard for him; from all accounts he was a generous man, which is often the way of those with little to give. As a night-watchman, he must have found it soul-destroying as well as health-destroying to spend so many hours walking around a dark, fume-laden factory.

The gravity of his illness was effectively concealed from his children, and his death came as a great shock. I remember being taken with my two sisters, Helen, seven, and Mary, three, to a nearby sweet shop the day he died. 'Your dad's dead; come and have a bag of sweets,' said our aunt. The stab of fear and insecurity sank deeply.

It must have been a much deeper wound for my mother. I learned years later that after he had been taken to Whiston Hospital, five miles away, the police called at our home a few days later and advised her to go immediately. This was a signal of impending death. Having no money for transport, she had to walk to the hospital, not knowing whether she would be in time to see him alive again. On that sad trek she knew, however, that she would have to bring up her children alone. In the mean days of the 1920s, this was a daunting prospect.

'Mam' was a small, quiet woman with soft, brown eyes reflecting a gentleness which remained unaffected by the vicissitudes of widowhood and poverty and the responsibility of bringing up a family on a tiny income of just over £1 a week. It was astonishing that so gentle a person could command the courage she displayed throughout such years. Fearful that the family would be broken up when my father died, she worked morning and night shifts scrubbing floors. She usually came home exhausted. When we went to the end of the street to meet her, as we often did, the sack she used as an apron was always soaking wet; I carried this symbol of her drudgery home for her.

One of Mam's jobs was cleaning in a public house. To her horror one day she knocked a bottle of white wine off a shelf and broke it. Afraid of the wrath of the landlord, she found an empty bottle and filled it with water as a replacement. It was probably the only piece of deception she ever carried out in the whole of her life. What a pity we never saw the face of the person who bought and drank the 'wine'.

Even in those early days, I was struck by people's attitudes to widows and their children. With a gush of initial sympathy everyone was helpful, but then, inevitably, they resumed their normal lives, and the widow was left to fend for herself as best as she could. As I grew older, I saw what loneliness meant to Mam when other families in the street had husbands and fathers around.

In our childish way, we were anxious to help, although there was very little we could do. Sometimes we bought her a great luxury – coconut iced cake costing a penny a slice. We used to buy it out of whatever pocket-money we had and we would hurry home eagerly with it. We probably gained more pleasure from the giving than she did from the eating, particularly as she always shared it among us. The gentle affection she lavished on us lightened the poverty of our lives, binding together our warm, close-knit family.

Our dependence on Mam was total, and I always feared that if she were to die we would be sent to an orphanage. Everyone felt sorry for the local orphans who played in a band at civic and social functions. Dressed alike in grey jerseys and dark short pants, they seemed robbed of their individuality. It never occurred to me that our shoddy clothes reflected an individuality which they would hardly envy. My feelings for Mam, although tinged with fear of the consequences if she were to die, were based on a deep love for her. Despite our poverty she gave us a happy childhood. Her quiet devotion, combined with a lively sense of fun, enriched my life. She lived until she was seventy-two, and today, many years after her death in 1969, I still feel a profound and incomparable sense of loss.

No doubt she was distressed by the conditions of our home, but I accepted them as I was young and knew nothing different. We had no electricity and, with a meter for payment, we relied on gaslight. The shout 'The gas is going!' was a signal for one of us to jump to the cupboard where a few pennies were stored. After the first flicker the gas faded quickly. If there were no pennies in stock – by no means unusual – the family groped around in darkness until a coin was found. No money meant no gaslight, and we settled for bleak candle-light. Sometimes the light would not return after inserting a penny, which meant that the gas pressure needed regulating. For a reason I never understood, filling a section of the meter with water usually solved the problem. If this did not work, we drained the water by unscrewing a stopper at the bottom and, the moment the light came on, replaced the stopper quickly.

Sometimes the gas mantle would begin to burn out, often after the shops were closed for the night. This meant sitting in half-light until bedtime. In the bedroom our only light was from a naked gas jet. Part of the natural order of things, it hardly made for easy living.

I went one day to meet Mam at the ICI offices, but as she hadn't finished the scrubbing, and no office staff were around, I wandered around the huge block. It was then I first discovered that electric lights could be magically flicked on and off with a switch. I had to be dragged away from the switches, then it was back to old-fashioned gaslight at home.

On cold days, Mam was exasperated when the fire would not light. It may have been due to lack of firewood, poor coal containing

(4)

too much slag or too many cinders. Later, when I was allowed to try, I learned the art of covering the entire grate with a newspaper to create a draught, then withdrawing it at the last split second as growing flames singed the paper. On rare occasions when the paper caught alight it would be flung on the fire and sucked up the chimney – with anxious warnings from Mam to 'be careful'.

Coal for the fire was bought from a merchant about a quarter of a mile away. Mam collected it herself, but when I was about twelve I took on the job of wheeling it home on a small hand-truck which had then to be returned. The customers had to shovel their own coal on to the scoop of an old, heavy weighing machine. The eagle-eyed owner weighed the quarter of a hundredweight himself. It took as long to get a balance that suited him as it did to shovel the coal on to the scales. Pieces would be taken off or thrown on by the owner until he was satisfied. When he took coal off he was careful, but when adding to the weight he casually tossed it through the air; this brought the scales into balance just momentarily, but it was enough for him.

No doubt the greengrocers used to play the old trick of putting their best fruit at the front of the display and mixing less savoury pieces when they served customers. This didn't worry us because we could not ordinarily afford fruit, but as children we used to buy 'fades' – faded bananas, apples and oranges. No wonder throughout my childhood I had no enthusiasm for fruit.

Poverty imposed its bleak discipline on our lives, and we wasted nothing. We ate bread and margarine or sometimes bread and jam but never all three together. No jam jar was ever thrown out with the slightest trace of jam; I was so skilful at scraping a jar with a knife that it would be left almost transparent. Damp coal dust could prolong a fire for hours; cinders would double its burning time – I could tell by a glance at the ash pan below the grate how many cinders could be sieved from the ashes with my fingers. Shoes with holes could have their life extended by inserting a piece of cardboard cut to the shape of the foot. I carefully avoided puddles in the street – not to keep my shoes clean but to keep my feet dry.

As we children grew older, we helped as best we could. But for some years, tasks like cutting the cardboard for our shoes and darning holes in our socks, besides the other chores of cleaning, washing and cooking, were all done by Mam. The weekly wash was an extraordinary affair. She had to coax alight a coal boiler in the scullery with newspaper, wood and coal or cinders, to heat the water. The clothes would be lifted from the boiler to a tub and laboriously agitated with a dolly. This was a wooden stool-like structure attached by a thick rod to a crossbar handle. Twisting and turning it was heavy work. The sodden clothes were then put through a mangle consisting of two wooden rollers on a metal stand which were revolved by cogs attached to a large wheel at the side. This had to be turned by hand, which was difficult if the clothes were folded too thickly, and useless if they were spread too thinly.

After Mam had completed the washing and hung the clothes on the line in the back yard, she would swill the ground and brush it clean. A special treat for us, watching through the window, was when she threw some of the water from the bucket at us.

Clean clothes were a high priority of Mam's, and she was just as punctilious in keeping the house clean. We had an open fire grate which she black-leaded regularly. The hob at the side, which served as a stand for the kettle, was also black-leaded, and the brasses of the fire-guard were brightly polished. Even the doorstep was cleaned with sandstone and water, and the pavement was regularly brushed. Neighbours chatted as they did these customary jobs.

Respect for authority was a tangible factor in our lives. Mam was anxious about any contact with people such as priests, doctors or employers. For the priest's weekly 'collection' visit, she always gave some money, no matter how impoverished we were. This was a practice I resented from a very early age. The priest, who lived in a fine, large house, would knock at the door, smiling and confident, and she hastened to hand him her money. A brief word of thanks, or a casual comment on the weather, and he was gone.

Before the doctor called, the house would be thoroughly cleaned, regardless of how clean it was already, and fresh sheets were put on the bed. I never knew where they came from; perhaps they were borrowed from neighbours. It is hard to believe that the doctor noticed, but that was the ritual, always tinged with anxiety and deference.

Doctors' visits were for the normal childhood infections, but on the whole we were healthy. I was blessed with abundant energy. The moment I awoke, I was alive and looking for action, which was readily found in the street. It was always bustling with activity and, with virtually no traffic in the 1920s, was a playground for children. We played rugby with a piece of sacking tied with string. As we were short of coins to toss with, the 'kick-off' was determined by the leader of one team cupping his hands to his face and moistening one with his tongue. The opponents had to guess which palm of the hand was wet, but a skilled observer would notice that one side of his opponent's lips was moist; this was usually, except with subtle double-thinkers, an excellent guide.

One of my friends once suggested we should pool our Oxo coupons and get a real leather rugby ball. I agreed, not thinking that I would be depriving Mam of whatever she was saving the coupons for. After months of patient saving we waited expectantly for the football to be delivered. I was not present when it arrived, but my friends quickly organized a game in the street. By the time I got there a lorry had run over it and we were back to the sacking tied with string.

Soccer was much less popular than rugby, though we played it occasionally with a small rubber ball or a tin can. A favourite game was 'bungout' in which one of us threw the can as far as he could and while another lad retrieved it we all hid. Sometimes when the can went through a window we stayed hidden for a long time.

None of us owned a bicycle, but nearly everyone acquired a 'gooch' – an old bicycle frame minus wheels, pedals, chain and brakes. A pair of small wheels from an old pram could always be found and a bent six-inch nail served as an axle. With these home-made scooters we achieved considerable speeds, though braking was hard on the shoes. These were our staple games, though there were diverting fashions – tops and whips would come and go for no apparent reason, and 'trundles', thin hoops of steel or thick bicycle wheels without spokes, would be ferried around with great dexterity.

The competitive urge dominated; we would compete as readily with tops and whips as with trundles or our tied sacking.

One of our great luxuries was to visit the local Picturedrome on Saturday afternoons. We cheered the stars of the Westerns – Tom Mix, Hoot Gibson and Ken Maynard – and when the villain was creeping up on the hero we would bellow, 'Look behind you, Ken!' If the hero was not so well known, the shout would be respectfully amended to 'Look behind you, mister!' The film was preceded by a local talent show, which meant half a dozen hopeful young vocalists rendering old favourites such as 'Sally, Pride of Our Alley', 'Nellie Dean' and the perennial Irish songs, 'Danny Boy' and 'A Little Bit of Heaven'.

These 'turns' and our response enlivened the atmosphere and the singing, clapping and cheering buoyed us. We were appreciative participants and excited judges. It was an interesting display of values. No singer was ever booed or jeered. That would have been too unkind to amateurs. People we did not know, but who sang well, were applauded. Yet when our close friends sang we banged our hands together, whistled and shouted.

If we did not have money for our cinema visits, we would try to slip into a side door beneath the stage and surreptitiously emerge in the darkness of the auditorium to join the audience. Eventually the ploy was discovered and we were locked out. We resorted to another trick which was equally successful for a limited period. As the audience entered, the attendants would tear the tickets in half and throw them into a narrow, deep box. With crowds of youngsters pushing in, some untorn tickets were thrown into the box and we scooped out what we could as we left the hall. We sifted through them to find the untorn ones, which we used the following week. After a while this too was discovered and the attendants began threading the used tickets on to a string.

The cinema was a rare opportunity to escape from reality – and from each other. People lived closely together in their poor surroundings. In streets which were seldom deserted, neighbours talked in groups for hours on end; in summer they brought out their hard wooden chairs to sit gossiping. Children played out at all hours. Even after dark, games continued, punctuated by the plaintive calls

(8)

of mothers that it was time for bed or the strident demands of fathers that someone should get home 'this minute'.

Outside a public house near the end of Wellington Street we waited every Saturday night at closing time to watch the inevitable arguments and occasional brawls. The fights were vigorous though rarely malevolent – people who had been fighting one Saturday night would be drinking together the next. Sometimes families bickered as they left the pub; one couple were particularly prone to loud, abusive language. Although they had four children and were very poor, both parents went to the pub every Saturday. One night after quarrelling all the way from the pub to their home, about a hundred yards away, they continued shouting for some time until the husband pushed his wife outside and locked the door. In her anger, and no doubt conscious of the spectators' amusement, she smashed the window with her shoe. Her hand went through the glass, cutting an artery in her wrist; the farce turned to tragedy when she died a few days later.

Her remorseful husband went to Mass every morning after her death and died himself not long afterwards from what the neighbours called a broken heart. Sentimentality overlaid family tragedy but it was of no help to the orphaned children.

Another eccentric couple, living a few houses away, were an Irishman and his wife. He was violent, given to blasphemous fury at the drop of a pint, while she was kind and sentimental, utterly devoted to their only daughter, a chronically sick teenager. When she died, her mother turned her room into a shrine, and no one, not even her husband, was allowed to touch or move anything in it. To raise money for the church, she held pathetic jumble sales in her back yard but she was so generous that she found it difficult to accept even a few coppers for the old clothes and trinkets on sale. 'Ah, go on, sure you can have it,' she would say in a thick Irish brogue to someone who asked her the price of an old dress. So, standing oriental bazaar procedure on its head, a somewhat embarrassed dialogue would ensue with the neighbour insisting on paying something and the seller depreciating the offer before accepting the absolute minimum.

(9)

Many years later, when I was the chief shop steward at a local factory, I worked with her husband, a great ally, who would curse the bosses with terrible vehemence. Unfortunately, he did the same to anyone who disagreed with him, and during one strike I had difficulty in dissuading him from physically attacking a striker who wanted to return to work. All his hard work, heavy drinking and angry clashes with other people ended when he committed suicide. Characteristically, he did so in a primitive and violent way, cutting his throat with an open razor. His wife lived to be 100 and received a telegram of congratulations from the Queen.

Our close community shared both celebrations and tragedies. One woman in particular specialized in helping the bereaved. When people died they were dressed in a shroud, laid out in their home for a few days, then taken to the church before burial. The laying-out was not a job to be undertaken by a deeply affected relative, so this plump, helpful woman would always be called in to perform the necessary service. It was customary for relatives and friends, including children, to see the dead after they were laid out in their home. Even though I was so young, I clearly remember being lifted up to look at the face of my dead father, and my sense of finality and sadness when I saw it.

During my childhood I saw many dead people in their houses when I went to pay my respects. It often struck me that both the smooth wooden coffin and the immaculate white shroud must have been very expensive. I sometimes reflected wryly on the Poles and Lithuanians who dressed their dead in their best Sunday clothes and, we were told, placed money in their pockets to help them with their journey in the next world.

When we went to visit the dead, the procedure was to look at the body and kneel by it to pray for the soul of the departed. In retrospect, I don't know whether we made these visits out of curiosity, a desire to show respect or simply an uncritical acceptance of a long-standing tradition; probably a combination of all three. But death was an important, almost ceremonial, part of life. On the funeral day, neighbours crowded outside the house, respectfully watching as the coffin was carried to the hearse, bedecked with wreaths, and the mourners filed out to the carriages. When I was very young, these were horse drawn, later replaced by motor vehicles. As the cortège wended its way to Widnes cemetery, people would stop whatever they were doing. Men invariably took off their caps, and women crossed themselves as it passed.

Our next-door neighbours were a childless couple who were comfortably off because the husband had a regular job. We were friendly with them, though we could not afford to share their pleasures – the most we could afford for a holiday was a once-a-year day-trip to New Brighton, twelve miles away across the river from Liverpool. The neighbours spent a week at Blackpool every year, and when they returned we were regaled with descriptions of these odysseys; the sun was twice as warm as in Widnes, sands were golden, shows were magnificent and hotels luxurious: every meal was described in mouth-watering detail. What we were missing of life's real pleasures! As a result of these tactless tales I spent my childhood visualizing Blackpool as Shangri-la – an illusion not dispelled until I visited it years later.

Unemployment was the prime cause of the surrounding poverty. Any man with a regular job was regarded as an aristocrat. Idle groups loitering on the street corner were part of the daily scene; some were tempted to supplement their dole by irregular means – the most common was to steal coal from wagons in nearby sidings. To see a group of men moving off at twilight with old sacks and shovels simply meant to me that they would have a fire in their grate the following day whereas we might not. Some went further and sold the coal. My mother would not touch it, preferring to do without a fire. This was partly her honesty – she was anxious that I should always keep to the straight and narrow – but partly because she was afraid the men might be caught and implicate us. Occasionally they were arrested by the police, but then the neighbours discussed their luck rather than their morals.

Near the end of Wellington Street was a grubby pawnshop. It was an institution in the area, a place where people went only when they were desperate for cash. I came to know it well. The man behind the small wooden counter was familiar with everyone and everything. Behind him were hundreds of parcels, boxes, garments and bric-à-brac of all kinds. He instantly assessed the value of anything shown to him and unhesitatingly made his offer. A coat might be threepence, a clock sixpence or a suit a shilling. But to get them out again meant paying substantial interest. As a child, I felt it was unfair. After pawning something I was usually elated taking the money home, but I felt defeated at paying over the odds to regain it. The poorest lost heavily when impelled to seek the self-defeating support of pawnshops.

In Wellington Street lived the only man I've ever met who begged with dignity. The legless grandfather of a school friend, he was a quiet, grizzled man who, every Saturday morning, swung on his crutches to a patch of spare ground a few hundred yards away. He sat there, upturned cap beside him, composed, friendly and at ease chatting to passers-by, who dropped coins in his cap before walking on. My friend and I took him his midday meal, a bowl of hotpot, known locally as scouse. He always left some and, with a twinkle in his eye, asked if we could 'finish it off' – an invitation we never refused.

Some people tried to relieve their poverty by gambling. Off-course betting was then illegal, but any chance of making easy money was eagerly grasped. Tipsters walked cockily down the street to encourage the triumph of hope over experience. They always claimed to have 'inside information' and for threepence would write the names of two fleet-footed certainties on a small slip of paper. The buyer was enjoined to 'keep it to y'self' and having paid the money he was inclined to play along with the tipster's game.

Once in a while Mam bought the tips. When she opened them I always had a sense of confidential conspiracy. The horses were duly backed for threepence each, though, of course, some mishap usually prevented their certain victory. Oddly enough, the tipsters were never unwelcome. Perhaps they gave the names of different horses to different people – or maybe they were eloquent and persuasive apologists for reported failures. But throughout my childhood they enlivened Wellington Street, especially on big race days, when they raised hopes that the bookmaker was at last ripe for plucking.

The bookmaker was the most smartly dressed man in the street – or rather at the back of our street – perhaps because he was never plucked. Dapper, brisk and unfailingly friendly, Jimmy Walker had a wooden leg which neither troubled him nor spoilt his appearance. It emerged like the end of a crutch at the bottom of his trousers. As a child I felt this must be better than two ordinary legs for a man who had to stand for so long. He was in our back entry, taking bets every racing day, from noon until 4.30 p.m. and then paying out at 6 p.m. The long, narrow entry ran between the back-to-back houses, and a slight bend in it, outside our gate, provided a niche for him. His look-out man, who was disabled, crouched at the near end of the entry while the bookie attended to his customers.

At six o'clock a small crowd would be waiting, and the bookie settled his debts as rapidly as he had taken the bets, paying out efficiently from a huge pocketful of silver and copper coins. Though we rarely got more than a few coppers back, I learned to read his long book upside-down to spot the pseudonym 'E. A. Ash' that my mother used; when my turn came I would point it out immediately. He worked quickly not to satisfy impatient customers but because there was always the possibility of a police raid.

These raids occurred periodically, but they were gestures, showing the flag rather than making a realistic attempt to catch him. If the police approached from the far end of the entry 200 yards away, a client would spot them; and if they tried the near end just behind him, the look-out would give a loud, almost hysterical whistle. The smart bookmaker would simply push our back gate open, walk into the lavatory and wait until the police had gone. If we wanted to use it, we had to wait until he had left.

The other popular gamble was 'pitch and toss'. On a patch of spare ground near the local docks a crowd would gather to bet on whether two tossed pennies would turn up heads or tails. The betting money was casually thrown in heaps on the ground before the coins were tossed. I never played because my mother persuaded me that this was gambling by people who were heading for trouble. I did not question the moral distinction between this form of gambling and backing slow horses but took it for granted that players of pitch and toss would get their deserts. They often did, because the police raids were dramatically successful. Dozens of men would be caught by intrepid police who either disguised themselves or hid in dirty wagons which were shunted nearby. When the names of the guilty appeared in the local newspaper, this was clear proof that those who played this heinous game got into trouble. The harsh lesson appeared indisputable; the only question was which of the gamblers grabbed most of the money when the police pounced.

It was surprising that there was not more gambling and crime in the area. Across from our back door was Paddy's Lodge, a dingy lodging house for vagrants, mainly Irish, with a few permanent residents. I ran errands for some of the men, but always wanted to leave the house as soon as I could. In a large gloomy room smelling of stale cabbage, the men, sad and depressed, sat on long wooden forms. The lodge was run by a small, spry man named Andy, who maintained strict order. The atmosphere was probably due to his inflexible discipline. Although he rarely raised his voice, there was no argument when he spoke. The lodgers included some strange characters: Nicholas hummed all day and spent most of his time in church; a tall, stooping man we called Uncle Tom never stopped talking aloud to himself, but seemed harmless enough; another, whose identity we never knew, occasionally left cats hanging by their tails and sometimes by their necks.

The Roman Catholic Church was influential in the area, and the power of the priest was more important than that of the policeman. When trouble occurred, the natural reaction was to send for the priest. His presence defused any explosive situation, as much because of his authoritative attitude as of respect for the cloth. The Church was strong because many Irishmen, Poles and Lithuanians lived there. Irish families had emigrated during the great potato famine in the middle of the nineteenth century, and in the late 1880s the Poles and Lithuanians had come to escape Tsarist religious persecutions. They had settled in the Wellington Street area, many of them finding work in Bolton's nearby copper works. Some of the most common names in our streets were Karalius, Rooskie, Steponevitch, O'Neill, Redmond and Murphy.

These were also the most common names in St Patrick's Catholic elementary school, a blackened old building adjoining the church, just a few hundred yards from our house. Boys and girls were separated, but this was the only segregation in the school. All the boys from the age of nine to fourteen were taught in one long room divided by curtains, and in the middle the headmaster sat in state – a terrifying figure.

Peter McKenna was small but in anger appeared ten feet tall to us. When he bawled, five forms quivered. Forms three and four were at one end of the room, five and six at the other, with his form seven placed majestically in the centre. His class was the centre-piece of our school lives: on its success or failure our tranquillity depended. No wonder we were apprehensive at the prospect of going into 'standard seven'. Even when the head was silent it did not necessarily mean all was well; only that he might be poised to assault a victim with roars of anger, a cuff on the head or strokes of the cane. To this day I can recall the sound of his favourite epithets – 'fool', 'idiot', 'jackass' – thundered at an unfortunate pupil. His rage would reverberate around the room. Yet he was also a sentimen-tal man; few things pleased or soothed him more than to listen to his class singing the Scottish ballads he loved. 'Vair me o, o ro van o – sad am I without thee', we sang uncomprehendingly. Or more briskly, 'Oh, the far Coolins are putting love on me, as step I wi' my cromak to the Isles.'

I never pondered the mystery of why the headmaster of an Irish Catholic school made us parrot these Scottish ballads. His wish was our command. Perhaps he felt it his duty to remind us of the other parts of our British heritage, though he never taught us a Welsh song. Or maybe he was displaying a streak of perversity which was perfectly in character.

The school's rugby and swimming feats were a source of great pride to us. It had a particularly good record at swimming and frequently won the town's school shield and the Catholic schools' shield. To us, the Catholic trophy was the more desirable, and there was jubilation in our streets when the team ran through in triumph. Being a poor swimmer, I had special admiration for the team as they carried off successive trophies. I was discouraged from swimming because of an ailment which seemed minor at the time – a perforated ear-drum.

I was never outstanding in examinations at school and usually came about tenth out of some forty boys. My best subjects were arithmetic – we just about learned decimals and vulgar fractions before leaving – and English, though this never went beyond the stage of identifying nouns, verbs and adjectives. In subjects I disliked – history and geography – my standard was low, but I was never unduly bothered by this, nor was anyone else.

Some teachers were rough on boys who, they felt, were undisciplined or lazy, and the cane was used frequently. We were always caned on the hand, which could sting painfully. The choirmaster in particular was strict; although never unfair, we feared his displeasure. It was possible to exercise the fine art of withdrawing an outstretched hand at the last split second, as the cane reached the fingers, while wincing with simulated pain, but it never worked with the choirmaster: he simply increased the number of strokes. Other methods of countering the punishment were often discussed. Some claimed that rubbing resin on the skin beforehand gave great protection; others said that laying a hair on the palm would reduce the force of the stroke. I was caned sometimes for unpunctuality or talking in class. I never managed to get hold of any resin but I remember my disappointment after unsuccessfully experimenting with the hair a few times.

When we were eleven we moved into the form of a teacher who enjoyed using the cane. Austin Gilfoy, a small, hectoring man, upset one of my best friends by constant caning, though some of it was provoked. Resin and hairs on the hand were useless, so my friend decided to enlist the help of his father, a tall, gangling Irishman with a violent temper. He hit his son much more often than the teacher did, but when he heard of his son's 'victimization' he was furious and lay in wait for the teacher at the corner of Wellington Street. We watched from a distance as the teacher was swung round almost off his feet. A long argument ensued, and the following day the teacher greeted my friend like a long-lost son. Later he was made a prefect, almost becoming the teacher's pet.

Our music lessons, which I enjoyed, were conducted by a senior teacher, Joseph Ludden, the strict choirmaster. Although tough with the cane, he was respected by the boys as a fair, intelligent man who loved music and demanded high standards. Many school hours were spent perfecting the singing of hymns for Mass or Benediction. The teacher's love for music communicated itself, and he fired us with his enthusiasm. He discreetly helped this along by saying that singing hymns was twice as good for our souls as saying prayers. We sensed the mood and message of the hymns and sang accordingly.

The Good Friday lament was sung in sadness, while the Easter hallelujah was delivered with high-spirited rapture. I had a strong, clear soprano voice and I was one of the small choir of four boys who sang verses between the general chorus. I loved the singing and was proud of my role in the small choir.

The relationship between the school and church was close, with regular visits from the priests. We were expected to attend Mass and Benediction regularly. Missing a service was worse than muffing a lesson. One enterprising teacher, trying to stimulate enthusiasm by establishing the 'house' system used in public schools, divided the form into four groups and named each of them after a saint – we called them St Pat's, St Mick's, St John's and St Joe's. Points were awarded to each for scholastic and sporting achievements, but most points were earned by going to Mass and Communion. St John's was rarely beaten because some members of its team attended Mass and Communion every morning. I was not a bad churchgoer but I could not compete with that. Sunday-morning Mass was compulsory. To miss it was considered a mortal sin; in addition one had to report it to the teacher on Monday morning.

I sang in the church choir on Sunday at morning Mass and evening Benediction. Each had its own distinctive atmosphere. The Mass was austere, dutiful and solemn, the priest's sermon a long lecture to the silent congregation. Benediction was a more relaxed occasion which I enjoyed; there was a musky warmth about it, the sweet smell of incense heavy in the air and clusters of candle-lights flickering in the church. It had an aura of sanctity, and when the

(17)

blessing was bestowed it seemed the culmination of an act of genuine piety. At Benediction I sang from the heart.

Although I was pious I was also flippant. The choir occupied a high balcony at the back of the church, and every Sunday night a bald-headed man sat directly below me. I used to compete with a mischievous friend to see who could form a bubble on his tongue then blow it down on the inviting head. Though we became competent marksmen he never complained. Choirboys took it in turn to pump the organ, which meant working up and down a sort of oar at the side. Two of us would pump together, watching an indicator that showed the air level; after an energetic bout of pumping we would sit back and watch the indicator slide down. Each of us waited to see if the other's nerve would break first, and only then would the handle be grabbed. If we were both too late, the organ wheezed discordantly, and we were in trouble with the choirmaster.

The choir had also to be present at more solemn ceremonies; before a burial the coffin would lie in the aisle surrounded by candles while mourners knelt nearby. The sight of the candle-lit coffin induced solemnity. Entering the church, as I reached the top of the curved wooden stairway at the back, and peered over the choir's balcony, I felt sombre. Singing the requiem made me even more melancholy, and after the ceremony came the most touching moments. The relatives would leave their pews and walk slowly down the aisle, touching or even kissing the coffin as they went. Their expressions and tears would bring a catch to my throat. I was easily moved.

I did not understand the mournful dirges I sang, because they were in Latin. 'De profundis clamavi, ad te Dominum' was beyond my understanding – yet during the sad ceremonies I shared the grief. In church I was touched by sorrow and reflected it in my singing, but it was quickly forgotten when I went outside.

Awed respect and even fear were felt on special occasions when missionaries visited the church. These great men were praised by the parish priest for weeks before the event and we were urged to attend the sermons to be inspired. Missionaries were always men with mighty voices. They addressed packed congregations – thanks to the efforts of the parish priest – and thundered their warnings of hell and damnation. Sin was all our fault. Man – never woman – was alone responsible for the evils of the world, and it was high time we prayed more and lived better lives.

While a missionary spoke, the churchgoers trembled. Then, suddenly, after his peroration, we were into the gentleness of Benediction. And at the end of these special occasions, the congregation always sang the stirring hymn, 'Faith of our fathers . . . we will be true to thee till death'. It was as if they had been inspired, and cleansed, by the missionary, and were now singing in celebration. The men's voices always dominated. Every time I heard this mass male choir I was deeply impressed with their combined, deep-throated power and authority. It made me feel wonderful; perhaps it was a fleeting substitute for my own father.

In 1933, Mam remarried and had another daughter, Margaret. Her second husband, Jim Dooley, had poor health and he died in 1940. We three older children loved having a younger sister, and her bubbling personality enlivened our youth. Mam was in hospital for several months when Margaret was born, and Helen ran our home. As the older daughter she had always taken the lead in helping Mam. Calm and capable, she was highly intelligent and forthright in her views. At St Patrick's she had always been top of the class and could easily have won a scholarship to the local grammar school; but it was not a Catholic one, so the opportunity was denied her. At fourteen she went 'into service' in a house in Liverpool, cleaning, cooking and doing odd jobs. She was paid only 5 shillings a week for this – 25 pence in today's money – and was, of course, unable to save anything. Although she hated the work and her isolation from home and friends, she could not leave until her maid's uniform was paid for; at the rate of a shilling a week deducted from her wages, it took five months.

Returning to Widnes, Helen subsequently married one of my friends and worked in local factories. For several years she was cook in a chemical factory canteen preparing hot meals for hundreds of workers, before she left to have twins.

Mary, two years my junior, had a lively personality. Although she did her share of chores, and was always quick to see what was required, she enjoyed conversation and company. Despite her excellent school record, she left to go to work in a nearby bag factory, a prison-like building with small windows that were always closed, even in the summer; they were barred and covered by wire mesh to keep vandals out but looked as if they were designed to keep the girls in. The work entailed long hours for low pay. The only alternative was unemployment. Mary married a local boy when she was nineteen. Her first child, a daughter, gave Mam her first grandchild. After having two more daughters, Mary subsequently took a course for mature students and qualified as a teacher, a job which gave full rein to her warmth and imagination.

Margaret, the baby of the family, missed our early very poor years. But she, too, was restricted by her educational experience, spending most of her working life as a shop assistant. With her sensitive, energetic personality she was capable of much more. She married a town hall employee and later had two daughters.

My three sisters were as deeply affectionate to Mam as I was, but they gave more effective practical assistance in the home. In my early teens, I began to take on the substitute role of father-figure, carrying out odd jobs and helping with the decorating. I was not very expert and, on one unfortunate occasion, trying to repair the mangle, I could not put it back together. Despite this, Mam and the girls let me take on the leadership of the family – indeed they welcomed it. We loved and respected each other; and they developed an easy and lasting tolerance of my foibles.

2

Off to Work

My fourteenth birthday, 6 December 1936, marked the end of my
school education. Although I stayed at St Patrick's for a few weeks
longer, boys attending school between birthdays and the end of term
were regarded as visitors rather than pupils. Applying for the local
grammar school was out of the question for me as for my sisters
because it was non-Catholic. Economic pressure often reinforced the
sectarian prejudice against the school, and many youngsters from
our neighbourhood went to work as soon as possible to assist their
families.

Most boys became labourers in the chemical factories which dominated the town, although a few lucky ones were given office jobs or
promised apprenticeships to craftsmen when they were sixteen.
Fathers usually spoke for their sons, and boys were unlikely to be
apprenticed without this informal nepotism. There was no one to
speak for me, so I decided to apply to ICI myself for an office job.
Anyone who held one of these was envied for his security and
reasonably good wages. After waiting in vain for some weeks for a
reply, I sought a job at a large asbestos factory across the town, a
branch of the Turner & Newall Company. Taken on as a labourer, I
was tersely instructed to present myself at 7.30 on the following
Monday morning.

I felt a sense of adventure, tinged with apprehension, as I left 34
Wellington Street at 6.30 one cold January morning to catch the bus
to my first job. I carried an old tea can containing tea, sugar and

condensed milk, and a packet of bacon sandwiches which had been lovingly prepared and wrapped in old newspaper by Mam. Although she was proud that I was starting work, she was also a little anxious. We were both conscious that this was the beginning of a new era in my life, with new relationships and new responsibilities. I wore long trousers for the first time and a pair of leather clogs with metal reinforcements – like horseshoes – on the wooden soles and heels. With an injunction from Mam to 'be careful', I clattered down Wellington Street in the darkness to join queues of workmen at the bus stop.

It was a jolting change in my way of life, but I felt no deep sense of unease on the crowded bus. There was an air of purposeful activity, and although the atmosphere was earthy it was by no means unfriendly. I was alert and curious. On that first journey I began to catch the moods of industry which I came to know so intimately in the years ahead: bawdy banter, passionate arguments about football, dogmatic assertions about the job and the bosses, and an underlying sense of comradeship, a feeling that we were all in it together. At the factory I joined a group of young boys to be shown around a vast shed where asbestos was moulded. Our job was to supply the work-men with tools collected from women at a store. It soon became apparent that new boys were butts for old jokes. One moulding tool was called a baby, and the men had as much fun ordering us to ask for one as the women had in responding to our requests. The ribaldry caused me more embarrassment than it would any fourteen-year-old today. When the men had exhausted their standard repertoire of jokes about babies, busts and bottoms, left-handed spanners, sky hooks and barrow-loads of steam, we settled down to the humdrum work of the factory. Despite the dirt and noise, I soon adapted to the routine, glad to be earning money for the family.

My wages were 12s 3d a week (about 62p in terms of today's money). I felt proud taking them home, though by the time I had deducted bus fares and a little spending money, they did not provide much support for the family. I was soon dissatisfied by the poor pay and sought a better job. Mam, anxious at these early signs of a rebellious nature, urged me to settle down, but a few weeks later I received an unexpected reply to my application for a job at ICI. After an interview with the Labour Officer I was accepted.

Although my new job was not specified, I was delighted with the idea of working in an office. Presenting myself wearing a collar and tie, I found that I was to be a labourer in a long, wide shed full of carboys and tanks of formic acid. The carboys were large bulbous thick glass bottles about two feet high and nearly as wide. They were filled by men from six large tanks of acid nearby. A team of boys prepared the carboys and helped to dispatch them after filling. The work was hard and dangerous, and only slightly better paid than at the asbestos factory.

My first job was to hammer the corks tightly into the necks of the bottles, then to tie pieces of sacking over them. The corks – nearly three inches in diameter – soon became saturated with acid, so that when I hit them with a large wooden mallet they sent up a fine spray. This burned the skin, but there were worse hazards. One day, trying to hammer in a badly fitting cork, I hit the glass and shattered the carboy with a tremendous crash. It was unnerving, but my instinctive reaction caused some amusement. 'It must have been cracked,' I claimed.

Before the glass containers were filled I had to pack them into the metal cases. A protective layer of straw, on the bottom and all round the casing's interior, ensured a tight fit. The bottles, placed inside, had to be forced down as low as possible, for if they were above the casing they broke when stacked on top of each other. I held the container with my left hand, gripped the neck of the bottle with my right and levered both high in the air with my knee before banging them down on the ground. Too much straw on the bottom made it impossible to force the bottle in; but the first time I used too little and shattered the carboy as I hurled it down. This was even more spectacular than breaking it with the wooden mallet. Other workers began to warn each other, with mock solemnity, of the grave danger to life and limb from flying glass when I was busy.

They looked at these mishaps with a tolerant eye, as well they might because they were scarred from their own earlier experiences. But when I progressed to become a 'filler' of the carboys I sometimes upset them. The supply tanks from which the carboys were filled had to be replenished as they emptied. I had to open the taps of large pipes connected to the containers above where the acid was produced and, as acid gushed into the tanks, I had to check the level to avoid an overflow. But having to fill carboys at the same time as the supply tanks, I was neither as concerned nor as vigilant as I ought to have been. My tanks began to overflow with alarming regularity.

The fumes were noxious and even after hosing water and sprinkling sawdust they remained troublesome for hours. My workmates were as unconcerned as I was about the loss of acid, but in their own interest one of them reported me to the boss. After a severe reprimand I was more careful. It was one of my earliest lessons as a worker in industry that you could damage yourself or your firm if you wished but you could not damage your workmates and get away with it.

Already I was accepting values shared by workers in that and other factories. The bosses – a pejorative term – were out to screw us for all they could get and keep our wages as low as possible. The employers in turn believed that watchful, firm oversight for our work paid the best dividends. So suspicion bred suspicion. The hard, dirty work could not be avoided but, with discretion, it could be minimized. Yet the minimum was very demanding with hundreds of carboys to be filled in the fume-laden shed every day, then manhandled on to hand-trucks, wheeled away, stacked six high and eventually loaded on to lorries or railway wagons. We were unwilling to work harder.

There were exceptions. Some men felt an obligation to the firm and behaved accordingly; but they were regarded as bosses' men. In their presence, other workers were always wary about what they did and particularly about what they said. An incline of the head in their direction would warn anyone criticizing employers that a potential informer was nearby. By and large, there was no great sense of loyalty to the firm; yet, as I learned later, ICI was one of the better employers, and many others were far worse. Nevertheless, neither side made any real effort to understand the other.

For the next two years, I worked in that shed. The work was drab and uninteresting, but I was not unhappy; I accepted the job as a necessity although I took it at my own pace. On one occasion I miscalculated. The foreman told me to sweep the floor of the shed, a job I particularly disliked because it added thick dust to unpleasant fumes. He watched through a window in his office as I ambled the full length of the shed – several hundred yards – brushing slowly as I went. When I got to the end I strolled back to my starting point and began to sweep another strip. Striding from his office, the angry foreman reprimanded me for wasting time, and demonstrated how to do the job by sweeping briskly across the width of the shed and back. I had to submit to the rebuke and I swept vigorously for a few moments while he stood and watched, but when he was out of sight my work rate fell again. Nevertheless, I was embarrassed by his angry demonstration before my workmates.

The foreman was stern, and I regarded him with wary hostility, though it was he who had good reason to be wary and hostile. No doubt he knew that many of us could work much harder if we tried, and he often caught us playing football in the road outside long after the end of our midday meal break. He turned a blind eye to many of our tricks and even when we practised judo on the straw during working hours he would walk past apparently without noticing. But he could not overlook such unpardonable occasions as when he found one of my workmates giving an acrobatic display, dangling by his legs from a girder high above the straw; he sacked him on the spot.

Most of the men were tolerant of the boys, providing they were not kept waiting for essential supplies of carboys. We had no production line with a stop for an official tea break, but we drank plenty of tea during the day. Each man or boy made a brew in his own tea can. A regular pattern was established so that we knew whose brew was available at a given time. The shout of 'Brew up!' meant that the tea was ready.

I had an old, chipped tea can which my mother found somewhere and gave to me when I started work. It never occurred to me that this might not be acceptable to my workmates. In any case I could

(25)

not afford a new one. One day, after one of the boys thanked me for his tea and walked away with it, I happened to follow him round a corner. To my astonishment, I saw him pouring it down a drain. Embarrassed, he admitted that the condition of my old tea can was too much for him and he poured my tea away every day after pretending to sip it. Apparently one of the other boys had told him that my grandfather had some dubious uses for the tea can. The incident illustrated to me the relative nature of poverty; I felt like a pauper among the poor, but I gave in to this pressure and bought a new can.

When I was sixteen years old I decided to leave ICI and seek a better-paid job elsewhere. The idea of abandoning the security of a job with ICI caused consternation at home. My stepfather, an unskilled, unemployed man, was incredulous and indignant when I told him I intended to give up my job, but I would not be dissuaded. It was 1939, and with the war imminent, more jobs were becoming available.

I took a job delivering coal for a local merchant; it was heavy work, filling hundredweight bags, carrying them on my back from a lorry into houses and emptying them in cramped spaces beneath stairs. The pay was few shillings more but I certainly earned it. The coal merchant laid down 'heads I win, tails you lose' conditions, so that if I had time off I was not paid for it, but if I did overtime I received no money for that either. I missed the comradeship of the factory. The work was dusty and dirty, and I used to go home looking like a miner, but without a miner's pay.

I soon left and wandered from one casual job to another. Most of them were hard, with a high labour turnover, so that it was impossible to make worthwhile friendships, though the pay was generally a little above average. Finally I got a job at the copper-smelting works a few hundred yards from Wellington Street. It had a reputation for tough bosses and heavy work, but the wages were reasonable. In this sprawling factory with over four hundred men, there were half a dozen furnaces each smelting up to fifty tons of copper a day.

I was now a high-spirited sixteen-year-old, slim but strong. Two years of hard work had developed my body, and some practice in

(26)

judo and boxing had given me self-confidence in the rough no-nonsense atmosphere of a gang. I settled down and made some good friends. Although our job of wheeling copper bars to the furnace on long-handled trucks was hard work, we never made heavy weather of it. Naturally exuberant, we often raced each other with the trucks, though we were careful to return more slowly so that no more bars were wheeled than was expected. As we dragged the trucks up and down the factory we discussed girls, Rugby League football, the bosses and local gossip.

Before knocking off work at 5 p.m. we dispersed into the most unlikely parts of the factory. The first boy to get a good truck or wheelbarrow at 7.30 a.m. could have it for the rest of the day; heavily laden rickety ones were harder to pull. So when work was finished we hid our prized trucks in dark sheds, under old sacking, behind railway wagons and even inside unlit furnaces. We were supposed to begin work immediately after clocking on in the morning but we invariably spent some time recovering trucks or searching for better ones.

The meal break was from noon till one o'clock; many of us went home because we lived near the factory. After a quick meal, I was back at 12.30 to enjoy the company and whatever fun was available. One of our favourite tricks was to creep to a three-wheeler vehicle which stood outside the garage where the foreman had his sandwiches. We would release the brake quietly and gently push it a few hundred yards away. Out of earshot we would start the engine and career around the factory at hair-raising speeds. We were careful to return the vehicle, with the engine switched off, just before one o'clock when the foreman would emerge. Although we were never caught red-handed, our joy rides were suddenly ended by an order that vehicles should be locked inside the garage during the midday break. We then had to rely on football, wrestling and cards to occupy us before resuming work.

Apart from our unofficial tea breaks, there was little respite from the work. I disliked the foreman's attitude and often clashed sharply with him. A curt, sharp-spoken man, he always wore a black suit and a dark cap. His word was law, and I was surprised at the submissiveness of the men as he issued instructions. Every morning at 7.30, as the factory hooter sounded, the foreman approached the waiting men who had to stand near one of the furnaces. Pointing to each man in turn he barked out his orders: 'Load this furnace ... Load that one ... Unload two wagons of coal ...' and to the boys: 'Get the bars down to the furnaces.' After allocating jobs to everyone he stood awaiting latecomers. I was usually among them, and when I arrived breathless he would give me a job coupled with the threat 'I'm not standing for this.'

The men looked like cattle as they waited to be allocated their work, but this method was an improvement on the one used in the earlier years of mass unemployment. Then labourers waited outside the gate, hoping for a day's casual work, and the manager would point to the strongest, who were duly grateful for the favour. Although I understood the history, I was surprised that the men should still allow themselves to be treated in this way – especially as it was 1939 and, with the country preparing for war, unemployment had been much reduced.

Gradually I began to take on the heavy work of loading the furnace with copper scrap. Four men using long-handled spades threw the metal in diagonally through two hatches, one on each side. The furnace was about twenty feet long and ten feet wide with the hatches about three feet square. It required strength and physical rhythm to throw heavy spadefuls far and accurately. Occasionally the scrap would go in one side and out the other, provoking a loud and angry reaction from the men on the receiving end. I concentrated on mastering the technique of flinging spadefuls with precision. It was not only safer but easier. If the scrap was allowed to build up in the centre of the furnace it had to be laboriously pushed and prodded back to the far corner before more scrap could be shovelled in. Aiming at the corner first and stacking towards the mouth was simpler. There was no question of slacking, because it created unacceptable tension in the team. Every spadeful was hard work, and the heat and exhaustion were so great that when each pair of men had sweated through a spell of ten minutes they were replaced by two others for the same period.

(28)

The furnace was also loaded with slabs of copper weighing three hundredweight. Too heavy to be lifted by hand, each one was winched on to the flat end of a fourteen-foot-long iron paddle which rested on the base of the hatch. Four burly men held the paddle at the other end and propelled it into the furnace. The sweating men running in and out of the blinding heat, swinging heavy slabs from the paddle, made an impressive spectacle.

Another man had a crucial role in the operation. When a slab was winched high enough, he had to swing it so that, when lowered, it landed squarely on the paddle at the mouth of the furnace. Then he had to tug away the claws holding the bar. Incredibly, this job was done by hand in the blinding heat of the furnace, and where I worked it was always done by a very small man, Billy Tippett. He had a heavy drooping moustache which was permanently singed yellow. This job was especially well paid and so in great demand, despite the heat. Tippett kept it even though he wasn't particularly good at placing the bar in the precise position. The main reason, I assumed, was that he was friendly with the foreman and usually left toffees for him in his jacket pocket hanging nearby. One or two cocky workers took advantage of this and helped themselves, but the inoffensive little man merely shrugged his shoulders. I liked his quiet, philosophical attitude.

The most common method of discharging the molten metal was to hand-ladle it. Six men, with no more protective clothing than a long pair of thick gloves up to their elbows, circulated before a hatch cut waist high, just above the level of the molten metal, and ladled it into a row of moulds. Their job was even more difficult than loading the hot furnace. The ladle handles were only as long as the average golf club, and the men had to dip them continually into fifty tons of searing liquid copper. If moisture was inadvertently left in the moulds after cleaning, the molten metal exploded and cascaded in the air like some fearful fireworks display – and everyone ducked or ran for cover.

Within minutes of starting work, the ladlers were lathered in sweat, but they drank more than sufficient beer to compensate. Just before opening time a boy went to the pub with a basketful of bottles of all shapes and sizes. Despite these being unlabelled, the boy easily identified the owners. The furnace – and the bottles – were empty at 1 p.m. when the men went to the pub along the road for more beer. Some claimed that they drank fifteen pints a day, but they never seemed wildly drunk.

As soon as the metal solidified, the moulds were kicked over and the pieces of red-hot copper, shaped like artillery shells, were knocked out with a sledge-hammer. Even after the copper was ejected, there were risks, because the shells had to be loaded six at a time on to a hand-truck and pulled out of the refinery. One day the man pulling the truck slipped and fell, and the red-hot shells rolled down on to the back of his legs.

I was uneasy pulling scorching shells. The job I liked, apart from loading the furnace, was swinging the sledge-hammer at the punch, held by another man. To begin with, I could raise it only to knee height, and several blows were required to loosen and eject the shell. But my swing gradually improved until the sledge-hammer was high in the air and the shells dislodged with a single blow.

In winter, after mornings bathed in sweat, we were often instructed to work on an exposed, outside chilly platform, loading railway wagons with heavy slag, the waste products of the furnaces. In rain or gusting winds, the dead weight of cold slag, the squealing of our shovels between the slag and paving, and the effort of heaving it into wagons made for a depressing afternoon.

Sometimes we had to unload wagons of coal dust, called slack. Though not as heavy as slag, moving it was still hard work. Two of us would be allocated to one wagon and I had more difficulty with my workmate, Andy Naughton, than with the slack because he took his job very seriously. We shovelled vigorously, throwing the slack clear of the wagon, digging deeper as we went and keeping to our own halves of the wagon. When my back was aching, or sometimes to catch my breath, I paused – but my mate simply carried on. Consequently, his half, precise to the inch, would be empty long before mine, and he stood and watched while I laboured. I occasionally tried competing with him, but as I sweated and swore, my anger got the better of me and I cursed at him for being stupid. He carried on quite unmoved, with a legitimate air of injured innocence, regardless of my outraged and outrageous comments.

By this time my gang of friends was a mixture of neighbours and workmates. In our spare time we went out dancing, playing football on the spare ground near Wellington Street and boxing. Our interest in boxing was aroused by the pugilistically inclined family of one of my friends. They had a set of gloves, and the four brothers practised regularly, two of them fighting amateur bouts. We regarded the eldest brother with some awe, and he could have pulverized us if he had wished. I learned to box reasonably well, although I was unable to handle two of the members of our gang. The first, one of the boxing brothers, was too fast and experienced for me. The other was utterly fearless; he came out of his corner with arms flailing like windmills. My straight lefts, hooks and upper-cuts were all demolished by the windmill, so I tried to persuade him to change his style and to box in the normal way. He wisely declined my invitation.

The boxing family suffered terrible tragedies. Their only daughter was drowned in the nearby canal when she was about five years old, and one brother, who was one of our gang, died of meningitis when he was sixteen. Later the father, who must have been unbalanced, cut the mother's throat and served a long gaol term. Luckily she survived.

We enjoyed our evenings, often dancing in church halls or the Conservative and Liberal clubs. We made no connection between these dances and the political parties. We wanted the company of girls, not political discussion. I became master of ceremonies at one of our favourite halls, and the presence of the boxing brothers ensured that trouble-makers behaved themselves.

Although I went out with girls, I did not have a steady girl friend. It was all platonic. The mores of that period and the teachings of the Catholic Church affected the attitudes of most, but not all, of us. Their somewhat puritanical attitude did not affect our enjoyment of music, dancing, laughter and general bonhomie, however. We enjoyed our youth, paying scant heed to events in Europe and the gathering war-clouds of 1939.

At that time our jobs were the central focus of our lives, and we were preoccupied with them. Although I did not closely follow the political events of the Munich period, by mid-1939 I was aware that war was inevitable. Some years earlier the Irish father of my closest friend in Wellington Street had emotionally and confusingly reiterated his conviction that war was 'sure to come when Itly and Muscolina get together'. I had not been able to puzzle this out, because I vaguely understood that Italy was under the dictatorial rule of Mussolini anyhow – but we never dreamed of challenging my friend's father. Much later the riddle was resolved when I discovered that by 'Itly' he meant Hitler, and despite his flamboyant mispronunciation his prophecy was not far out.

The older men of Wellington Street and the surrounding area had suffered grievously in the battles of the First World War, and we were brought up on blood-curdling tales of Passchendaele and the Somme. The Irishman who forecast war used to rant the most vivid and compelling descriptions of these bloody battles. Tall, gangling, excitable and aggressive, he would shout when he was aroused, 'Bejasus! You've no friggin' idea of what we went through. The friggin' men wus friggin' terrified.' When we were young he never used the original four-letter word in our presence. 'The friggin' men wus shot to pieces. Christ almighty! They used to scream in agony an' cuss God an' cuss the day they wus born. I'm telling ye. They used to cuss their mothers for having 'em and bringin' 'em into the friggin' world. By Christ they did!'

His eyes would turn up to the skies as he shouted and repeated this at us. It was almost as if he was accusing us, but we listened silently and respectfully and tried to nod at the right places.

I was nearly seventeen when the Second World War broke out and I looked forward to fighting in the Air Force when I was eighteen. In the meantime I was doing a man's job at the factory. I demanded a man's wages, to no avail. But like my friends I was less concerned with the work than I was with joining the armed forces. Shortly after my eighteenth birthday I was called up and applied to be an air gunner in the Royal Air Force. I did not know what the requirements were, but my qualifications soon proved inadequate. Sent to a camp at Padgate, near Warrington, I was to have three days of intensive tests, but as I knew little mathematics I was dismissed after the first day. Bitterly disappointed by this rejection, I joined the Army shortly afterwards and served in the Royal Army Service Corps.

After less than a year I was discharged on health grounds. A slight difficulty with my hearing had not seriously disturbed me while I was working in the factories, but during my Army service my hearing deteriorated, and after a series of medical boards I was discharged. When I returned to Wellington Street I discussed the problem with a local doctor, who arranged for me to see an ear, nose and throat specialist at Widnes Accident Hospital. One of my eardrums had a serious perforation as the result of an early infection, and the consultant was able to patch it up. I did not understand the rest of his treatment, but he improved my hearing. Although the army did not want me back, I was able to return to work without fear of the increasing burden of deafness which had seemed probable during my spell in the services.

3

Shop Steward

When I returned to work at Bolton's copper factory I was again given the heavy job of loading furnaces. Work and discipline were still hard, and the only change the war had brought was to make plenty of overtime available. This meant more money, though the foreman refused overtime to anyone who displeased him. He gave it, and some of the less exacting labouring jobs, to the most docile, as 'carrots' for conformity.

It was remarkable that in a factory with domineering management, old-fashioned processes and poor working conditions most workers were not members of a trade union. Although the craftsmen belonged to their craft unions, only four out of about four hundred unskilled workers were members of a general union. This was the more surprising as trade unions had been established in Widnes as long ago as the 1890s, and they had been strong before the inter-war Depression.

Although I was always prepared to argue with authority in the factory, I had never given any serious thought to trade unionism. My attitude changed after I had an emergency operation for appendicitis. I tried to return to work after a few weeks' convalescence. As I was unable to load furnaces until fully recovered, but needed money, I asked for a temporary light job – such as sweeping the factory floor – which was sometimes given to men who had been ill. The foreman refused; I could start work again, he said, when I was able to load the furnaces and not before.

Resenting this brusque response, I walked out and immediately began inquiring about trade unions. The same day, a friend told me that one of the best was the Chemical Workers' Union; within twenty-four hours I met the secretary of the Widnes branch to discuss the best means of organizing Bolton's. Although the connection between copper smelting and the chemical industry was not obvious to me, I accepted his assurance that we were eligible to join his union. When I eventually returned to the factory I was fit, broke and bitter – and supplied with hundreds of application forms.

The response of my workmates when I asked them to join was encouraging; they were willing and eager to take action against an employer who had never been seriously challenged. They were ready for action, but it had to be planned, organized and unexpected. Moving surreptitiously from one department to another, I contacted men who were able to influence their workmates. Before long, the management suspected my activities, but this was a spur rather than a deterrent, because the sooner we had a strong organization the less likely I was to be picked off. In each department, I selected the strongest and most articulate people to be shop stewards. Some of them became over-enthusiastic about recruiting and applied pressure against reluctant workers, but I stopped any strong-arm tactics. Apart from this, each steward was encouraged to develop his own approach to those who refused to join. Most tried persuasion and force of argument; a few used ridicule or contempt.

It is always difficult to differentiate between a worker who objects to joining a union on conscientious grounds and one who is prepared to undermine the organization to ingratiate himself with the employers while taking advantage of the benefits it has won. The shop stewards respected genuine objectors but they had little time for the bosses' men. Apart from a handful of these, the men were eager to join, and within three weeks we had organized over four hundred workers.

I had been contacting the shop stewards individually until the time came for our first meeting in the factory. It had to be a secret one, because we were not recognized by a hostile management. One of the shop stewards, a crane driver, arranged for us to meet in a

shed which housed the mobile crane. As the men slipped in one by
one I took stock. They were a tough bunch, and if they could be
welded into a team, the management was in for a shock. I asked
each of them in turn to report on the membership and organization
in his own department. Sid Hillier, a lantern-jawed Hercules who
spoke rarely but incisively, was responsible for transport. He simply
said: 'All in, no problems.' Jim Ratcliffe, representing the ladlers,
reported that all his men had joined without question. Tom Cosgrove, a burly furnace loader, said: 'Most are in – the rest will soon
follow.'

It remained to elect a leader as spokesman and to formulate
demands. Although I was only twenty years old, with no experience
of trade union organization, I was unanimously elected chairman of
the Shop Stewards' Committee; we decided that our first demand
should be for recognition and negotiating rights.

Later that day I went to see the Labour Relations Officer.
Although more of a diplomat than the rest of the management, he
had to express their policy, which was to maintain an existing
agreement with the other general union and refuse recognition to
ours. My argument that the other union had less than half a dozen
members in Bolton's left him quite unmoved. The company's other
factory in Staffordshire employed many members of the other union,
and this determined the management's attitude. I was angry but not
surprised. The personnel manager expressed regret, saying he knew I
would appreciate that he must accept management's decision. I was
aware that fulminating would not affect him; power lay elsewhere.
But remembering those tough figures in the shed, I said he should
tell management that they were now dealing with a strong and
unpredictable group – and I knew he would appreciate that I must
accept their decision.

The management's refusal to recognize us was a potentially lethal
blow to our organization. Although the immediate effect was to
anger the men, I knew that if we failed to win recognition and were
unable to represent them they would eventually lose heart. I raised
the issue in the Widnes branch of the union to which I had now
become an accredited delegate. Its members supported our claim,

and so did the North-West Area Organizer, Bob Edwards, a full-time official. Edwards, who later became General Secretary and then a Labour MP, wrote a strongly worded letter to the company. We decided to wait for the response, but when it came, the management were firm and unbending. Many of the men demanded a strike, but after serving in the Army I was uneasy about one while the war was on. Yet the employers were exploiting an empty agreement with the other union to reject our claim for recognition. At our next meeting I argued that the threat of a strike should be enough to get the management to reconsider and meet our demands. My words were unheeded, and the men voted almost unanimously for a strike, conceding only that we should give twenty-one days' notice.

Although we were taking unofficial action, we had the tacit support of the union. The management's attitude began to soften a little, but they still refused to negotiate, insisting that our committee should recommend calling off the threatened strike. We refused and called a mass meeting in the refinery near one of the furnaces. I told the men of the management's decision, but before we could discuss it the General Manager walked in.

Everyone stared as the hitherto unchallenged boss faced his workforce. I was sure of the line he would take but unsure as to how the men would react; it was not easy for them to repudiate decades of deference. He warned them that they were being led by irresponsible and destructive militants. 'Get back to work at once' was the gist of his message.

The men responded as they had never done before. Someone switched on a large fan used for cooling molten metal; adding to this noise, other workers began scraping their spades on the stone floor. The General Manager turned and stalked out.

Delighted by their unprecedented defiance, the men listened cheerfully as I addressed them again. It's time, I said, to confirm your decision to strike, and so they did with an overwhelming show of hands. I suggested we should all meet the following day, outside the gates, and the meeting broke up. Workers put their tools away, damped down the emptied furnaces and headed for home.

Next day in an atmosphere of near disbelief the men found

themselves outside the gates for their first dispute. A strike in Widnes was a rare event – a strike at Bolton's was unheard of. Brinkmanship had failed to move the employers, but it had certainly moved the men. Inside the factory the previous day, I had been talking to workmates. Now, outside the gate, I was addressing a public meeting of strikers. They listened attentively as I told them they deserved credit for their stand, that the shop stewards would press hard for recognition, and that they should stay out that day. No one demurred, and the meeting broke up as men drifted away from the factory after a further unanimous show of hands.

When we saw the Labour Officer later he was placatory, and said the management had agreed to negotiate with us at any time. What they could not do was to accord technical recognition, because that would provoke an inter-union dispute.

I told the shop stewards afterwards that I felt this was as much as we could get at the moment. They all agreed that we should recommend a return to work on this uneasy compromise and see how it developed. I knew that the men would expect more than we could get across an unofficial negotiating table; but at this brittle stage of building our organization I wanted to avoid pushing the new trade unionists too far.

That night, the strike committee's recommendation was discussed at a meeting of the union's Widnes branch in a local public house near the factory. Tempers soon flared. One of the shop stewards, supporting the proposal to return to work, was attacked by the angry Irishman from Wellington Street who years later committed suicide with his razor. I sought both to pacify them and to persuade the branch to support our recommendation. This was difficult because some of those employed at other firms were eager for us to continue the strike. Nothing is easier than cheering from the sidelines. But the branch eventually supported our recommendation, and at the next day's mass meeting the men agreed to return; their protest had been made.

My life in the factory was now transformed, and every kind of grievance was brought to me by groups and individuals. Each day I discussed them with the Labour Relations Officer and foremen in various departments. My own foreman was predictably disdainful and determined to ignore the union. I soon got to know who was hostile and who was responsive. Although the Labour Officer proved to be more tolerant than I had expected, senior management remained inflexible.

Our members were not blameless – but neither were some of the factory staff. I occasionally worked with a cross-eyed labourer whose every third word was a swear word. Having served time in gaol, he boasted to me that it was easy to steal from the works stores. 'But it's easier still for the bosses and they're worse,' he said. One day he had stolen some wood from the stores, and he said that while he was hiding there he saw a guard creep in and steal some tins of paint. At 5 p.m. as we walked to the factory gate, he made no attempt to conceal the wood and when challenged by the guard he replied, 'It's only wood, not bloody paint.' After a few face-saving comments by the guard, he was allowed to walk out – in his own view, vindicated.

Union activities began to affect my work as a furnace loader, which was unfair on my workmates as we were on piece-work. Through the influence of the shop steward in the garage department, I became a crane driver. This gave me greater freedom of movement, and more opportunity for making contacts. I drove it all around the factory wherever heavy lifting was needed; sometimes I was merely 'on call'. I wondered if it was a subtle managerial sop, but they were not subtle employers and remained rigidly opposed to the union. Still denied recognition, the Shop Stewards' Committee continued to meet in the secrecy of the shed.

The management set up a works council, a device for informal union recognition because all our shop stewards sat on it. Here we discussed long-standing grievances such as working conditions, safety, protective clothing and hours, but the employers insisted that pay should be excluded. A few months later Pay-As-You-Earn Income Tax was introduced, and pay became an issue.

It was already standard practice for management to keep a week's pay in hand, but suddenly they announced their intention to keep a further two days' pay to give them more time to assess the tax. Their decision, made without consultation, provoked an immediate response. The men, already angry at management's attitude to the union, demanded a strike, but this time we played it differently. Instead of giving twenty-one days' notice, we decided to seek negotiations and, if they failed, stage a lightning strike.

I told the Labour Officer that the committee intended to meet the General Manager next day to discuss the new pay arrangements and pay for annual leave. He was doubtful whether the Manager would accept the request; I told him that it was not a request but an ultimatum. Left in no doubt of our intentions, he promised to pass on the message; the committee then arranged for each shop steward to prepare his men for possible strike action.

Each department was run by a manager and foreman. We saw the General Manager only on rare occasions when he made a quick visit to a particular furnace or process. A tall, angular man with a sharp nose and an authoritative manner, he was never seen without a brown trilby hat, even in summer; in winter he also wore a short mackintosh. He walked with a sense of urgency, as if he had just heard of some disaster, and then would stop suddenly if he spotted workers idling. No words were needed; the icy gaze was sufficient to send them scurrying. If I was caught idling or drinking tea, I stood up and walked, very slowly, to my job. The movement was a surrender to his authority but it was grudging.

The General Manager spent most of his time in his office in a large block about twenty yards away from the furnaces. This short distance separated two worlds. The office staff men wore clean suits, collars and ties, and the women neat dresses, whereas we all wore dirty overalls. They came in at nine o'clock in the morning while we clocked in at seven-thirty. They were given sick-leave pay; we were not. It was to this citadel that the shop stewards went to put our demands: we headed for the General Manager's office at the top of the stairs.

The office staff were surprised when twelve working men in overalls and heavy boots appeared among them. No one spoke to the uninvited guests as we entered, but near the top of the stairs the General Manager's secretary appeared and said he would not see us. A prim, well-groomed woman, she was brave enough to criticize us for threatening to strike, but we were not interested. As she was speaking, the General Manager appeared behind us and pushed past, pausing only to tell a shop steward at the rear of the delegation that he had no right to be there and he was sacked. Then he vanished into his office, leaving us on the stairs. None of us knew why he should discriminate so oddly against one man, a long-serving craftsman. Knowing that it was up to me to make a move, I proposed that we should call the strike immediately and make the reinstatement of the sacked man another condition of our return to work.

There was a chorus of approval, and we marched back to the factory where each shop steward went to his own department to give the prearranged signals. The effect was startling. Within two minutes every man had stopped work while the factory processes ground to a halt. The railway engine, hauling wagons through the factory, stopped. Men ladling molten metal left it in furnaces which were cooling rapidly: a few who had already filled their ladles poured the molten metal back; for good measure one of them threw the ladle in as well. On another furnace, with a different system of discharge, molten metal was gushing out and filling a series of rapidly moving trucks. Within seconds the trucks stopped moving and molten metal overflowed on to the floor.

The men were jubilant. It had taken only a few minutes to produce chaos. For the first time the management's nerve broke; the departmental manager came running, urging me to ask the men to clear the molten metal before it solidified on the floor and in the neglected furnace. He assured me that the management would 'do something' about our claim. As I wanted to avoid permanent damage and an urgent decision had to be taken, I agreed. Later that day, after endorsing my decision, the Shop Stewards' Committee recommended a full resumption of work when the management reaffirmed their assurance. This was the result I had hoped for – a short, sudden strike which would shake the employers' complacency. But when I put the strike committee's recommendations to a mass meeting, strong objections were raised. Men who had been docile for years were now aggressive and some wanted a specific promise of money before returning to work. Eventually the majority voted for the proposal, accepting my argument that, if the employers double-crossed us, we would stay out next time.

Soon afterwards we were given our two days' pay and the dismissed craftsman was reinstated. The union became highly popular, as well as increasingly influential. With more co-operation from management we achieved greater success in what were still called unofficial negotiations. Relationships, however, were more difficult to change. Foremen on the shop floor, whose power had never previously been challenged, were particularly bitter; my own foreman rigidly maintained his cold, contemptuous attitude towards me personally.

One man, a commissionaire, who was violently anti-trade union, made no attempt to disguise his feelings. He had the additional job of selling tickets for the factory meals – a week's ticket cost 3s 6d, and I occasionally bought them. Whenever I appeared, he became engrossed in his work, leaving me to stand waiting a long time for my ticket. One day, when he had played his usual trick, I paid with a pile of coppers – eighty-four halfpennies. He refused to accept them, but I insisted that he must as they were British currency. Reluctantly he counted the coins and said there were only eighty-three; I maintained there were eighty-four. There was a silent and angry recount until, just before he reached the eighty-third, I tossed the additional halfpenny casually on to his desk, indicating that I too could play games.

Within six months of joining the union I became one of the main spokesmen of the Widnes branch and represented it at various conferences. At one large regional conference in Manchester, attended by delegates from all other unions, I tried to criticize the union which was impeding our recognition at Bolton's. The chairman ruled me out of order on some technicality but I persisted, and after a barrage of encouragement from the delegates I was allowed to speak. The union I criticized was the National Union of General and Municipal Workers, later the GMB, which later sponsored me as a Member of Parliament. The chairman of the conference was Ellis Smith, then MP for Stoke-on-Trent South, whose seat I was to inherit many years later.

When I became a delegate of the union to the Widnes Trades Union Council, I found a man who became a guide and mentor to me on trade union affairs. Gus Roberts, a very tall, rosy-cheeked railwayman, was secretary of the council. I had read reports of his comments in the *Widnes Weekly News* and always respected them, but at my first meeting I was astounded when he spoke. He had the worst stutter imaginable. For five, ten or sometimes fifteen seconds he would struggle to get a particular word out. Once over that barrier, he would speak normally until the next one came and the stutter would be repeated.

At first hearing, most people were embarrassed, and so was I. But everyone got over it. It was a rare example of general acceptance of an intrusive disability. The reason was that Roberts, extremely intelligent and blessed with good judgement, commanded respect. He dominated the Trades Union Council, not by hectoring but by genuine leadership qualities. He became a great friend, quietly discussing issues with me at his home and never reluctant to tell me frankly when he thought I was going too far. We remained very close friends until his death some years later.

Some of the delegates were bus drivers, members of the Transport and General Workers' Union. As my friendships with them developed, they stopped their buses whenever they spotted me walking, to see if I wanted transport. This hardly pleased the passengers but it certainly impressed anyone accompanying me.

I was delighted when I was appointed a delegate to the union's annual conference in London. Now twenty-one years old, I had never been to London, far less to a national conference. Studying the agenda eagerly, I found it a little daunting, with resolutions on important national issues, but I was not too concerned. In the Blue Room of the Bonnington Hotel in Bloomsbury, where the conference was held, the leading officials sat at the main table, and the delegates from all over the country at branching tables. The atmosphere stimulated me, and before long I was on my feet speaking on a resolution about workers' control of industry. The response of the conference delighted me. During the week I spoke in a number of debates and although I was often on the losing side I invariably had a good reception.

(43)

One of the visitors to the conference was a Widnes-born journalist living in London, Jack Carney. The London representative of an Australian newspaper, he wrote a regular column for the *Widnes Weekly News*, so although I had never met him he seemed a familiar figure. That evening he invited the Widnes delegation to his flat in Clifford's Inn, off Fleet Street, and we chatted about our home town. He was particularly friendly to me, and for years to come he wrote me typewritten letters, some as long as twenty pages and all of them thoughtful. He took an interest in me, wrote about current political affairs and urged me to read, study, keep my feet on the ground and keep faith with the ordinary people of Widnes. My very brief replies must have disappointed him.

The dominant figure at the conference was the General Secretary, Arthur Gilliam, a white-haired cockney who, as a speaker, combined an urbane manner with explosive matter. His habit of stating, with apparent affability, that he would deal with a recalcitrant firm by taking the factory to pieces 'brick by brick' was always well received by the delegates. They delighted in his militancy.

I did not know that in the preceding months the reports of my activities in Widnes had been noticed by a very attractive young woman who was Arthur Gilliam's secretary. We met at one of the social functions of the conference and developed a mutual affection rather like a shipboard romance. Both of us were sorry when the conference ended, and when we parted she said that 'fate' would decide whether we met again, while I felt it would be 'circumstances'. In the ensuing elections for the National Executive Council I just missed being elected. Shortly afterwards I received a letter from the General Secretary saying that a member had suddenly retired and as I had more votes than any of the other candidates, according to the rules, I was now on the Executive Council.

This meant regular meetings at the London office. Inside the envelope was a personal note on which was written the single word 'Fate'. With my formal reply to the General Secretary I enclosed the note with the word 'Circumstances' written on the reverse side. The day my letter arrived was one of the rare occasions when Arthur Gilliam opened some of his mail himself while his secretary was busy. He must have thought he had a odd new member on his Executive Council.

Bob Edwards, the North-West organizer, had growing power in the union and he was favourite for the leadership when Gilliam retired. The comradeship displayed by both of them earlier soon evaporated when Gilliam's leadership was challenged by Edwards. A special conference was convened to consider charges of malpractice against Gilliam, but his supporters fought strongly with ingenious manoeuvres. The day before the conference I received a telegram saying it was cancelled, but I was suspicious. A quick check with Edwards proved the message false. My telephone call enabled him to advise all delegates to ignore similar messages. Although Edwards had my warm support, I was saddened when I arrived at the door of the conference hall to see Gilliam, the former rumbustious leader, sitting silent and dejected outside, forbidden to enter. Delegates trooped past, but I stopped to have a word with him. He knew I was one of his most vigorous opponents, yet I think we established a personal rapport.

The chairman, a Gilliam supporter, played his last card at the opening of the conference, announcing it out of order, invalid and closed – all in the space of three minutes. Of course, we had anticipated this and an immediate nomination was proposed from the floor for an alternative chairman, who conducted the rest of the business. Many charges were made during the rancorous dispute which ended with Edwards being elected General Secretary. The trouble was not of his choosing, and he handled a difficult situation admirably. But such clashes were bound to weaken the enthusiasm of shop-floor workers, leaving a sense of bewilderment. Internal strife is always debilitating, and our union was weakened by it, although once the struggle was joined it had to be fought through to the end. It was my first experience of internal power struggles and it revealed both their necessity and their unpleasantness.

The members at Bolton's were relieved when the trouble was over. As we had been advocating unity on the shop floor, the lack of it at headquarters was not helpful. We had enough problems in the factory without worrying too much about disputes elsewhere. The management had mellowed a little since our successful strike, but they were still sufficiently difficult and obstinate to keep us occupied with our attempts to improve the wages and conditions of our members.

4

Town Councillor

Our old house in Wellington Street, one of the typical two-up-two-down type, had never been repaired since being built at the turn of the century. It was in a deplorable condition. Although I was busy with trade union activities, I constantly complained to the landlord. In the bedroom the rain came directly through holes in the roof and we used buckets to catch it. A hole in the gable-end wall was large enough for children to reach inside and steal things. The landlord, prosperous and pompous, owned many other houses nearby, as well as two confectionery and tobacconists' shops. He rejected my repeated requests for repairs as 'uneconomic'.

Argument was unavailing, so I went to see the Town Clerk at the Town Hall. James Wallace was punctilious and formal but not unfriendly. Watching me warily through rimless spectacles, he listened as I complained about the conditions and the landlord's attitude, and demanded to know what he would do. He disclaimed responsibility but suggested, I thought somewhat wryly, that I might be interested in the Rent Act, a copy of which was available in the Town Hall. This provided, he said, that if a house was not in a fit state of repair, a 40 per cent reduction in the rent could be made. That information triggered me into action.

When the public health authorities received our application form, they inspected the house – a derisive formality – certified 34 Wellington Street unfit for habitation and reduced the rent by 40 per cent. Mam was pleased but a shade apprehensive. Sure enough, it angered

(47)

the landlord, who was sarcastic and insulting when he saw her. Infuriated by this, I went to his shop to blast him with army and factory invective, but he simply grinned, impervious and arrogant in the belief that I could do nothing more. He was wrong. As I couldn't dent his pride I decided to damage his pocket. From the Town Hall I got hundreds of application forms for rent reductions and delivered them to every house in and around Wellington Street. At first people were a little sceptical, which was not surprising because tenants were expected to pay regularly and promptly or be threatened with eviction. Many were surprised by my assurance that they could have their rent reduced so easily.

I had grown up with these people and knew nearly all of them, yet I was taken aback by the conditions of their homes. They were bad enough in my own, but some I saw were wretched. Hundreds of houses needed repairs and many had leaking roofs, cracked walls and draughty window frames. One woman showed me how, no matter where she placed her bed, the water would drip on it. In one case, part of the roof had collapsed on a woman in bed expecting a baby. Bedrooms, living rooms and parlours were all badly affected by damp. One parlour had eight or nine holes in the bare floorboards, some so big that I could put my foot through to the damp earth beneath. The occupant of the house, an old lady, could never use the parlour, and a nasty smell there was traced to a dead cat under the boards.

Coalmen would walk through the kitchen and tip coal under the stairs against crumbling parlour walls. One man said, 'I don't mind the hole so much, but old Jones next door comes in at night and pinches my coal.' In some cases it was possible to crawl from one house to another through large holes in the walls, caused by damp and the impact of coal tipped against them. A woman complained, 'I've lived in this house for forty years and never had one repair done.' Under the door, where the floor had sunk, she had stuffed sacking into a four-inch gap to keep the draught from her husband who lay dying in the icy room. He was too ill to be moved to hospital, and the bedrooms had been unusable for five years. The woman was chosen as a member of our deputation to complain to the local authorities the following week, but she did not turn up: she was attending the funeral of her husband.

This new insight into an old problem changed my attitude. Instead of merely trying to damage the landlord, I sought constructive help for local people. Even simple amenities such as dustbins were lacking and dumped rubbish added to the squalor. I urged people to complain, but it was difficult to persuade them to act. Poverty had stultified activity, especially among those who had endured it all their lives. These people never dreamed of challenging the landlord or the officials at the Town Hall. They were expected to keep their place and nearly always did so.

I wrote to the Town Clerk asking if dustbins could be provided. He replied that none were available, because of a wartime shortage. I checked and found there were no dustbins in the Widnes shops. I decided to hitch-hike to London at the weekend to try to find some. Before long I came across an ironmonger's shop with dustbins on display. I explained the purpose of my visit to the manager, who was amused but willing to discuss it. He invited me to have a cup of tea and sandwich at a nearby café and promised to reserve a gross of dustbins until he heard from the Town Council; but he warned me to expect problems when I notified them of our agreement.

Afterwards I called on Jack Carney, the Widnes-born journalist. He wanted the details of the order and the name and address of the manager of the shop, and he asked me to let him know the Council's response. He and his wife were generous, inviting me to dinner and to stay the night at their home in a block of flats that seemed to me a place of great luxury. They appeared pleased with my trade union work and housing campaign and encouraged me to continue. I began to feel that my journey to London had been worthwhile.

Back in Widnes, I hastened to see the Town Clerk to tell him that dustbins were available and I gave him the details. He received my report with interest and wry amusement, promising to inform the appropriate committee and tell the shop in London of their decision. This was done, but the councillors refused to buy on the ground that the cost was 'prohibitive'. The Council obviously hoped the matter would soon be forgotten. Jack Carney had other ideas. He wrote about it in the local newspaper, applauding my 'idealistic' efforts and describing me as 'the Knight Errant of the dustbins'.

His article drew public attention to my activities, and many people in the area began to discuss their problems with me. One day the local parish priest, Father Heyes, visited my home to tell me that he was calling a meeting of tenants to discuss their grievances; if I would be the main speaker he would act as chairman. I readily agreed.

At the meeting a large and enthusiastic crowd listened to the priest's opening remarks, and then to my own vigorous speech demanding action from the landlords and Council. The local newspaper's report of the meeting quoted the priest's words extensively, and briefly mentioned at the end that I had also spoken. This surprised and disappointed me, but it was my first lesson that for the media what usually matters is not what is said but who says it.

Labour councillors for the ward were understandably cool towards me, since my campaign was an implied rebuke to them. Instead of placating them, I reacted against them and looked elsewhere for support. At that time Bob Edwards, the regional leader of my trade union, was the national chairman of the Independent Labour Party, and I took an interest in it. I had only a vague idea of the historical divisions which had racked the ILP and the Labour Party, but naturally Edwards and his colleagues justified their own party's stand.

They told me that the ILP – small, militant and dedicated to the purest ideals of socialism – was unsullied by power and behaved responsibly. It regarded the Labour Party more in sorrow than in anger, and felt it was misguided in accepting an electoral truce during the war. The struggle against Tories, capitalists, speculators and landlords had to be carried on at all times. It sounded fine to me and in 1944 I joined. I helped to organize a Widnes branch, became secretary and called periodic meetings which were badly attended. Between times I sold copies of the *New Leader*, the party's newspaper, but few people were interested; the membership never increased, and we merely limped on until the General Election of July 1945.

(50)

The war in Europe had ended in May but its shadow remained; shortages, rationing and controls were part of normal life. To the electorate, the major question was which party would manage the difficult transition from war to peace and build a better society. It was the first election in nearly ten years, and as the Widnes branch of the ILP did not want to split the Labour vote we supported Christopher Shawcross, the Labour candidate. I was disappointed when I was not asked to speak in support of him but I was invited to appeal for funds at one of his meetings. This small gesture of goodwill neatly avoided any risk of ILP policies being advocated – and illustrated the local Labour Party's lurking suspicions of me and the ILP.

Polling day was 5 July 1945. Because of the large number of postal votes from the armed forces, the results were not declared until 26 July. That day, as we worked at the furnaces, everyone was excited as massive Labour gains were reported by radio. The latest figures, chalked in large letters near one of the furnaces, indicated the Labour landslide.

Despite their national success and our co-operation in the election, my personal relations with local Labour councillors in my ward did not improve. Fighting Tories on national issues in a General Election was exciting, but once it was over we were back to the perennial problems of slum housing. The Widnes branch of the ILP was fine in theory but weak in practice, so I left it soon afterwards and continued my campaign alone.

The municipal elections were due in November, and I was asked by neighbours to stand for the Town Council. In my ward, there were two vacancies for which two Labour and two Conservative candidates were nominated. Although the Church played no formal part, it supported the Labour candidates, who were both devout Catholics. I decided to fight all of them, standing as a local man without any political label or philosophy, wanting only to improve, or preferably remove, the slums. My organization, consisting of a dozen friends, had its campaign headquarters at 34 Wellington Street. Despite a gift of £5 from Jack Carney we were desperately short of money, so we raffled packets of cigarettes in the factory to help to pay for the printing of an election address and some posters. Without a car or loudspeaker, I had to address people by standing on the street corners and speaking up. At my first meeting in Wellington Street, the only people present were the twelve members of my campaign committee. They appeared self-conscious before I began but when I addressed them as my audience they became positively embarrassed. Gradually people came out of their houses to listen, but they did not crowd around.

The atmosphere changed when two of the other candidates appeared. They drowned my voice with their loudspeaker, and their chairman, who chatted up a gathering crowd, introduced them as great local statesmen. I could not compete with the loudspeaker but I took advantage of the crowd they attracted. As soon as their chairman ended the meeting, I began a tirade against the councillors and the landlords. This time I won a favourable reaction.

From then on, whenever I saw the other candidates with their loudspeakers, I repeated the process. They were nonplussed. If they moved off when I appeared at their meetings it looked as if they were running away, and I said so. If they kept talking, I waited until they had finished and then criticized them – always emphasizing their failure to deal with the slums. It worked so successfully that my supporters would come running to tell me where the other candidates' loudspeakers were operating.

Gradually I began to win strong support in the ward. Crowds of children paraded, chanting and singing and making as much noise as they could with tin cans or anything else. One of my opponents was named Trayner and he was not pleased with the children's chorus:

> Vote, vote, vote for Jack Ashley,
> He's as steady as a rock.
> We'll put him in a ring and crown him as our king,
> And we'll throw old Trayner in the dock, dock, dock.

This was chanted in all the streets and, with appropriate variations on the name, whenever any of my opponents appeared. Once again they were at a loss for a suitable reaction; those who listened to the chorus appeared acquiescent, yet any loudspeaker bombardment seemed crude and was almost certainly counter-productive. Their supporters chalked slogans on the walls and roads, but no sooner were they written than the children obliterated them and replaced them with mine. When my opponents escalated from chalk to white-wash, the children went further and used white paint. Years after the election the slogans were still visible.

I canvassed every house in the ward with encouraging results. Inevitably I met the tenants whom I had helped during the housing campaign; they needed no persuasion. Many people were confident that I would win, but I wasn't so sure, although I tried to appear as confident as my opponents seemed when I walked with my supporters to the count. The ballot boxes were opened in a large hall, crowded with civic dignitaries, councillors, candidates and their supporters. Because it was different from the usual two-party clash, my contest became the centre of attention as the votes were counted. To the delight of my friends and myself, I topped the poll.

That Council election gave me great pleasure because I had been supported by my own people. At the age of twenty-two I was eager, and intent on extending the housing campaign I had begun. The atmosphere matched the occasion. Hundreds of people crowded in the town centre, many from my ward; they were not the party activists usually to be found at the count, but ordinary people who realized their lives could be affected by the election. Some of the old women among the delighted crowd walking back home with me did a little jig in the street. We celebrated at 34 Wellington Street that night with a party which ended with one of our more exuberant supporters having to be carried home at about 7 a.m. At 7.35 a.m. I walked to the factory, a little late as usual, self-consciously treading over slogans of 'Vote for Ashley' painted on the roads as well as the factory walls.

I was rarely tired at that stage of my life. Neither loss of sleep nor my additional work for the trade union and Council weighed heavily on me. When I took my seat on the Council I found myself in a cosy, sedate atmosphere which discouraged vigorous debate. The chamber was flower-bedecked as if in floral homage to former

(53)

Mayors whose portraits hung on the walls. Councillors sat around a polished semicircular table facing the Mayor, in his elevated chair, with aldermen on each side. Proceedings were formal, courteous and even pleasant; I looked forward to tossing a few stones into this tranquil political pond.

At the first opportunity I spoke of the urgent need for better houses and repairs to slums. Apart from the discomfort and misery caused by bad housing, the infant mortality rate in my ward was 10 per cent – more than twice as high as the national average of 4.5 per cent. I made housing my main theme. Most Labour councillors were friendly when I spoke, but the Conservatives and a few Labour councillors treated my more outspoken attacks with disdain. In one debate, a local Tory elder statesman said he strongly objected to my 'boy talk'. My rejoinder about 'living monuments of senility' hardly made for good relations with him and his colleagues, but enlivened the proceedings. People from my ward came to listen to the debates with a growing awareness of their rights. I was accused of being repetitious by some councillors. They were right, but I knew it would take more than an isolated comment to generate a new sense of urgency and improve housing conditions.

As my relationships with councillors gradually improved, we had fewer acrimonious exchanges. Now I needed allies to back up my campaigns and when one of the Council seats in my ward became vacant a few months later I tried to get one of my supporters elected. Ken Merrifield and his wife, Nancy, were two of my closest friends. Ken was gifted with a happy blend of integrity and humour. He was one of our shop stewards and although I felt he was rather old – he was about thirty – I thought he would make a good councillor.

We fought a campaign similar to my own. Ken and I arranged to canvass every house in the ward and speak at street corners. Our closest supporter, a Welshman named George Davies, worked on the furnaces with us at Bolton's, and his enthusiasm was limitless. Although his capacity for public speaking was nil, he was to act as chairman at our street-corner meetings. At work, he would write out the most glittering introductions to Ken Merrifield and myself, and practise them by the furnaces. Bathed in its golden glow, elevated on a copper slab, he was Demosthenes personified. But when he came to address the street crowd he would perspire nervously, take off his cloth cap and say, 'Ladies and gentlemen . . . Jack Ashley.'

At the end of a campaign lacking in sparkle, Ken Merrifield received fewer than 100 votes, much to the disgust of Nancy. The gloomy walk back from the count was lightened only by her passionate diatribe about the lack of gratitude in politics. 'The rats!' she concluded as we laughingly consoled her. I shared many joys and sorrows with Ken and Nancy – that night was one of the sorrows, and it showed me that political support is not easily transferable.

Despite this set-back, I continued to press for improved housing. My speeches were always fairly reported in the *Weekly News*, which was read by nearly everyone in Widnes. I became friends with the chief reporter, a small, mild-mannered Scotsman who listened with understanding to my sometimes extravagant requests. As a result of my public work I was becoming well known in the area, and so deeply involved in its problems that all my spare time was taken up with Council work and trade union responsibilities. I lived and worked in drab surroundings but I was happily absorbed in the battle to change them. Suddenly by chance the whole scene was transformed.

At work one day, as I waited in the garage for the meal break, I glanced through a newspaper and saw a report of scholarships to Oxford for working men. I showed it to a friend who agreed that it looked interesting, but we did not discuss it at length; I went home for a meal and promptly forgot all about it. A few days afterwards, thinking about it again, I wondered if it might just be worth applying – but I had forgotten the name and address of the college in Oxford. Had my friend not remembered I should almost certainly never have applied and I might have stayed at Bolton's all my life. But he did remember. It was Ruskin College, Oxford. I wrote to the Secretary asking for details. Apart from an essay, which I presume they wanted in order to prove that I was not wholly illiterate, the scholarship seemed to depend on an interview in Oxford at which practical experience and academic potential would be taken into account. I felt that academic potential was not my strong point but I hoped my experience in local government and the trade union movement would be of some value.

While my application was being considered, one of my Catholic friends, a teacher in Widnes, heard about it. Although he knew that I was questioning my religious beliefs to the point of rejection, he asked me if I would like to go to the Catholic Workers' College in Oxford. Perhaps he felt that a spell there would revive my flagging enthusiasm for the Church. Some time earlier, anxious about my loss of faith, he had arranged for me to talk to a Jesuit at his home. At this meeting, which was friendly, the Jesuit had an answer for every objection I raised, but to my friend's regret, and no doubt to the priest's disappointment, I was not convinced. However, I agreed to see the Principal of the Catholic Workers' College, Father O'Shea, when I went to Oxford, although I made it clear that I was not committing myself to go to the college even if invited.

I took the train from Widnes and made straight for Ruskin College for an interview which turned out to be simply a pleasant conversation. The Principal, Lionel Elvin, in his book *Encounters with Education*, called me an unorthodox applicant. He recalled that when the chairman of the interviewing board, Sir Walter Citrine, invited me to sit down I said that I had a statement to make first. Elvin said that Citrine was a little taken aback at this but agreed to hear it. Then I told him that I knew that many of my rivals would have been trying to persuade them to award a scholarship because of all the reading they had done. But, I said, my claim was the opposite; I had read practically nothing and thought I should.

Possibly in view of my work in the trade union and on the Council they were prepared to tolerate this. At any rate, I was not asked about any of the great national issues of the day, which was just as well for I was completely bound up with the local problems of Widnes. I talked about my activities and my hopes for the future; it all seemed friendly and civilized. I could not make up my mind if they were being open and frank, and a scholarship was easier than I had imagined, or if this was a kindly façade for a hopeless applicant.

Later I went to see Father O'Shea at the Catholic Workers' College nearby. A slim, greying man with a gentle manner, he gave me tea in his room and treated me like an old friend. There was nothing artificial about this. The priest exuded natural warmth, albeit with an attractive diffidence, and told me that I would be welcome to his college if a Ruskin scholarship was not offered. As he clearly wanted me to be one of his students, I reflected that it was to his credit that he did not try to outmanoeuvre Ruskin. A place was assured for me at his college but only if and when Ruskin rejected me. I received the offer with some misgivings. I had made sure that he knew of my near rejection of Catholicism, yet he still wanted me as a student, possibly with a view to reconversion. As that was out of the question for me, and I would therefore be going to his college under false pretences, the discussion had a strange air of unreality. Yet we both understood the situation perfectly and it was a very friendly discussion.

A few weeks later, as I walked home from the factory at midday, I saw Mam and my sister Helen waiting outside 34 Wellington Street. A letter had arrived from Oxford. I was now excited about the prospect and quickly opened it to find a message from Father O'Shea congratulating me on winning the Ruskin scholarship and regretting that I would not be joining him. I was delighted with the news but puzzled that the college had not yet officially informed me. After the meal Mam gave me a large envelope which she had put aside assuming it was some kind of advertisement; it was the official notification from Ruskin that I had been awarded the scholarship, together with information about the college.

Mam and my sisters were delighted for me, yet I knew they were also sad. My activities had made 34 Wellington Street one of the busiest and liveliest houses in Widnes. They had shared and enjoyed the excitement, but now it was ending. So too was my wage packet with which I had helped Mam. It was probably a bigger blow to her than I realized at the time. Yet she was full of encouragement and showed not the slightest reservation. Soon afterwards, in October 1946, I left the factory, gave up my official position in the Chemical

(57)

Workers' Union and resigned from the Council. My regret was mingled with excitement at the prospect of an entirely new life at Oxford.

5

Oxford and Cambridge

The train journey from Widnes to Oxford, by no means a long one, spanned two worlds for me. At that time, before the eleven-plus and the relative mobility in education, it was rare for anyone to go from a factory to college. Delighted at the opportunity, I was confident but a shade wary because of my lack of learning.

I did not intend my move to Oxford to be the end of my working life in Widnes. I intended to acquire knowledge and qualifications if possible, then return to the town, preferably as a full-time trade union official. If my experience in Bolton's factory could be combined with academic qualifications, I felt I would be well placed. But at that stage of my life, I had only a broad outline in my mind and no fixed ideas. I would adapt to the future as it unfolded.

One of the passengers on the train was a small, chunkily built, dark man. I could not define his quality but he interested me and I wondered if he, too, was going to Ruskin. Fortunately he was. We immediately liked each other and established a friendship which has continued to this day. A shipyard worker from Belfast, David Bleakley had a background similar to my own. On the short walk from the station to the college we agreed that if possible we would share a room.

Ruskin had none of the expansive, manicured quadrangles or historic cloisters of some other colleges. A small building with a plain exterior, it struck me as an academic workshop. Yet the other university activities – art, politics, sport or social life – were as available to us as to other students.

Scores of bicycles lined a passageway from the gate to a simply furnished common room; newspapers and periodicals lay on comfortable settees and armchairs. The adjoining library, well stocked and intimidating, was a reminder of all the books I had not read. Across the hallway was a large lecture room, and on the floor above were the students' living quarters.

I assumed, like many other students, that the college was founded by Ruskin but oddly enough it was established on the initiative of two Americans. They admired Ruskin and, being interested in the Labour movement, established the college in Oxford to provide educational opportunities for working-class students. For me it provided a unique opportunity for a two-year course of study and the opening up of a new and unexplored world.

Although I liked the friendly and unaffected atmosphere of the college, I was disappointed to learn that we would only live there for the second year. I left reluctantly – with David Bleakley – by bus for Headington, two miles outside Oxford, where we were to live for our first year. My mood changed when I saw The Rookery, a spacious building with clean, white-painted woodwork, set in lovely meadows. There could hardly have been a greater contrast to 34 Wellington Street with its cramped conditions and outside lavatory. I was stimulated by the new surroundings, feeling a sense of adventure and pleasure at the prospect of living there, studying at the college and meeting other students. The Rookery was primarily residential, although there was a library for private study; lectures and tutorials took place at the college. David and I moved from the separate rooms provisionally reserved for us into another which we shared with two other students; one was a serious draughtsman and the other a tubby steelworker with the unlikely name of Claude.

That evening, when we met the rest of the students, I found that most had worked in industry as I had, but they were different in a way I did not appreciate at first. Although mainly manual workers – miners, lorry drivers and from the shipyard – nearly all had taken courses of study before coming to Ruskin. Some were impressively well read, though they had few academic qualifications. I had not studied at all since leaving St Patrick's elementary school eight years

(60)

earlier. All my work had been practical; the only books I had read were a handbook of regulations governing the Town Council and Jack London's *The Iron Heel* – hardly adequate preparation for a university diploma in economics and political science.

Lionel Elvin, the Principal, was my tutor in political science. With him I embarked on a study of philosophers who were totally unfamiliar – Plato, Aristotle, Marx, Locke, Hobbes, Rousseau and Green. Dark, slim and athletic, Elvin was a former running Blue. He took my lack of learning in his stride, but there was no easy familiarity with him. I was always conscious of his stature, yet the acknowledgement was probably more in my mind than in his. He was friendly, enlivening our discussions with humour and encouraging questions and even criticism of his views. He gave me encouragement rather than good marks. I rarely got above B-plus, and often it was B, which was far from brilliant, but I always felt that Elvin appreciated the profound difficulties facing working-class students.

Every week I wrote a political essay which I discussed with him in an hour-long tutorial. It was rather like boxing with a far superior opponent who wants to encourage you and will not take advantage of his greater skill. Yet he never patronized or pretended ignorance; he treated students as his equals in intelligence, if not in knowledge.

The Vice-Principal, Henry Smith, was a cherubic economist who stalked up and down the rostrum seeming to enjoy baffling students with paradoxes. He was nevertheless a fine teacher because his manner and enthusiasm immediately excited interest and having caught it he held it throughout. Anyone unable to grasp a particular point would be invited on a long walk to discuss it. I once rashly accepted his invitation and found myself scurrying in the countryside around Oxford, trying to keep abreast of him and his erudite explanation of economic theory. I would have been wiser to stay in college with a book, learning the fundamentals before approaching him with more advanced problems.

One other noteworthy teacher, Stephen Schofield, the social history tutor, spoke slowly and reflectively. His favourite ploy was to debunk historical myths. 'The Peterloo massacre?' he would ask innocently, extending his arms widely. 'But only a few old men and a dog were killed that day, so I don't know why they call it a massacre.' He was one of the most amusing lecturers in Oxford. I thought that history would be taught as in St Patrick's, Widnes, with numerous names and dates of important events. In our old elementary school, it had been mainly monarchs and battles; but at Ruskin, Schofield dealt with the great social and economic trends of the past. He brought them to life, analysing, interpreting and assessing people and events with verve and humour.

Although Ruskin was not part of Oxford University we were able to attend university lectures and use its libraries. Lectures in Ruskin, by men we came to know well, were more relaxed than those in the university; these seemed formal and the dons remote.

I was impoverished in comparison with the undergraduates, a few of whom flaunted their extravagance. As I was sending part of my allowance to Mam I had great difficulty in managing. I was so short of money that I answered the advertisement of a middle-class couple who wanted a girl to clean their house. They were astonished when I applied, but as no girls volunteered they accepted me. Three or four times a week I went to clean their living room, bring coal in from a shed in the garden and light the fire at about four o'clock. It was a far cry from the tough, rumbustious atmosphere of the factory where I had loaded furnaces. As I kindled the little fire I felt lonely and gloomy. They were a genteel old couple who retired to bed after lunch and came down later for afternoon tea. They were grateful for my work, but I disliked it, feeling that I was misusing my time.

As I had to find money from somewhere, I wrote to my Member of Parliament, Christopher Shawcross, seeking help with my application for a further education grant. The condition of such a grant was that an educational course broken by war service was being resumed. A great flight of imagination was necessary to identify me as a scholar before I left Bolton's, but the cliché of learning in the universities of industry and life helped to make it airborne. A generous Minister of Education, giving me the benefit of what must have been monumental doubt, awarded me the grant. It meant leaving the old couple, and I felt so sorry for them that I kept extending my notice to quit until they found someone else.

Dress was the most visible sign of the difference between Ruskin students and the undergraduates. They wore gowns and we did not, but the differences went deeper than that. Starkly contrasting backgrounds were reflected not only in clothes but in attitudes. Not every undergraduate was a dilettante, nor every Ruskin student a thoughtful citizen, but many undergraduates seemed to have boyish bonhomie, or even flippancy, that was not shared by students at Ruskin.

Their accents differed from ours, reflecting long-established class divisions in British society. With our backgrounds in factories, mines and shipyards we had a sense of surprise that we were at Oxford, whereas they seemed settled in their natural habitat and fitted in snugly – we sometimes thought smugly – with the cloisters and spires. The impression may have been false but it was powerful, and it prevented me from ever feeling completely at home in Oxford.

I liked the lively Ruskin student body, earnest at its work, humorous in its social life. Occasional concerts at the college had a faint echo of the singing competitions of my childhood at the Picturedrome in Widnes. Local talent flowered; students proved to be fine sopranos, impressive baritones or amusing mimics. Once a tutor's lecturing eccentricities were caricatured so perceptively and devastatingly that he changed his style (for a few days).

David showed his strength of character when, with his Irish brogue, he was referred to as 'Paddy'. He mentioned, apparently casually, that his name was David, but when he was called Paddy again he said pointedly: 'I've already told you my name is David, not Paddy. If you can't understand that I'm prepared to repeat it for you until you do.' Never again was he called Paddy. A gifted student, he had high academic standards and an almost puritanical outlook. He could moralize without preaching. Early in our student days he got into a discussion with a cockney student who was fond of what he called 'the birds'. A quiet but vigorous denunciation from David about promiscuity left the cockney pledging that he would be different in future. David was not seeking converts, merely expressing his own views; he happened to make a big impression.

I never found the work easy, and I took a long time to master the

(63)

basic elements of the course. Rather belatedly I realized that it was essential to study in the first few months or one was left behind and could never quite catch up. Lecturers would naturally go ahead on the assumption that the preceding lesson had been understood. Ploughing through Marshall's vast tract on the *Principles of Economics* tested me sorely; it did not help when others praised its simplicity and lucidity.

I was much happier with political theory. Although I was more interested in current controversies than the ancient ones, these gave philosophical depth and understanding to fundamental political problems. Later we moved on to theories of more modern political thinkers; some Ruskin students were dedicated Marxists, but I disagreed with them. Despite my past confrontations with employers, I rejected Marxism and the theory of inevitable revolution, preferring democratic, rather than revolutionary, change.

By this time I had become a Labour Party supporter. I had always been opposed to the Conservatives on class grounds. In Widnes they favoured employers and landlords against trade unionists and tenants – to me they were natural opponents. My studies at Ruskin provided theoretical justification for my socialist instincts. I learned to appreciate the historic significance of the Labour movement; my differences with the Labour Party, caused by my association with the ILP and conflict with local councillors, fell into perspective.

At Ruskin I saw, for the first time, direct clashes between the democratic socialists of the Labour Party and the then revolutionaries of the Communist Party. The communists, assertive and dogmatic, used political jargon and patronized the socialists. Nothing pains a radical more than to be told he is only a milk-and-water reformer, lacking the rich red blood of a man of action. The revolutionary fervour was so much in evidence in my early days at Ruskin that I felt almost apologetic for being a socialist – but I soon learned to overcome these feelings as communist diatribes were met with equal ferocity, and sometimes derision, by the socialists.

Personal friendships survived political differences, though extreme views could disturb a relationship. I once went to an Oxford bookshop with a friend who was an ardent communist. After selecting our books we were about to return to college when, instead of going to the till to pay, he left by a side door. Later, when I asked him if he had stolen the books, he told me not to be so naïve. The printers and publishers, he said, were making vast profits by exploiting the workers; they were unjustly supported by laws made by the ruling class, so his action was a justifiable retaliation. We argued, without animosity, about morality, the rule of law and the ends not justifying the means, but his views remained unchanged.

At the end of the academic year I returned to Widnes and, despite my need to study, I soon put my books aside and resumed campaigning for better housing. This time, instead of acting on my own, I went to see the local Labour councillors. Willing to co-operate, they called a special meeting in St Patrick's church hall to shake up the authorities.

At this crowded meeting the councillors spoke first. I was about to make the final speech when the lights went out. No one knew whether it was an electrical failure or, as we suspected, sabotage, but before long some candles were produced. In this eerie setting, I made an emotional speech quoting the high death rate of babies and condemning the landlords as having 'blood on their hands'. Given warm support, I promised to amass evidence and seek urgent action from the Council.

After only a few days at home I felt as if I had never been away. Oxford seemed distant and irrelevant, and I was happier resuming campaigning. In the next few months I visited hundreds of slum houses, collecting evidence of overcrowding and of people living in abysmal conditions. I accumulated a formidable dossier. Scarce building materials were being used to repair and renovate cinemas and football grounds while houses were neglected. I also found that new council houses had not been allocated to those in greatest need.

When I had compiled all my evidence I told the Town Clerk, who invited me to appear before a special joint meeting of the Health and Housing Committee of the Council. Before I addressed the councillors he warned that there would be a verbatim report of my speech, with possible legal action if I slandered anyone. The joint committees had obviously decided to give me enough rope to hang myself; and apart from one or two pointed questions from the Town Clerk, there was no discussion. Eventually all my demands for an inquiry were rejected, but my efforts were not in vain. The number of housing repairs and the allocation of council houses were significantly affected by the campaign.

The Town Clerk had behaved impeccably throughout. Peering through his spectacles, he had said, rather primly: 'May I remind you, Mr Ashley, of the standing orders of the Council concerning the point that you seek to raise.' Yet this formal exterior disguised a deep humanity. He told me later that when he read the transcript of my evidence he was impressed by it. I heard that he spoke against all my demands, as he warned me he would do, since he had to defend the Council's policy. His opposition did not alter the deep friendship we developed and I always appreciated his guidance and the kindness he showed me. I was deeply saddened by his death a few years afterwards in a car accident.

When I returned to Oxford for my second year I lived in the college and spent more time at my studies. I was acutely aware of the need to make up time after the leisurely first year but I found it hard going. As the year progressed and examinations loomed large, our work became a frequent topic of our conversation. At The Rookery we had been a diverse collection of individuals taking a course of study, whereas in the college we were now a corporate body of students approaching a searching test. Not only was our personal standing involved but so also was the reputation of the college; it had provided workers with opportunity, books, lectures and tuition, and we were anxious not to fail it. I was by no means confident, since formal examinations were wholly unfamiliar to me.

The tension must have been even greater than I thought, because when I walked out after the final paper, Oxford looked brighter to me. I was seeing it without the cloud of anxiety which had hung over me for months. That night I celebrated with my friends. All we could do now was sit back and wait for the result. A few days later, I heard that some Ruskin students were applying for extramural scholarships: two at Oxford University, two at Cambridge and ten state scholarships. I joined the throng, thinking that if I won one, I could then decide whether to go on with academic study.

The first stage of the scholarships was a written essay on any subject we chose. I decided on an imaginary conversation between T. H. Green, the Social Democrat, and Karl Marx. Although I was fairly familiar with the political views of both, I spent a few weeks intently studying their works. It was strange that I should find myself totally absorbed and enjoying concentrated study only at the end of my two years in Oxford. I began to regret that I had left it so late. My long essay reflected the clash of philosophy and political theory between these two men who naturally debated fundamental political issues – but I felt that a lighter ending was needed. Marx concluded by saying that they did not seem to have reached any agreement in the discussion. 'No,' said Green, 'but if it has only enabled this bright young man to get a scholarship to Cambridge, surely it will have been well worthwhile.' Despite this cheeky ending my essay secured me a place on the short list for all of the scholarships.

The first interviews were for Cambridge. I travelled there with two other short-listed Ruskin students, David Bleakley and Eric Linfield. On the journey no one spoke about our prospects, but in Cambridge, as we were walking by Fenner's playing field, David put my thoughts into words when he said: 'I wonder whether this will be our first and last time in Cambridge or if it will become familiar to any of us in the next three years.'

We were interviewed in turn by the board. They questioned me about my essay, my background and my hopes for the future. They were informal and friendly with all of us, so there was no realistic way of evaluating the impression each had made. If the criteria were to be academic standards, I had no doubt that David Bleakley and Eric Linfield would be chosen. But the board members had seemed interested in my activities as a local trade union leader and town councillor. Back at Ruskin the following morning I was congratulated by a smiling student who had just heard that the college had carried off both Cambridge scholarships and that I had won one, Eric Linfield the other. I was delighted, for I had taken an immediate

(67)

and instinctive liking to Cambridge. The Principal of Ruskin, himself a Cambridge man, came to congratulate me, and we had a celebratory drink.

When I visited my future tutor, Stanley Dennison, at the Cambridge college I was allocated, Gonville and Caius, I liked him, although I sensed, correctly, that our political attitudes were different. I still had a lurking doubt about passing the Oxford diploma examination, so I asked him what would happen if I failed. It would make no difference, he said. My Cambridge scholarship was safe regardless of the Oxford results. When they were published soon afterwards I was relieved to find that I had passed. It was no surprise to anyone, least of all to me, that David Bleakley got a distinction. I wondered if that result would have affected the Cambridge scholarship decision had it been known at the time. I was delighted when within weeks he won a scholarship to Queen's University, Belfast. He subsequently had a distinguished career, becoming Minister for Community Relations in Northern Ireland.

In my final few weeks at Oxford, I became involved in another public controversy. In the *Widnes Weekly News*, regularly sent to me by Mam, I read the report of a speech by the leader of the Council's Conservative group, Dr Baxter, a senior ICI chemist who later became a professor at Sydney University. He said the trade unions should end their affiliation to the Labour Party and become politically independent. I believed the unions and party should work closely together, so I challenged Dr Baxter to a public debate. Rather to my surprise, he accepted. This created great interest in the town, and within weeks the Trades Council arranged the debate under the chairmanship of the Town Clerk.

I studied the history books for all the relevant Acts and significant dates, compiling an imposing array. Just before I left Ruskin for Widnes I met Stephen Schofield, the laconic social history tutor, and told him about the forthcoming debate. He was agreeably interested and I was encouraged enough to show him all my data. Glancing through my notes, he said to me with a slow smile, 'I'd chuck 'em away if I were you. All you need is three or four points. And debate, don't recite.' His advice rang true. I also took the precaution of writing to the Conservative Central Office for their views about the unions and the Labour Party. They probably assumed I was a supporter and their reply, prompt and comprehensive, enabled me to study my opponent's case for what was to be the first formal public debate of my life.

Even some of my warmest supporters in Widnes felt I had bitten off more than I could chew. The most that a worried Ken Merrifield would allow himself to say, as we walked to the debate together, was, 'Well, he's a very clever man, you know.' This, coming from a close friend, was a little ominous, and I began to share his qualms. As the debate had attracted wide attention, hundreds of people were swarming into the hall when we approached. I noted with dismay that many of them had come in cars, and these were probably Conservative supporters. I spoke first, and although my speech was well received I thought Dr Baxter's was better. Polite, well spoken and intelligent, he put an effective case. But I was relieved that he followed exactly the lines I had expected so that when I wound up the debate I was able to quote and deride the sources of his quotations, and even some of his phrases. Then I subjected them to what I hoped was withering criticism. My best line was in response to his claim that Conservatives wanted co-operation with trade unions. I described how they had robbed trade unions of rights over the years and said, 'If a burglar breaks into your home six days a week, then offers co-operation on the seventh, would you believe him?'

The Town Clerk took a vote by a show of hands. It was evident that I had won by a wide margin, but he diplomatically announced 'a narrow majority' for me. Of course, the vote was meaningless, because I noticed that my people voted solidly for me and Dr Baxter's supporters voted for him. As the hall was overcrowded, it was really a question of whose supporters had arrived first and were able to cast their votes within sight of the chairman while the overflow in the corridors went unseen. Nevertheless I was delighted with the result – the occasion whetted my appetite for debate.

Although I had been happy at Ruskin I never loved Oxford; its atmosphere, which many students found heady and inspiring, did not affect me in that way. Despite my youthful confidence, the

overnight change from factory to college and my unfamiliarity with
books, compounded by my failure to concentrate on them until the
end, created a lurking doubt. I went to Cambridge as a full member
of the university, acclimatized to an academic atmosphere, and it
filled me with an exhilaration which was to last throughout my stay.

In 1948 the mixture of undergraduates was particularly interesting. Some had come straight from school, and others had been in
the forces during the war. Most were middle class, and many were
public school boys. In Gonville and Caius College, there were no
workers or factory labourers to provide instant companionship as at
Ruskin. At the first informal assembly for freshmen, where many
students seemed to know each other, they grouped together amid a
buzz of animated chatter. No one spoke to me. Although I made a
few attempts at light conversation which quickly faded, I did not
feel uncomfortable. I looked forward to my years with this cheerful
crowd, knowing that our class and backgrounds were different but
not expecting them to cause insuperable difficulties.

I had heard about college servants, known as scouts, who looked
after students and addressed them as 'sir'. Perhaps they were some
kind of civilian batmen, waiting hand and foot on busy undergraduates. My scout turned out to be a middle-aged woman whose job
was to clean and tidy the rooms; she called me 'sir', but in an
unaffected way, accepting it as part of the normal verbal currency.
Far from being deferential, she had a sense of humour which
ridiculed any idea of a personal 'batman'.

I was allocated attractive rooms in the forecourt – a sitting room
and an adjoining bedroom – to be shared with a fellow student.
Another David Bleakley, perhaps? But when he entered I knew that
we had nothing in common; it was not just a difference of class or
character but a disturbing combination of both. He was tall, elegant
and self-assured, with an upper-class accent – when he spoke at all.
No doubt he resented a rough, working-class character sharing his
rooms. Either the authorities had an odd sense of humour or they
calculated that I could gain, and he could lose, a little polish to our
mutual advantage.

For some time we lived together without developing friendship, although discord was muted by his impeccable manners. Even the small gestures at mutual accommodation seemed to emphasize rather than soften our differences. One day he received a parcel from his mother containing Stilton cheese, which I had never seen before. When he offered me some I cut a hefty chunk, rather like hacking a piece of Cheddar in the factory canteen, and made a sandwich. He murmured that the best way to enjoy Stilton was to eat a little at a time. Remarkably enough, we did become friends eventually as we slowly got to know each other and found that underlying our differing attitudes we both had a sense of humour.

Despite these uneasy months with my room-mate, I never found that class alone prevented friendships. Some of the few working-class students at Cambridge felt bitterness about class and the inequality it reflected, but I did not share these feelings. I knew that some upper-class students enjoyed, and took for granted, wealth and privilege unknown in Widnes. But they, with their cut-glass accents, were as much the product of their environment as I, with my Lancashire accent, was of mine. I did not want my strong political opposition to class privilege to degenerate into personal animosity.

Nevertheless financial differences could create awkward situations. One night as we walked downstairs from the dining hall a group of friendly students invited me to have a drink at the 'buttery'. This turned out to be a small wines and spirits bar below the dining room which I had not noticed before.

'What will you have – a glass of port?'

'Well, yes, certainly,' I replied, reflecting that port wine was something we had with mince pies at Christmas in Widnes.

It was a pleasant drink and an enjoyable conversation. Later, when I bought a round of drinks for the group, I was stunned at the cost. Apart from very special occasions, I kept away from the 'buttery' after that.

Many pleasures at university cost nothing. The tolling of bells has always affected me; as a child in Wellington Street, on tranquil Sunday afternoons, I used to listen with pleasure to the church bells pealing in the Town Hall Square a quarter of a mile away. The bells of St Patrick's Church, just before Mass, were a solemn and welcome

(71)

call to duty. In Caius College the bell tolled for five minutes before the evening meal as gowned students and tutors made their way across the quadrangle to the dining hall. This bell symbolized for me the traditions and academic spirit of Cambridge more than all the buildings.

In hall we stood in long lines at the tables. When the bell stopped, silence fell – to be broken by the intoning of a Latin prayer from the high table. I sometimes wondered, as I stood with bowed head, what my friends in Widnes would be doing at that moment, and what robust and irreverent comments they would have made seeing me gowned and at prayer.

Life at Cambridge was organized to ensure maximum opportunity for study. We had our own college rooms, splendid libraries and regular daily lectures. Although there was no compulsion to attend lectures, I was encouraged by my tutor to go and listen to the many world-famous economists who taught in Cambridge. Each lecture started punctually on the hour and finished a few minutes before the next, so that students rushed from one lecture room to the other. I rushed a little more than most to get a front seat as I could not hear clearly if I sat at the back.

It was interesting to note the individual characteristics of the lecturers. In the Economics faculty Professor Denis Robertson was sardonic and witty, Joan Robinson authoritative and clear, Stanley Dennison intellectual and informative. I liked Dennison very much. A dark, handsome man with aquiline features and a gentle voice, he was my tutor in college, and each week I spent an hour with him discussing my essay on economics. In social economic affairs it is difficult to draw an exact line between economic theory and political argument. Dennison encouraged me to analyse my own assumptions and was prepared to discuss his own without attempting to persuade me to accept them.

In the first few weeks I visited various university clubs and sporting groups where some of the games were unfamiliar to me. I had never played tennis before and did badly; at squash I was unskilled; when I tried rowing I became bored. I decided to try my old game, rugby, and as the first college game was a sort of Probables versus Possibles I went along to play. Unfortunately the referee did not arrive. Since no one seemed to want the job, I volunteered. I was an expert at this game, having played Rugby League often in Widnes, and I knew the rules well. Soon after the start the ball was kicked ahead over the touchline without first bouncing inside. This meant no ground was gained and I ordered the teams back to the kicking point; they were obviously astonished, but obeyed my instructions. Next time this happened the man who kicked the ball argued. Gradually I felt a sense of incredulity spreading among both teams.

I had assumed that the rules of rugby in Cambridge were the same as those of rugby in Widnes. But Rugby Union at the university had many different rules to Rugby League in my home town. Before long the teams were playing to their own rules by common consent; players would stop without my whistle or go on in spite of it. It must have been the first time in the history of the college that two teams worked in such harmony with total disregard of a referee. It was clear from uncomplimentary remarks that I should confine my football activities to Rugby League.

Although I got to know fellow students at the college first, it was in the University Labour Club that I made most friends, some of whom were from my college. As a former councillor I had practical experience of the politics they talked about and this inevitably gave me an advantage. We spent much time together, discussing and arguing. The animated meetings were sometimes addressed by MPs who, if they were wise, entered into the spirit of the occasion. Sonorous MPs were not accorded a deferential welcome.

I played an active role in the University Labour Club and just before the end of my first year I was elected Chairman. The leaders of the University Conservative Club, our main opponents, included some interesting characters, later to make their way, and their names, in Parliament. The most flamboyant, and one of the wittiest, was Norman St John Stevas. His dress, manner and speech all seemed calculated to provoke, but when attacked he was usually ready with a sparkling riposte. If on occasion he appeared foppish, with a yellow waistcoat and cravat, he proved in debate that appearances were deceptive: he was one of the most able men in the university.

He later became Leader of the House of Commons and then a member of the House of Lords.

My direct counterpart was Geoffrey Howe, Chairman of the Conservative Association. After one explosive first meeting, I grew to like him, and our friendship has endured over the years. There was an interesting contrast between him and the leader of the Labour Club who preceded me as Chairman, Percy Craddock. Howe was amiable, diligent and astute, and although he never became President of the Union, the university's famous debating society, he was an able debater. Craddock was dry, sparkling and satirical. He was the most scintillating debater I heard. Although he gave the appearance of not working, he, too, must have been diligent because he got two double Firsts, in English and Law.

Later, Craddock was to become British Ambassador to China and then foreign affairs adviser to the Prime Minister. Howe became Foreign Secretary, and for a while was Craddock's boss.

My arguments with Conservative student leaders were passionate. Geoffrey Howe gave some indication of this many years later when, as Foreign Secretary, he hosted an official lunch for the Chinese Ambassador in London which I attended. An amused Howe told the Ambassador that the first time we met at Cambridge we had an angry political argument which ended when I stormed off saying, 'I'll never speak to another bloody Tory again.'

Of course, I did so, and I met most of them at the Union Society. I joined at the suggestion of the administrator of my scholarship who believed that I would get much interest and pleasure from the debates; I also recalled my debate with Dr Baxter in Widnes. Before joining the Union I attended the opening debate of my first term as a visitor. It was a crowded and lively occasion, the President and officers in evening dress and packed students opposed on political lines for a motion of no confidence in the Labour Government. The opening Tory speaker, fluent and impressive, was enthusiastically acclaimed by his supporters, and acknowledged by the opposition. I didn't envy his opponent. But it was Craddock, then unknown to me, who rose, swirling his long graduate gown and smiling at the opposition. Within moments he had the audience laughing at his barbed mockery, the prelude to a brilliant speech.

My own first speech, a few weeks later, was on the Irish question when the legendary De Valera was the guest speaker. I knew little about the subject but that did not deter me and I won a reasonable reception. Shortly afterwards Craddock, whom I had met at the Labour Club, told me that I would be invited by the President to be one of the two main speakers to open a forthcoming debate. I hoped for a political subject, but Craddock said it was to be 'The scientist and artist must accept responsibility for the social consequences of their work'. He looked at me wryly when I asked who my opponent was to be; then he admitted with a smile that he himself was. The occasion was, as usual, an auspicious one for Craddock, though not for me. Yet I made good progress during the year, and in my second year I was elected to the committee and then to the Secretaryship.

I was now set fair for the Presidency if I won the Vice-Presidency first, but some of my opponents criticized the clothes I wore. Unable to afford evening dress, I wore my lounge suit at debates, even when sitting in a prominent position at the Secretary's desk; this was unprecedented. Shortly before the election for Vice-President a personal attack on me was printed in the Oxford *Isis*. The anonymous critic wrote: 'No one would object to an officer appearing at debates in a lounge suit through financial necessity, but to do so (as no other officers who were Socialists have done) on account of perverted political principle seems to many to amount to a gratuitous insult to the dignity of his office.' The article, timely for my opponents, was given much publicity in Cambridge.

My natural reaction was to fire off a strong rejoinder, but I was dissuaded by some of my colleagues, including Craddock, who were generally regarded as the elder statesmen of the Labour Club. Instead of an angry retort, I said I was sorry that so violent a personal attack should have been launched upon me in an election which, I had hoped, would have been conducted along very different lines. I never knew whether my reply was effective or if the original attack backfired. Perhaps it was regarded as irrelevant by members of the Union; in any case I won the Vice-Presidency with a comfortable majority of over ninety. The following term I was returned unopposed as the first working-class President of the Cambridge Union Society – still wearing a lounge suit.

My guest speakers included personalities such as Hugh Dalton, Selwyn Lloyd, Gilbert Harding, Donald Soper and Jeremy Thorpe. Some care was exercised pitting one against another. Inviting a politician with a comedian, no matter how attractive a proposition, would have insulted the one and discomfited the other. Two people I thought would make good opponents in a debate on world peace were my friend Bob Edwards of the ILP and Chemical Workers' Union and Randolph Churchill.

Although Edwards was an emotive and effective platform orator, the Cambridge Union Society was not the place for his particular talents and he did not adapt his style. His speech, which would have electrified a political conference, was received with some banter by unimpressed though friendly students. When he was speaking of the horrors of war, Churchill baited him by waving his handkerchief as the white flag of surrender; in fact, Edwards was no pacifist, having fought in the Spanish Civil War. But it was an example of misplaced oratory by Edwards and a caricature of it by Churchill.

Near the end of my Presidential term I was invited to make a debating tour of universities in the USA, along with Ronald Waterhouse, my predecessor, later Sir Ronald, a High Court judge. A well-groomed Liberal lawyer, he came from a middle-class home. Although our backgrounds were different we enjoyed each other's company. We lightly agreed to speak on any of six motions which were sent to twenty American universities – each one choosing the subject it preferred. The two most popular subjects were that we 'deplored the banning of Communist parties in free, democratic states' and that we 'regretted the American way of life', although one of the others – 'that democratic socialism is the most effective barrier against Soviet communism' – was chosen by a few universities. We combined on the first two issues and opposed each other on the last one.

I was to be away for two months. As my final examinations were due within a month of my return, I took a case full of books. It was never opened; I had simply given myself an added weight to carry around the States. Because of the pressure of time, neither Waterhouse nor I had prepared speeches on any of the six subjects when we embarked on the *Queen Elizabeth*. We intended to work on them during the voyage. It was a silly idea; the entertainments on that magnificent ship, together with the excitement of our first trip to the United States, induced us to enjoy a frivolous and relaxed voyage. Originally we had been allocated berths deep in the ship, but Waterhouse had a well-connected friend in the Cunard Line. As a result we were promoted to a top-deck cabin, invited to the Purser's receptions and placed on his table for meals. The menus were magnificent, and we enjoyed the food as well as the ship's recreational facilities including music, dancing, books, games and sports.

When the ship berthed in New York we faced a tour of twenty universities beginning the next day, a journey from the Atlantic to the Pacific, and no speeches prepared. Our first debate was at St Joseph's College, Philadelphia. I expected it to take a similar form to our own in Cambridge, though perhaps in a more modern building. We were accustomed to speaking in a small debating chamber, with a few hundred students around us interjecting in the debate. At Philadelphia there was no audience participation in this sense, although they listened. Instead we were elevated, with our opponents, on a stage in a vast stadium – the Union Jack draped behind us, the Stars and Stripes behind them – facing 3,000 people. Advertised as an international debate, it was adjudicated by a panel of judges which included a Federal Court judge, a Congressman, a professor and the president of an insurance company. The British Consul turned out to give us moral support.

Doubtless the organizers intended it to be a serious occasion, but Cambridge debates were liberally spiced with humour and we decided to stick to our style. The audience readily responded, although I suspect they were laughing as much at our accents as at our wit. The American team were more solemn, adopting the formal pattern we were to recognize throughout the tour – introduction, facts, interpretation of facts, conclusion and peroration. This rigidity made our opponents predictable targets, and we took full advantage.

(77)

They were particularly vulnerable when opposing our motion that we deplored the banning of Communist parties in free democratic states. American students arrived with detailed notes about the iniquities of communism, assuming that we would be supporting it. We usually caught them off balance – to our delight and their discomfiture – by immediately agreeing on the iniquities but arguing that the principle and tactics of banning were wrong and counterproductive.

The Americans treated us like visiting celebrities. After the debate, a crowd of teenagers would ask for autographs before we left for late-night parties. After the debates, we were rushed on to the next university. It was a rigorous schedule which was to take us to the Pacific coast and back. During the next few weeks, accepting warm American hospitality, we maintained in debates that we deplored their way of life – but they were tolerant and generous hosts.

After our intensive debating across the USA, we hoped to resume studying for exams on the return voyage. I achieved very little, arriving back in Cambridge to find most students revising material I had not even heard of. It was near the end of April and, with exams in less than a month, a friend helpfully brought his notes to my room. We were interrupted by an undergraduate who was working on the university newspaper *Varsity* – a lovely young woman with dark brown hair and blue eyes. She wanted to ask me about the debating tour, but I was too busy so I asked her to return the following day. Unable to do so, she said that she would ask the editor to send someone else. I told her that since this was the first time *Varsity* had ever sent me a pretty reporter, if she would not interview me no one else could; she accepted the compliment and came back next day.

I was more interested in her than in the interview so I talked light-heartedly about the tour. Waterhouse had spoken to her at some length, but when her report appeared his views were secondary. I joked about it when I met him and warned him not to be too critical as I was now going out with the young woman, Pauline Crispin. A first-year student, she was a mathematics scholar at Girton College. I knew we would be parting soon because I was at the end of my third year. But having met her, I did not want to part. After being away from Cambridge for two months, I had to work hard for my examinations, yet I wanted to see more of her.

I maintain that I cycled the three miles to Girton regularly, but Pauline claims that she more frequently cycled to Caius College. We probably did a lot of each, but one way or another we met often and grew even closer. We hardly seemed compatible as she was quiet and shy while I was rumbustious and extrovert. She was the scholar; I still found it hard to concentrate on books. Her sports were swimming and hockey, in which she represented Cambridge; mine were rugby, soccer and boxing, in which I represented no one.

The days were passing all too quickly. As my examinations grew closer I was remorseful at neglecting my studies. No doubt this was a feeling shared by many undergraduates, but they had not spent the preceding two months away from the university. I was relieved to get a second-class Honours Degree and in June 1951 I left Cambridge to set about finding a job in the trade union movement whence I had come.

6

Labouring – and the Lost Election

As a result of a misunderstanding, I returned to Widnes with an Oxford diploma, a Cambridge degree and no job. Although I had not been promised a post in the Chemical Workers' Union, Bob Edwards had talked about the possibility of my becoming his assistant. He was, no doubt, thinking aloud and speculating. I unwisely assumed a job would be waiting when I left Cambridge, but I was mistaken.

Anxious to work in the Labour movement, I got in touch with George Woodcock, then Assistant General Secretary of the TUC, who suggested I should approach individual trade union leaders. He offered to speak to Tom Williamson, leader of the giant National Union of General and Municipal Workers. This was the union I had fought when I organized the Chemical Workers' Union at Bolton's, but Woodcock, speaking highly of Williamson, felt he might have a job for me. I wrote, hopeful but doubtful.

Meanwhile, I went to stay with Pauline for a few days at her home in Ewell, near Epsom in Surrey. There I met her mother and her sister, Barbara. Her father had died eighteen months earlier in a road accident. We left Ewell to go to Widnes for Pauline's first visit to this highly industrial town, replete with chemical factories. The mainline train stopped at neighbouring Runcorn, and at that time people crossed the River Mersey to Widnes by the old Transporter Bridge. From an enormous superstructure dangled a platform which held about 20 cars and 60 people. On windy days when this shaky contraption was attempting to cross, it sometimes had to turn back; on stormy days it was wisely docked. Pedestrians then used a footpath across the adjoining railway bridge, and car drivers had to detour through Warrington, a town some five miles up river, approaching Widnes from the other side.

Pauline crossed the Mersey, saw my home town and met Mam and the rest of the family. Diplomatically perhaps, she made no comment on the environment, although she told me later that she was taken aback by the chemical smell in the air, particularly in the evening when the area reeked with fumes. She was warmly welcomed and instantly accepted; although her background was different from ours, her human values were the same. Shortly afterwards we got engaged, and she quickly became one of the family.

While Pauline resumed her studies at Cambridge, and I needed a temporary job, I applied to the Council building department, where I had worked as a labourer during two long vacations. They took me on again. Laying concrete foundations on a new housing estate, I worked with two old friends, strikingly different in physique, character and outlook. In very different ways, they made light of heavy work.

Tom Cosgrove looked like a bull-necked prize-fighter. Of medium height, he was barrel-chested and stocky, with powerful arms and shoulders. When I tried to wrestle with him, he would simply lift me off my feet and hold me in the air. We had been close friends since he had been one of the shop stewards at Bolton's. He worked hard and expected others to do the same, though few could keep up with him when the pressure was on.

Our other workmate was a man who loved to loaf. Billy Knott, a small, thin man, elevated avoiding work to a fine art. He was one of the downtrodden characters of this world – a Charlie Chaplin figure, buffeted by authority. His clothes were always a bit too big for him and he shuffled rather than walked. His careworn, deeply lined faced contrasted with a twinkle in his eyes, reflecting a whimsical sense of humour. No man derived more pleasure from the simple act of leaning on a spade. With one foot resting on the blade and his arms folded over the handle, he would address a stream of comical remarks to Cosgrove and me as we worked. We protected him as best we could from being caught standing idle by the foreman. This did not happen very often, not because he was never idle but because he watched constantly for the boss. I enjoyed and shared the banter between this little man who joked and shirked and the burly Cosgrove, who tolerantly did his own 'fair whack' and a bit more.

We had a trick for punctuating Billy's conversation which rarely failed. One of us would look sharply over his shoulder and mutter, 'Look out!' To be caught idle and unaware by the foreman was sacrilegious to him and he had a sixth sense of when authority was nearby. But he could never be sure whether we had raised a false alarm, so the flow of chatter would stop as he worked his spade feverishly before furtively glancing round. If no one was there, we had to endure a stream of oaths as we laughed, then he would resume his stance and chatter. One day, after some false alarms, we muttered urgently to him when the foreman really was behind him. Instead of looking round, he snorted defiance, abusing the foreman, assuming we were pulling his leg. After the foreman had finished with him he was a crestfallen little comedian.

During this happy summer I had a great sense of well-being. Even on wet days our spirits were rarely dampened. It was understood that we would not work outside in heavy rain. If the sky clouded over and we felt a few spots of rain, Billy would announce that he was 'soaked to the bloody skin' and retire to a shed. If the rain increased I followed, to be joined later by Cosgrove, who always brought a set of draughts for this contingency. Billy would smoke a Woodbine and watch this highly intellectual game in respectful silence.

One Friday I asked the foreman if there was any weekend overtime as I needed the money. He told me of a reception to be held the following day at which councillors were to watch a special film, in a municipal building with a glass roof. I was to pull tarpaulins over the roof just before the film and remove them afterwards. While I waited for the civic party to assemble, the Leader of the Council, who was a friend, came over and urged me to join them. When I told him about the tarpaulins, he said, 'Pull the damn things over now and let this lot talk with the lights on.' I did so and joined the party. This incident was to affect the course of my life for the next fourteen years.

At the reception James McColl, the MP for Widnes, was one of the people who asked about my future plans. He recalled an advertisement he had seen for a radio producer's job in the BBC where one of the qualifications was some experience of the USA. I had been there only on my debating tour, but the job seemed worth applying for. McColl promised to send me the advertisement; it arrived three days after the closing date for applications. I telephoned Kenneth Adam, the Controller of the Light Programme on BBC radio, whom I had met at the Union Society in Cambridge, and asked him how rigidly the Corporation adhered to these dates. He advised me to apply at once, explaining the delay and apologizing for it. I sent off the letter and received a formal acknowledgement.

In the meantime I was invited to see Tom Williamson at the London office of the National Union of General and Municipal Workers. I knew of him as a mighty trade union boss who thundered at the TUC conference. Of course he could be tough when necessary, but he was warm to me and offered a job in the research department. Williamson admitted that the pay was poor but said that it was determined by the Executive Committee and there was little he could do. It was September 1951. After five years at college and three months labouring, I felt it was time to make more constructive use of my qualifications. The new job marked the end of my old life in Widnes, and although I was excited about the future, I left my birthplace with many regrets. I had known many happy years there and I knew that I would be returning often to see the family and my friends.

In London I took temporary digs in a drab bed-sitter in Belsize Park and went to work in the union office. I had to prepare information on diverse subjects such as gas, water, rubber and chemicals. Although much of the work was new to me, I found it intensely interesting. There I made some good friends, one of whom was David Basnett, later to become General Secretary of the union and an influential figure in Labour politics in the 1970s. A quiet and

(83)

reflective man, he would relax over a pint of beer after work and display surprising warmth and humour, in contrast to his rather serious demeanour at work. Together with Colin Chivers, a diminutive jester in charge of research, and Marie Butler, the capable and humorous secretary to Tom Williamson, we formed a close and friendly group.

My enjoyment of the job was marred only by concern over money. I was helping Mam and planning to get married, but my pay was very low. I had almost forgotten about my application for a job with the BBC. Quite unexpectedly, I was asked to go for an interview. It reminded me of the scholarship boards; everyone was friendly and easy-going. An obvious question, which I should have anticipated, caught me slightly off balance. I was asked to imagine producing a radio programme at short notice about an unfamiliar town – how would I go about it? I had no idea until I suddenly visualized Widnes; then I talked about all the interesting contacts I could think of, including civic leaders, employers, trade unionists, landlords, slum dwellers, local journalists and other characters. My blunderbuss approach would have produced a programme lacking in direction but so comprehensive that it must have included some good material. I was offered the job. Perhaps my debating tour of the USA influenced their decision, because my other qualifications were slight; I had no production experience, and my interest in radio was confined to news and music.

Soon afterwards the date of the 1951 General Election, 25 October, was announced. It would take place before I started my BBC job. The Labour Government had lived precariously since its majority had been slashed to six in the 1950 election. The vast post-war problems of the previous six years and the pressure of its minuscule majority had taken their toll; it was a tired and unpopular Government. Nevertheless I wanted to stand in the election. I had no idea how to get nominated and as telephone calls to Transport House drew little response I telephoned Hugh Dalton, with whom I had debated at Cambridge. I knew he was busy as Minister of Local Government and Planning, but he had asked whether I was interested in a political career and suggested contacting him if I

(84)

decided to try. It was perhaps taking him too much at his word, but he seemed pleased. 'So you want to have a go, eh?' he said, and the question seemed to express his satisfaction, though he could not promise anything. During the next week I received three or four letters from constituency Labour parties still without candidates, asking if I was interested in applying.

Dalton had worked quickly. They were political apprenticeships rather than Parliamentary seats, because in every case the Conservative majority was unassailable. Then I heard from Percy Clarke, a member of the Finchley Labour Party, who worked at the head office. He told me that Finchley would shortly be selecting their candidate and I could be nominated for the selection conference. It was a safe Conservative seat – later made famous by Margaret Thatcher – with a majority of over 12,000, but this was not as astronomical as some of the others. I agreed to have a go.

A few days later, I attended my first selection conference together with three other hopeful candidates. Huddled in a small room, awaiting our turn to address the delegates, we confined ourselves to small talk to avoid revealing any political gems to opponents. When my turn came, the chairman read out my credentials to a mainly middle-class group of about a hundred people. He talked about my activities in Widnes and gave an impressive gloss to my academic qualifications from Oxford and Cambridge.

After my speech I answered questions, then left to rejoin the other candidates in the ante-room. Tension mounted until the final speaker finished and we all strained to hear the counting of votes. I could not hear them, but suddenly one candidate leaned over to me and whispered that he thought I had got it – but he could not be sure. The finale was theatrically staged. We were led to the platform to sit facing the delegates while the chairman explained how difficult the choice had been. Finally he turned to me and said that I had been selected, whereupon I made a short speech of thanks. Aware of the other candidates' disappointment, I tried to disguise my delight at reaching the first stepping-stone to a Parliamentary career. But there was little time for self-congratulation. Polling day was less than a month away and we immediately had to prepare an election address and organize a series of tours and meetings throughout the constituency. It was different from my Council election; I had the support of a political machine, but I knew I would not top the poll this time.

The basic issues were full employment, fair shares, prices and nationalization. Some people expected the Labour Party to lose, but its Government had a fine record, especially in view of the immense post-war difficulties. Over a million houses had been built as part of a massive reconstruction programme. Prices had risen, but the cost of living compared favourably with that of our foreign competitors. Yet it was difficult to present price controls and food subsidies as an attractive electoral package. The magic of the 1945 campaign had worn off. In place of the euphoric war victory and the exciting challenge of rebuilding a new Britain was the hard, relentless reality of austerity and drabness. It was as if the national adrenalin was drained and the nation was pessimistic.

Although victory was almost impossible I fought an energetic campaign with strong support from party members. No one worked harder than an ardent Jewish socialist named Nat Birch, the local party's fund-raiser. Attending every meeting, he cajoled the audience with a fine mixture of special pleading and general flattery. If he knew someone was going to give a cheque, he would ask them to delay handing it to the platform until it seemed the perfect moment to start a flow of contributions. I always felt that he had just walked out of the bazaars of the Middle East; subtle, warm and kind, he added colour and vitality to the campaign.

I was lent an old car, covered in 'Vote for Ashley' posters, with a huge loudspeaker on the roof. It was more suitable for a carnival than an election, making a loud thumping noise like a drum when I drove it. I took the car to Cambridge when I visited Pauline. Her fellow students at Girton College enjoyed the fun, but we were all puzzled by the noise; it turned out to be the big end, which almost fell out on polling day.

Self-delusion is a political hazard, especially during elections. At the start of the campaign I knew there was no hope, but by the end I began to wonder. Party officials assured me that I would get the support of most residents in the new housing estates, and I allowed myself the luxury of thinking that we might pull off a surprise. It was a slight case of schizophrenia; basic political realities could not be altered by wishful thinking. On polling day the Conservative MP, John Crowder, retained his seat, winning 200 more votes than in 1950. The Liberals lost 2,500, and I increased the Labour vote by nearly 1,000 – a fair result considering the prevailing political mood. All over the country there had been a small and remarkably uniform swing to the Conservatives, and they took office with a narrow but decisive majority of seventeen. It was deeply disappointing. The prospect of a Conservative Government was depressing, but it did not affect my political zeal.

During the election campaign, and for some months afterwards, I lived in Finchley at the home of Percy Clarke, who had helped me to get the Finchley nomination. A bearded, reticent man, he was a Quaker with an interesting mix of moral principles and a lively sense of humour. He became Labour's Director of Publicity, playing an important role in the party's electoral battles. Percy never seemed to initiate conversation, yet he was the most agile and delightful conversationalist.

Although I was due to start work at the BBC shortly after the election, I still wanted to enter Parliament. This first Parliamentary election experience was a crossroads in my career. I discussed with Len Williams, the National Agent of the Labour Party, the possibility of getting another constituency. He said there were hundreds of bright young men seeking seats. I would be wiser to start work and acquire some kind of proficiency first, then consider Parliament later. His intentions were good, and, partly because I was shortly to be married, I accepted his advice and took up my BBC job. The man I replaced at the BBC was Tony Wedgwood Benn, who had resigned to become the MP for Bristol South-East – and subsequently a Cabinet Minister.

7

BBC Radio and Television Producer

I began work for the BBC in November 1951, in a cavernous building, formerly the Langham Hotel, opposite Broadcasting House. The North America section, which I joined, was part of the General Overseas Service – later to be known as the World Service. Its producers, a tightly knit though cosmopolitan group, were led with infinite patience by an experienced Canadian broadcaster named Rooney Pelletier.

Although head of the section, he himself used to broadcast in a rich, deep voice which seemed made for radio. My first job was to produce his weekly review of events and personalities in Britain. It must have been the easiest job in the BBC. Every Monday he would present me with the script of a ten-minute talk. Of course I could hardly improve his skilful work, but with deference to our professional relationship of contributor and producer, he accepted all but my most naïve suggestions. This was his diplomatic way of initiating me into my job. He was teaching me while I produced him.

I also produced a weekly four-minute talk on housewives' problems given by a motherly woman named Rose Buckner. It was an equally simple job. Mrs Buckner had been broadcasting for many years and needed no guidance from a producer for her cosy domestic chats. But I escorted her to the studio, suggested one or two minor script changes and carefully timed it to three minutes fifty seconds. Such were my early days in the BBC.

Most programmes expressed British views, but the impressions of visiting American tourists were of interest to their townsfolk at home. In the summer I went with a radio journalist, Stephen Grenfell, to Buckingham Palace, the Tower of London and Windsor Castle where we recorded scores of tourist interviews to be transmitted to their local stations. Stern and professional, Grenfell must have found the work depressing with its repetitive questions and predictable replies. The Americans were generous with their praise of Britain; they thought the Palace was terrific, the Tower historic and Windsor Castle great. The enjoyable part of these visits was drinking with Grenfell afterwards. An ex-soldier, he was a rumbustious character who recounted irreverent anecdotes about famous or pompous personalities.

The programmes were harmless, and the BBC was easy-going unless anyone transgressed the unwritten code of conduct. For a series about the monarchy, a Canadian woman, who had a transatlantic attitude to 'Queen Liz', wrote an amusing and breezy script. After some discussion I agreed to it with only a few changes, but I took the precaution of referring it to the head of my department.

Tolerant, easy-going Rooney Pelletier had been replaced by a new head, George Looker, who was astounded that I had even thought of condoning such blasphemy. After all, we were not talking about tourists' impressions or housewives' chores but the monarchy. I had obviously failed to appreciate the seriousness of the subject and ought to have immediately rejected everything but the most respectful account. The script was referred to the Service Controller, who, I was told, unhesitatingly decided that it was unsuitable and that I had made a serious error of judgement. There was some ruminative head-shaking at this; no doubt in the club and corridors people murmured that the new man was not up to it.

In response to my request for more creative programmes I was invited to produce a documentary about St Bride's Church, Fleet Street. I could not imagine the Americans rushing to their radios to hear the programme, but I had to accept. The vicar co-operated, describing the activities and history of his church. Did I know of the crypt? He ordered the caretaker to show me the depths – literally.

In a grisly tour I was shown human remains stacked in boxes being rearranged by the caretaker, who gave me a sepulchral commentary on his work. Perhaps the dismal atmosphere affected me, for my programme had a cool reception from the departmental head. Later, a more experienced producer was asked to 'tart it up a bit'. He added mournful music and echoing footsteps in the crypt, which were supposed to create atmosphere. It pleased the head but depressed me. Apparently I was not an outstanding radio producer. I wondered if it was time to seek a job elsewhere.

Near the end of 1951 I was less interested in BBC programmes than in my forthcoming marriage. Pauline and I hoped to marry in December, but understandably her mother felt she should wait for eighteen months to ensure that she got her degree. Just after the war, marriage had been tolerated for older women returning to college from the services, but conventional students were automatically sent down by all Cambridge and Oxford colleges if they married. I, too, was anxious that Pauline should not lose her university education and I went to see the Mistress of Girton, who agreed, after much discussion and some polite argument, that Pauline should be allowed to remain at college after our marriage. The decision was important to us – and it set a precedent. Future students at Girton no longer had to choose between marriage and a degree.

On 15 December 1951, we were married at Caxton Hall in London. My sister Margaret attended the wedding, while Helen and Mary helped Mam to prepare a party in Widnes. After the London reception at a nearby hotel with Pauline's family and many friends, we speeded, with Margaret, in a borrowed car up the dark roads to Widnes. There we held another reception in the evening of a hectic but memorable day. The first night of our honeymoon was spent in one of the most unromantic settings in the world – 34 Wellington Street. Next day we went to the other extreme – the serene beauty of the Lake District.

Our first home was the small room in Percy Clarke's house in Regent's Park Road, Finchley, where I had stayed during and since the election. It held little more than a wardrobe and a bed, but neither its size nor the sparseness troubled us. The next eighteen months were difficult, however. Pauline and I were apart for most of the time while she studied at Cambridge and I worked at the BBC in a job I now disliked. I was not interested in tourist interviews and housewives' chats, still less in skeletons, and my relations with the new head of the department deteriorated. He was unenthusiastic about my work, while I blamed him for insisting on fatuous programmes.

We had regular rows about trivial issues and a major one when I applied for a pay increase. My request astonished him, and I was summoned to his office where he sat behind a large desk, a small, grey man taking his responsibilities very seriously. It was clear that I had incurred his displeasure – again. He did not invite me to sit down but sternly asked how I justified the application. Did I not realize that salaries were professionally assessed and carefully reviewed by the BBC's administrative department? I justified my claim vigorously, if a little imaginatively and perhaps extravagantly; no one who heard the simple programmes I produced would credit the vast amount of thought and effort that went into them. He was unimpressed. When I had finished he replied, a little wearily, 'You know, Jack, I rather like you, but you make it difficult for me.' My application was rejected, but I persisted in pestering him. At length it was granted – it took so long that I was probably due for a rise in any case.

I decided to leave the BBC and applied for a job as personnel officer with the Philips electrical company, although with some misgivings. Having been offered the post after a series of interviews, I thought it would be useful to discuss it with the man who had held the job previously. Peter Parker, later to become a successful businessman and Chairman of British Rail, was known to mutual friends and they arranged for us to meet. We discussed the pros and cons. At the end of the conversation he said he had spent a year in the USA, and as I was unsettled that might be an option to consider.

Pauline had now left Cambridge. She had obtained a good degree, and we were fortunate in securing a small but pleasant flat on the fringe of Hampstead, near to Parliament Hill. As our first priority was to start a family, Pauline had not looked for a career, and she was pregnant when I met Peter Parker. We agreed, however, that I should try for one of the two highly prized Commonwealth Fund Fellowships (now called Harkness) that were reserved for journalists. I was just in time to apply. The interviewing board consisted mainly of university vice-chancellors and leading journalists. I was lucky because one of the vice-chancellors was Sir James Duff of Durham University, who had heard one of my debates in the USA. He was warmly disposed towards me, and to our great pleasure I duly got the Fellowship.

My fortunes were changing. A few days later, Stephen Bonarjee, head of the Current Affairs Unit in the BBC's Home Service, invited me to join his team. He was unperturbed when I told him that I would be available only for six months before my USA visit. Apparently the main obstacle to my joining the Home Service had been the attitude of the Controller, Mary Sommerville. She had opposed my suggested transfer because I had been a political candidate. But these misgivings had been overcome and I began one of my happiest periods in broadcasting.

BBC radio was at the time the most illustrious medium of communication, with large audiences for its programmes, including news and current affairs. Authority and reliability, established before the war, and enhanced during it, were its hallmarks. It was said that the head of News Division, Tahu Hole, refused to accept a news story, even from his own foreign correspondents, unless it had been confirmed by at least one news agency and preferably two. As a monopoly, the BBC had no need to be thrusting, and its pace was sedate. Some of its senior staff were chosen as much for their background and connections as for their ability. Producers were well informed, well spoken and well behaved. Their discussions were decorous and their language was restrained; they would sooner have dropped their salary than an 'h'.

Although announcers no longer wore dinner jackets, the spirit and some of the manners of the Reithian age still prevailed. In later years, and especially with the development of television, it was to become a shirt-sleeved, no-nonsense, competitive organization. But in 1951 the Corporation was touched rather than transformed by the pressures of the less deferential age.

At the daily morning meetings of producers, my outspoken comments may have caused a few raised eyebrows, and in discussion of other producers' ideas I could perhaps have been more diplomatic. But Bonarjee was unconcerned, welcoming frank criticism but demanding justification for it and constructive alternative suggestions. A skilled producer of current affairs programmes, he ran our disparate group with a deceptively light hand.

At Home and Abroad and *Topic for Tonight* were the heavy and light vehicles for current affairs. The former was a 45-minute programme, rather like a radio equivalent of television's *Panorama*. Contributors were politicians, industrialists, trade unionists and professional men and women who were making news. *Topic* was a five-minute explanation of a major news item by a journalist. It clarified and simplified issues without trivializing them. The journalists included editors of national newspapers and weekly journals, which meant that very few faults were to be found with their scripts.

At that time the BBC was forced to operate under the 'fourteen-day rule', which meant that we were unable to broadcast on any subject to be debated in Parliament within the next two weeks. The acceptance of this gagging device was astonishing in an organization rightly admired throughout the world for its independence. Eventually the rule fell into disrepute and was abandoned in July 1957, but during my early years in the BBC it constrained political discussion.

There was also a firm rule against advertising of any kind. This was understandable, and desirable, in public service broadcasting but it was taken to excessive lengths. Thus the chairman of ICI would not be named but described as the head of a large chemical company, which might have implied he was the boss of Boots. Nevertheless, this did not discourage employers from taking part in the programmes. Broadcasting on BBC radio seemed well worthwhile to them.

Trade union leaders were powerful figures then and none more so than Arthur Deakin, General Secretary of the Transport and General Workers' Union. Messages for him had to be sent through his secretary, a formidable frowning figure, and I had to accept this second-hand contact. Nevertheless I arranged for him to participate in a live studio discussion. He spoke well and turned out to be unpretentious and friendly. Not for the first time, the secretary of a public figure gave a false impression of the person.

Another trade union leader was of more direct importance to the BBC. In early 1956, the Musicians' Union was embroiled in a strike which seriously affected the Corporation's extensive musical output. As this became increasingly damaging we decided on an item for *At Home and Abroad* with the union's General Secretary, Hardie Ratcliffe, and the BBC's Director-General, Sir Ian Jacob. I was to be the producer. It was obviously important for me to be professionally impartial, neither permitting my trade union links to favour one side, nor my status as a BBC employee to help the other. I was angered at a suggestion that I should deal only with the trade union leader and a senior figure should handle the Director-General. The day was saved by Bonarjee, who arranged for me to handle both. The discussion went well. It clarified some misconceptions and cleared the air. After the broadcast Jacob and Hardie had a long private discussion. A few days later the strike was settled.

Now that I was doing different work and was a member of a team, my attitude to the BBC changed. Even the top brass were beginning to be friendly. During the lunch break one day, the aristocratic chief of my department, John Green, in pin-striped trousers and with rolled umbrella, was anxiously standing outside Broadcasting House, vainly trying to catch a taxi. My battered motor cycle was propped up outside this august building and, seeing his agitation, I offered him a lift. Late for an appointment at the House of Commons, he accepted. I got him there quickly, but he had to hold tight to his black trilby and umbrella on a hair-raising journey which became a hilarious talking point in Broadcasting House.

On 10 September 1954, our first child was born. Our daughter, Jackie, gave great pleasure to her loving but inexpert parents and we settled happily with her in our small flat. But before long it was time to take up my Fellowship in the USA. We decided that Pauline would follow with the baby in January. When I left, we gave up the flat and Pauline went to stay with her mother in Ewell in Surrey.

In those days it was usually cheaper to go by sea than by air. I went on an old ship, the *Franconia*. Unlike my first sea journey on the *Queen Elizabeth* with Ronald Waterhouse, on this one I was seasick and lonely. I missed Pauline and the baby and the journey took nine long days. When I arrived in New York I felt no sense of novelty. The skyscrapers, neon lights and breathless pace all seemed unexcitingly familiar. The only new sensation was loneliness.

Officials at the headquarters of the Commonwealth Fellowship made me welcome and readily assisted in making arrangements. The senior official, E. K. Wickham, known as Wick, a small, rotund man with a nimble mind, had a ready grasp of the problems of visiting English students. I was to study the relationship between broadcasting and politics, and he suggested starting in Louisville, Kentucky. There, a well-known newspaper proprietor, Barry Bingham, a cultivated and knowledgeable southerner, who was well disposed to the Fellowship, had a radio and television station.

Before leaving a few days later, I bought an Oldsmobile car from a friend of the BBC's New York representative. My first-ever car – it cost about $300, less than £100 – was enough to spoil me for any other. It had a radio, automatic gear-change and electric push buttons for the windows and sliding roof. Large, even by American standards, it was massive compared with British cars. I felt like a millionaire as I surveyed this sleek monster which I was to drive across the United States.

In Louisville the major radio and television stations were under the same ownership as the excellent local newspaper, the *Courier*. Bingham and the staff were friendly and welcoming. The newsmen invited me to chase the news with them. They did this literally, as their van was fitted with a police radio, and they raced police to the scenes of crimes. This helped them to make excellent news programmes since they caught people's first reactions rather than second thoughts. A man who has just been robbed speaks with more feeling when he has no time to reflect that the insurance company will make up his loss.

After some weeks in Louisville, I visited radio and television stations in Tennessee and Florida. I found the southerners remarkably generous. One person would recommend a visit to another, creating a chain of friendship. In Nashville, Tennessee, I stayed with a professor, a friendly man with a high regard for Britain. When I mentioned that I intended to go to Georgia he simply picked up the telephone and rang another professor, who invited me to stay.

In Georgia I nearly came to an untimely end when I went alone on a fishing trip on a huge lake. After fishing for a while, I went swimming, although I am a very poor swimmer. Wading deep in the water, I found I was suddenly well out of my depth. I struck out for the shore but as I reached the point of exhaustion it seemed as far away as ever; I was still in deep water so I put my head down and flailed away weakly. At the extreme limit of endurance, I sank, and to my unbelievable relief my feet touched the bottom. I staggered to the edge and lay exhausted, vomiting in the shallow water; instead of the idyllic lake I had seen on arrival, it had nearly been a death trap.

For the next few months I toured broadcasting stations, gradually working my way back to New York to meet Pauline and the baby. I was particularly interested in the influence of sponsors on television standards, though it was difficult to assess. Each network insisted that there was no sponsor control over their news programmes – but then each of them claimed it had the best shows and largest audiences. They were sometimes accused of committing sins of omission at the behest of sponsors; on one occasion a television news programme sponsored by a tobacco firm failed to mention an important report on the connection between smoking and lung cancer. I asked a producer if it was true that the sponsor had insisted on deleting the item. He said the cigarette–cancer relationship had been mentioned many times since. This evasive answer was interesting, especially when he added that he 'wouldn't lean over backwards to offend a sponsor'.

Yet the Americans, despite the pressures of commercialism and sponsorship, were creating television standards crucial to a democratic society. The producers, particularly those working in the networks, fought to establish important principles. One was that no matter how exalted the interviewee, he was not allowed to dictate the questions. Some sacrifices were made to defend this principle: during the United Nations anniversary celebrations, the Soviet Minister for Foreign Affairs, Mr Molotov, accepted an invitation to appear in a network interview. I saw how delighted the producers were with this scoop as competition was intense, but then Molotov sent in a list of questions he was prepared to answer. The network cancelled the show and lost their scoop rather than accept this restriction.

It was a happy day in January 1955 when Pauline and four-month-old Jackie landed in New York. After my tour of the southern states I was struck by Pauline's English accent. She was shocked by the high American prices. During the next six months we travelled from coast to coast, on average staying in two different bedrooms each week. The car became Jackie's home. Luckily it was large enough to carry her equipment, which included an English pram and an American pushchair complete with sunshade. As she grew older and needed solid food, we developed a simple technique for cooking her food in the car. As we drove through the humid heat of an American summer we simply placed a tin just behind the car windscreen. It was heated as effectively as on any stove.

On these car journeys I learned as much about American radio programmes as when I visited the studios. Some of the programmes were awful, especially those from the 'music, news and sports' stations. Garrulous disc jockeys introduced pop records with a string of superlatives matched only by stupendous adverts for soap and corn-flakes. The output of these stations was defended by one local manager who said, 'I give 'em lots of music because drama takes too much thought and concentration. People don't want that – if they do, they get it on television.' There were over 1,400 of these disc-jockey stations scattered throughout the States and apparently they all made a profit.

At that time, small American towns generally had half a dozen or so small competing radio stations. Nothing comparable existed in Britain. One of their main attractions was the friendly and intimate nature of the news, which in very small places was pure gossip. Local news bulletins had such items as 'Mr and Mrs Hiram K. Smith had four friends to dinner last night and they played bridge until midnight . . . Mr and Mrs Ed Jones returned early today from their holiday in Florida where they stayed with their daughter Jane, who settled there ten years ago when she married.' As I drove across the USA, I found this gossip amusing at first, but I quickly tired of the repeated parochialism. Yet the stations were taking advantage of local radio's greatest asset – its ability to personalize local events.

The scenery changed dramatically as we travelled westwards, but the towns, cars, clothes and food remained much the same; and nothing was more uniform than the broadcasts. Radio and television stations produced the same curious mixture of banality and occasional brilliance. Local stations in small communities were unpretentious but popular, while large ones in big cities were more impersonal, but still profitable.

In Berkeley, California, we spent two happy weeks with an American family. Jeffrey Cohelan and his wife, Evelyn, had been friends of ours in England when he was studying British trade unions. An articulate trade union official, he later became a Congressman. With their four children, they were due to move house while we were there, and most people would have diplomatically suggested it was time for their visitors to leave. In fact, we suggested it, but they turned the idea down. So we helped in a gloriously confused removal. Jeffrey insisted that I must speak to his trade union colleagues, tour the university, meet local politicians and, of course, visit the radio and television stations. He usually explained to local people, with tongue in cheek, that I was an expert in their subject in England. No matter how I tried to disabuse them I was expected to speak authoritatively about British trade unions, Oxford and Cambridge, and the BBC.

We left Berkeley with regret to start the long drive to Washington. There I went to see the radio and television operation in the Capitol. At that time there was no equivalent at Westminster. US politicians had recognized the growing power of television, and Senators and Congressmen had their own television studio in the Capitol. It

was a simple affair in the basement; the only 'props' behind a desk
and chair were bookcases with imitation book backs and a picture of
the Capitol behind a glassless window frame. But it was highly
efficient. As most Congressmen were unpunctual, schedules meant
little, and the atmosphere was relaxed and informal. I met and
chatted with many American leaders, including Vice-President
Nixon, Postmaster Summerfield and a host of Senators who were
awaiting their turn before the camera. Many of them were surprisingly effective with apparently little or no production. The interviews
were done with slickness and style, but the smoothness masked the
relative superficiality of the questioning. Each Senator was fed deferential questions and responded accordingly.

A novel feature was interviews between Congressmen and high-
ranking leaders. These lacked sparkle but they were designed to be
cosy. For example, Vice-President Nixon was interviewed by a Re-
publican Congressman while I was there, and it followed a typical pattern:

'Well Mr Vice-President, the folks I represent are proud to have
you come and talk to them.'

'Well, Jim, I only hope your folks know what a splendid job you
are doing for them here in Washington.'

The most dubious practice was the 'ghost' interview. From a
script of questions and answers an Administration member or high-
ranking official recorded a film of the answers only; days or weeks
later any Congressman could walk into the studio and ask the
scripted questions – and then the Administration member's filmed
answers were dubbed in. That was unsavoury canned politics.

In Washington I became aware that in some instances television
was merely mirroring the image which politicians chose to put on
public display. And occasionally the image was faked. The medium
was using politicians; but, more significantly, politicians were using
the medium.

We sailed for home in September 1955 on the SS *United States*.
The constant travelling had unsettled our baby daughter and we felt
the need for stability in our lives. We stayed with Pauline's mother
in Ewell for some months on our return. It was still very difficult to

find accommodation, and with a young baby we had little time for house-hunting. But we settled in a pleasant semi-detached house in New Malden, Surrey, where we lived for the next nine years.

I returned to Stephen Bonarjee's department at the BBC but not for long. He told me one day that a job had been advertised internally for an editor of a new radio programme of news and current affairs for London and south-east England. 'You ought to apply for it,' he said. 'I shouldn't think you have much chance as a northerner, but you should be seen to be trying.' So I applied, and a few weeks after the interviews I had a message from a surprised Bonarjee congratulating me on getting the job; I was to start in September 1956.

Sorry though I was to leave Bonarjee's group, setting up and editing my own daily programme gave me new opportunities. A great deal of organization was required and some battles had to be fought. The News Department, powerful and autonomous, was difficult to deal with, but as the new programme would include a regional news bulletin, close liaison was necessary. The first question was whether the joint daily discussions were to be held in the News offices across the road in the News Department or in mine at Broadcasting House. Territorial advantage was tactical advantage and I won it. Fortunately the man deputed to represent News, Maurice Ennals, was one of the most co-operative people in the department.

We got on well, but I was not always happy with the News announcers, a legendary breed with famous names: John Snagge, Alvar Liddell, Frank Phillips and Robert Dougall. I thought that one of them delivered our regional news nonchalantly, possibly feeling it was below his dignity, and I asked him to improve. This request was ignored and so was a further one. The announcer sent a memorandum to the Head of Announcers, John Snagge, objecting to my pressure, whereupon I sent one to Snagge complaining about him. The Controller of my department, Andrew Stewart, told me later that Snagge, at a meeting of departmental heads, slipped my angry memo to him to read. A meeting between Snagge and myself was arranged and I was unwise enough to complain about the announcer's memo to Snagge. 'Ah,' said Snagge, understandably defending one of his staff, 'so you mean it's all right for you to write memos complaining about announcers but it's not all right for an-nouncers to complain?' It was a good debating point, but at least the announcer improved.

The programme, *Town and Country*, covered a large area including London and much of the south-east coast. I travelled around it extensively, meeting Town Clerks, Mayors, trade unionists, employ-ers and, above all, newspaper editors. These were the contacts crucial to the success of the programme. Less helpful were public relations officers – especially those in seaside resorts. Their expense accounts meant I was assured of lavish hospitality but most of them were death to critical or investigative stories. Their co-operation was guaranteed only for cosy items.

The producers on my programme were constantly on the look-out for new talent. One tried a new interviewer and asked me to listen to the recording to see if I would like to use him regularly. I was not impressed. The man I rejected, Alan Whicker, later rose like a rocket and became a household name in television. Despite my misjudgement, he became a good friend.

Although the producers in my unit were highly professional, some of them enjoyed that relatively leisurely age of the BBC. Two in particular would stroll into the office at least fifteen minutes late, flick through the papers on their desk, then leave for a lengthy coffee break. This irritated me, especially when I was under pressure, and I made myself unpopular by demanding a sense of urgency. It was a far cry from my sullen resistance to pressure from the foreman in Bolton's. Nevertheless, they did co-operate and help to make *Town and Country* a successful and highly regarded programme.

News of *Town and Country*'s success must have reached Lime Grove television studios, because some months later I was invited to become a television producer by Leonard Miall, Head of the Talks and Current Affairs Department in television. Instead of entering as a trainee, I was appointed as a full producer specializing in industrial affairs. This was because, in 1957, when I went to television, there were no producers with first-hand experience of industry on the shop floor. Complaints had been made, with good reason, about the poor coverage of industrial affairs, and I was expected to remedy this.

In the late 1950s, BBC television was fighting a battle for its future – and apparently losing. Deprived of its monopoly in 1955, it was losing its audience. Commercial television claimed a 79:21 preference over BBC, and many broadcasters were wondering where the slide would end. Already some people were reluctant to pay a licence fee. As the BBC's audience fell, the volume of complaints rose. 'Why', viewers asked, 'should we pay for a service we never watch?' Many BBC producers still clung to the Reithian philosophy that the BBC's duty was to produce high-quality programmes irrespective of popular appeal; they thought that seeking mass audiences would mean abandoning cherished standards. But young men were challenging the old. New creative talents were fighting their battle on two fronts – against commercial television and against some of their own colleagues.

There were several clearly defined groups in the television Talks Department at that time, though none was formally organized. The liveliest consisted of bright young men eager to break new ground in blitzkrieg style. Talented and aggressive, they referred to the quieter, older people as having 'bomber-pilot' attitudes compared with their own 'fighter-pilot' approach.

Two of the most dynamic young producers were Donald Baverstock and Michael Peacock. Baverstock was an innovator; his programme *Tonight*, based on the earlier *Highlight*, made a decisive breakthrough in the previously more staid programme presentation. The equivalent of a tabloid daily newspaper, *Tonight* consisted of short, colourful items varying in pace and depth. Although this format is familiar today, it was then new and startling, with a persistent style of interviewing and an irreverent, sceptical approach. Baverstock's right-hand man was Alisdair Milne, later to become Director-General of the BBC. Peacock edited the heavier, equally professional *Panorama*, a weekly current affairs programme analysing major issues.

The older men like Richard Cawston, Norman Swallow and Hugh Burnett were no less able, although they generally had quieter and more reflective dispositions. While the so-called fighter-pilot producers bubbled and effervesced, exploiting controversial issues and personalities, the bomber-pilot group eschewed what they called 'argy-bargy shows' and preferred thoughtful and constructive programmes. Some of them were outstanding, such as Cawston's *This is the BBC* and *On Call to the Nation*, about the medical profession, and a later one on the Royal Family. Equally famous was Burnett's *Face to Face* series.

A third group was composed of men like Huw Wheldon and David Attenborough, outstanding producers who were above the battle, unchallenged because of their professional expertise. Wheldon had a shining and provocative intelligence, though he never used one word if a dozen would do. Attenborough, at home before and behind the camera, was one of the very few men in television, or anywhere else, who seemed to attract the affection of everyone who came into contact with him. Wheldon later became the Managing Director of Television, and Attenborough Director of Programmes. Neither lost his charm in the process, though they were as formidable a pair as could be found at the head of any British enterprise.

Some of the best performances of all were at the departmental meetings held every Thursday morning at Lime Grove. Into these post-mortems on the past week's programmes were tossed ideas, wit, banalities, epigrams, scorn, praise and sheer bloody-mindedness. The unenviable task of controlling these meetings, and organizing the work of this turbulent department, fell to the rather diffident Leonard Miall. He had a high reputation as a journalist, having served for some time as the BBC's American correspondent, but he never seemed completely at ease in his role as head of a department packed with personalities.

The person who bestrode this stage majestically, if uncrowned, was the assistant head, Grace Wyndham Goldie, an intense, birdlike woman, passionately absorbed in television. Producers divided their time between producing programmes and discussing anecdotes about Mrs Goldie. Some people regarded her as queen of the jungle, strong and cunning, with respect for those who could hold their own and none for the weak and vulnerable. She was certainly a very impatient executive with no inhibitions about exercising her authority; but if at times it included some hectoring of harassed producers, it was all devoted to the cause of better television. She always showed personal consideration to those she professionally attacked, trying to find suitable roles for them elsewhere if she felt they were inadequate. Proud of her successful protégés, she showed an emotional, almost maternal, concern for all her lively brood.

Mrs Goldie constantly pressed her producers to improve television standards and achieve better programmes. Greater imagination was needed; new ideas must be produced; more energy was required; costs should be cut; and magnificent programmes should be the rule rather than the exception. Of course it was impossible to keep up with her ambitious ideas, but they were never less than stimulating. Exceptionally knowledgeable, she was one of the most creative thinkers in television, and made a significant contribution to the BBC's quality.

My own relationship with her was mutually wary. As a new producer I deferred to her authority and knowledge but after a while I began to resent her hectoring. On one occasion when we were discussing one of my programme ideas and she had been excessively critical, she said patronizingly:

'My dear Jack . . .'

I interrupted, 'Let's get it clear, I'm not your dear Jack. Now what's your point?' Thereafter, we had a cool, but not altogether unfriendly relationship.

To widen my experience of television programmes, I was invited to work on *Panorama*, then the most important programme, with a regular audience of up to 10 million. Each Tuesday the production team met to review the previous night's programme, discuss ideas for future programmes and provisionally plan a filming schedule.

Most producers preferred to have a few days to organize their contributors and plan locations before filming later in the week, or indeed some weeks hence. This was a sensible approach, but if a camera crew was not being used at the beginning of the week I tried to help by going straight out on location with a reporter and camera crew. Although this benefited the administrators of *Panorama*, it did not assist me – it also led to strained relationships with some reporters. Their exasperation was understandable since I was sometimes trapped into directing the filming while sitting at a telephone making arrangements for the next location.

The relationship between a producer and a programme performer was and still is complicated. A producer has the final responsibility for translating the idea into a programme, deciding its shape and content; but performers are naturally much better known. The public identify with them and believe that the programmes are theirs. Sometimes they can be more experienced and knowledgeable than a young producer.

Robin Day has since written that the reporter, untrammelled by producers, should be responsible. A producer, he felt, should be a kind of administrative assistant. But in my experience the programmes were better when the man in charge was behind and not in front of the camera. In the years after I left the BBC, some clashes obviously occurred between Day and what he called 'young producers'; but while I was producing, these were the exception rather than the rule. When I produced some items with him for *Panorama*, we had an amicable relationship and no problems.

I found that television reporters rarely attempted to influence production techniques, but it happened when I was working with Woodrow Wyatt on a *Panorama* programme about changes in the law affecting prostitution. We filmed interviews with some prostitutes, then I arranged one with a publican to talk about the effects of new legislation on pubs frequented by prostitutes. On location I set up the cameras and waited for Woodrow to arrive. He turned up quite late after a lengthy lunch.

With no apology, he told me that he intended to start with an introduction to camera, then he would turn and begin the interview. I told him to start with the interview and that he would do the introduction live in the studio. After we argued about this at some length and he apparently agreed, I directed the camera to begin. He then turned to it and started on the introductory piece. I stopped the shooting at once. Wyatt then warned me that unless I agreed to his method he would go home, whereupon I handed him his overcoat. I had to admire the way he swaggered off with an air of injured innocence. I liked him, but that day I was angry. My anger dissolved into laughter a few days later when a woman telephoned the BBC's duty officer to complain that she was 'on the street and done a job' for Woodrow Wyatt but had not yet been paid for it. I hastily explained to the official that the job she had done was an interview for the programme.

Occasional differences between producer and reporter were inevitable, but they would unite if anyone else attempted to influence the content or its presentation. When I was filming an item in a northern steel factory with Robert Kee, I invited one of the shop stewards to be interviewed. He was Mayor of the town, but I urged him to come for the interview dressed in working clothes, in his role as shop steward. He turned up at the factory in his Sunday best, because his wife thought it would be undignified for the Mayor to appear before the camera in dirty overalls. Kee and I had a quick word together and with the cameraman; we couldn't tell the Mayor to push off, so we filmed the interview with him dressed as he was, in front of the furnaces. I later wrote to explain that he would not be in the programme due to a technical problem. In fact, there was no film in the camera.

I was fortunate in working with many professional reporters on *Panorama*. Chris Chataway, easy-going but highly competent, was still famous as a runner and drew crowds wherever we went. Jim Mossman, laconic, tall and handsome, only appeared to be easy-going. The appearance belied reality. He tragically committed suicide at the height of his career. Francis Williams, later Lord Williams, who had been Clem Attlee's Press Officer, was rotund, dignified and professional. I was very irreverent towards him, but we shared the same sense of humour and had tremendous fun together. It was also enjoyable to work with Robin Day, whose stern public appearance belied an impish sense of humour. Robert Kee was an outstanding and penetrating interviewer. In addition to our *Panorama* programmes we did many by-election specials and delighted in beating ITV every time to get the first interview with the winning candidate.

The best of all was Richard Dimbleby, the presenter of *Panorama*. For millions of people he *was Panorama*. A master of his craft, he was authoritative, relaxed and able to establish instant rapport with viewers. With outstanding natural talents, he nevertheless worked exceptionally hard on his briefs. He eschewed the hectoring, interrogatory interview, yet his questioning was incisive. Accused occasionally of pomposity, he was the least pompous of men. He had a quick, gentle and sometimes ironic sense of humour. In the hospitality room before a programme he would listen to my more flamboyant assertions and comment, 'Well, Asher, you *could* be right'; and in the laughter that followed we all knew he meant that he thought I was wrong. If I had produced a particularly good item for the programme he would raise an eyebrow and say, 'Not bad, Asher', which was valued more than fulsome praise.

When I produced my own documentary programmes, I wanted to show the real relationships between trade unions and employers and the atmosphere in industry, so familiar to those working in it but unknown to and misunderstood by others. It was not easy, because routine industrial matters were rarely dramatic enough for television, and when there was a dispute both sides were reluctant to take part. After it was over neither side wished to rake the ashes.

In 1961, I tried to assemble a programme on a major unofficial strike taking place at the Acton car works of the Rootes Group. The firm's directors and the leaders of the Amalgamated Engineering Union rejected my invitation to take part, and the pickets were suspicious when I sought to contact the strike leaders. Only after a long delay and many telephone calls did they agree to drive me to a private garage near the factory for a meeting. The leaders were cool and tough. They would take part in the proposed programme, they said, if I would accept some obviously prearranged outrageous demands for large fees to each member of the strike committee, and a guarantee that every word they uttered would be broadcast. It looked as if there would be no programme.

However, I was used to discussions with shop stewards and in a better negotiating position than them as I stood to lose only a non-existent programme, while their case would go by default. Eventually, after heated argument, they withdrew their demands and accepted a small, reasonable fee and my assurance of fair representation in the programme. Returning to the President of the AEU, Bill Carron, I told him that his critical, unofficial shop stewards were taking part in the programme. He decided he had better express the official union view. Armed with all my film I returned to the employers, and this time it wasn't too difficult to persuade them to participate. It was an unusual way of winning the co-operation of three conflicting industrial groups, but it worked.

The shop stewards had not been playing hard to get; they were genuinely hostile to television, expecting all kinds of tricks to be played on them. After accepting my assurances, they presented their case articulately. They were untypical. In other programmes I found that some trade unionists – if they overcame their suspicions and took part at all – would insist on reading a dull and unconvincing prepared statement, especially if they were on strike. It was years before a few eloquent people began to demonstrate that trade union- ists can be as persuasive as anyone else on television.

Two remarkable trade union personalities at that time were Les Cannon and Frank Chapple of the Electrical Trades Union. They played a major role in an unusual power struggle. A small group of men gained control of this union, the sixth largest in the country, with nearly a quarter of a million members doing work essential to most major industries. The 1 per cent of members who were commu- nists controlled the 99 per cent who were non-communist; they manipulated the union and maintained themselves in office by fraud until Cannon and Chapple exposed them.

Some clever tricks were used to ensure the election of leaders, including the disqualification of inconvenient votes from over fifty towns. The communists at the ETU head office produced envelopes displaying postmarks as evidence that the anti-communist votes they contained had been posted too late. But the further away from London these envelopes were posted, the later the postmark. Cannon and Chapple suspected that someone might have driven from London northwards, posting fraudulent envelopes back to head office, which were then produced as apparent evidence. To test this theory a private inquiry agent made a trip from London to Scotland, posting envelopes at boxes near to each main ETU branch centre; the time stamps on these envelopes were similar to those used by the communists to justify disqualification. Woodrow Wyatt was the reporter for an investigative programme on the scandals in the ETU, the first to expose ballot rigging and manipulation. With the ensuing publicity, the communists were ousted and Cannon and Chapple took control. I was not involved in the first programme, but subsequently I produced a follow-up programme, which was when I got to know Cannon.

He and I became close friends, perhaps because of our similar backgrounds. He was a working-class man from Wigan, near Widnes, and we often joked about each other's home town. An easy-going sense of humour contrasted with his hard and unrelenting attitude to his opponents. An ex-communist himself, he was a particularly effective opponent of the communists in the ETU. Although his sharpness offended some colleagues, his striking intelligence and personality made him an outstanding union leader. By his early death from cancer, the British trade union movement lost one of the few men who could have fanned the wind of radical change.

Difficult as it was to illustrate industrial attitudes on television, explaining class attitudes was even more complicated, as I found when producing a series of documentary programmes called *Does Class Matter?*. The narrator was Christopher Mayhew MP, public school boy, son of a knight and later to become a lord. Pedantic and addicted to detail, he had little in common with me. Mayhew was patient, but he must have been sorely tried by my refusal to accept many of his lively ideas and my intention to conduct the programme in a different way.

Eventually we sank our differences and pooled resources. He conducted a poll which showed that people believed the five things determining social position were education, accent, job, family background and wealth, and we allocated a programme to each.

One of the outstanding contributions to the series came from a brilliant young Oxford undergraduate who had been a miner. Refreshingly frank with us, he revealed deep feelings about class problems and the cultural differences between university and home. Before the programme was broadcast, a Sunday newspaper correspondent asked if he could see the transcript. I agreed without hesitation, but a few days afterwards the headline in this newspaper read: 'Miner's Son at Oxford Ashamed of Home. The Boy Who Kept His Father Secret'. The story misinterpreted the student and misquoted me. I was furious; so was Mayhew. We sent a telegram to the student, Dennis Potter – later a distinguished playwright – dissociating ourselves from the report. It was all we could do, but it probably did nothing to ease his embarrassment after giving a frank and mature interview.

I was taken for a ride by some trade unionists when Mayhew and I did one of these programmes in New York. We were illustrating class divisions in the USA. In a jeweller's shop I filmed, with an American camera crew, some of their most expensive jewels. I suggested to the cameraman that one of these would look better on a small, dark cushion. He agreed, made a quick telephone call and stopped filming. Aghast, I asked what he was doing. He said he had phoned the office for two 'props' men to place the jewels on the cushion. Union rules, he explained, required props men to do such work and it had to be a minimum of two. It made no difference when I said I had changed my mind, or when I condemned the camera crew. They had booked two men, and I had to wait for them to arrive and do the preposterous job at great cost. So much for my cherished trade union principles.

The BBC was right to try to use my experience of working-class life, but in some programmes it was valueless. A new programme called *Monitor*, dealing with the arts, was introduced, with Huw Wheldon as editor. The programme controllers, afraid that it might be too highbrow, thought that my down-to-earth approach might be a counterbalance. I was appointed associate editor, despite my warning that I was no expert on painting, sculpture or the theatre, and knew little of the personalities in these fields.

For one programme I was asked to invite the playwright John Osborne to discuss the theatre; when I spoke to him on the telephone he seemed indifferent and uninterested. His manner deterred me from trying to persuade, so I simply said, 'Right you are, then', and rang off. I was asked about our discussion by Huw Wheldon and the director, and I told them. When I had finished, their eyes met. Wheldon muttered savagely, 'Well done, Jack.' He brushed aside my argument that Osborne did not want to appear anyhow and said that I had not appreciated how important the playwright was.

Despite the occasional error, I was becoming an experienced television producer. When *Panorama* went off the air for a summer break I was made editor of a series about Europe that replaced it for six weeks. Unfortunately, the best and most experienced producers had gone on holiday and I was left mainly with new recruits. It was a desperate business as I sent raw producers all over Europe; they urged politicians to express their views, marched German regiments for their cameras and filmed in factories. They were seeking views of Europeans towards Britain and news of German rearmament and the development of trade and industry in Europe.

I heard nothing for nearly a week from one producer whom I had sent to France to get people's impressions of some important subject or other. He eventually phoned at a moment when all the other phones in the office were ringing.

'Where the hell are you?' I barked.

'In France.'

'Ha,' I said, 'I know damn well you're in France. Which part?'

A pause. 'The south.'

A snort. 'Which part of the bloody south?'

A longer pause. 'Well, actually, I'm in St Tropez but I've got some very good film.'

I banged down my receiver. But, true to his word, Phillip Whitehead brought home excellent film. He later became a distinguished television producer with a leading role in the industry. He also became a dear friend, a Member of Parliament, a politician of outstanding judgement and one of those who gave me tremendous help when I lost my hearing. I was saddened when he lost his marginal seat in the 1983 General Election.

I invited David Dimbleby, then in the early stages of his career, to present this series, *Outlook Europe*. He was a great success despite the pressures of constant and last-minute changes. For one programme, with thirty seconds to go before transmission I had to rush downstairs from the control gallery to tell him of alterations to the script. He coped with aplomb.

I was always conscious that my main responsibility in television was to feature industry, and I was anxious to try a documentary film of my own. In 1963, the rate of unemployment was 2.3 per cent, a cause of much concern at the time. I went to West Hartlepool to film *Waiting for Work*, a programme for which I was producer, director and interviewer.

I visited derelict shipyards, dole queues, slum homes and poverty-stricken families. It was just like Widnes all over again, except that Hartlepool had docks rather than chemical factories. Oddly enough, this deprived town had a high-class hotel at which I stayed. Living there, eating well and going to the slums and derelict shipyards for filming gave me an uneasy sense of unreality.

My opening sequence was film of the empty shipyards with a description of their former prosperity, followed by ghostly echoes of cheering the launch of ships and the music 'Rule Britannia'. Former workers and wives spoke movingly about the impact of unemployment, their poverty and disappointment, and their pessimism about the future. At the end, remembering that when I was a crane driver the swinging jib indicated a busy day, my final shot was of a motionless crane hook – a silent and eloquent symbol of unemployment.

Throughout the late 1950s and early 1960s, television was constantly seeking new ways of presenting political issues. The BBC interpreted the Representation of the People Act very cautiously and until 1959 its only role in a General Election had been to lend transmitters for party broadcasts. Once an election campaign began, the BBC did not transmit any party political material, even in news bulletins. Such restricted output satisfied neither viewers nor politicians. It was time for a change, and by the 1959 election the BBC's interpretation of the Act had changed substantially.

It was understandable that the BBC proceeded with caution. Politicians were, and always had been, jealous of its power, and for a few years in the very early days they prevented the broadcasting of any political controversy. The ban was modified in 1928, but even then the Corporation had to observe strict rules laid down by the political parties.

In February 1961, a new programme, *Gallery*, appeared. It aimed to reflect political controversy without histrionics. I worked as associate editor and watched at close quarters the love-hate relationship between politicians and broadcasters. Collectively politicians were supreme, since Parliament could change the BBC's charter and veto a broadcast. But Governments were fearful of exercising their power because of the outcry that would ensue and the precedent it would establish.

I became increasingly conscious of the differences between MPs and television producers. Both wield power; but whereas with his programmes the producer has regular and frequent access to a mass audience, and most MPs do not, he does not express his own views. He presents the views of others. The MP, able to operate directly in Parliament, presses for policies he personally believes in.

By 1965, our family was well settled. Our second daughter, Jane, had been born in 1958, a cause of much rejoicing as two years earlier Pauline had had a very premature baby who had not survived. In 1963, when Jane started school, Pauline became a part-time maths teacher, which she greatly enjoyed. A year later, we moved to a lovely old Edwardian house in Epsom. Typical of the period, it had a long narrow garden. With a park nearby and many trees in our and neighbouring gardens, it had a countrified feel, yet was convenient for my work. The house was roomy enough for us all to feel comfortable and relaxed. It was our daughters' home for the rest of their time with us, and is still home for Pauline and me.

In Widnes, my sisters were preoccupied with their young children, and Mam was happily helping them. We visited Widnes frequently, and my BBC colleagues would laugh tolerantly when I replied, 'Widnes', when they asked where I was going on holiday.

With my background now more secure, and with a growing appetite for politics, I decided to try for a Parliamentary seat. When I told the head of my department at the BBC, he warned me that permission would probably be refused. My request went through various levels of the hierarchy until finally I was told to see the

Controller of Television, Kenneth Adam, the man who had been partly responsible for my joining the BBC. He said that I could not be given permission to become a Parliamentary candidate. As he gave me the bad news he offered a large cigar. He smiled and did not inquire whether I still intended to seek a seat. I thanked him, went back to my office and started to look for a vacant Parliamentary seat.

The first one I applied for was Neath, in South Wales, reputed to be in the gift of Welsh miners and steelworkers. As I travelled by train through the valleys I did not feel at home. For me, Wales was the land of the Bevans and the Baverstocks, mercurial men who spoke English with a lilting accent and had been reared in a national-ist culture which, although British, was foreign to me. As a Lanca-shireman, I felt I could understand Yorkshire and the Midlands; Scotland perhaps; but Wales never.

At the selection conference it was clear that my prospects of gaining the seat were remote because of the importance attached to being a Welshman, mineworker or steelworker. But the reception I had from the conference was so warm and friendly that it gave me tremendous encouragement.

Within a few weeks, two other seats became vacant, and I was short-listed for both. The first selection conference was at Barrow-in-Furness. The Widnes Rugby Football team had played Barrow for years, so I felt no sense of remoteness as I had when I applied for Neath. At the selection conference my speech was well received. Question time presented no insurmountable problems until I was asked if I would give an undertaking to spend every weekend up to the General Election electioneering in the constituency. This was impossible because my job at the BBC often involved film locations at weekends, but I promised to campaign as often as possible. A section of the conference was not satisfied; as they magnified the issue, I could feel support for me ebbing quickly. I was not selected, but I was far from discouraged.

A week later, I went to Stoke-on-Trent for the second selection conference. I had passed through the town many times on my way from London to Widnes. It was an environment akin to Widnes, and I immediately felt at home. The candidates included Arthur

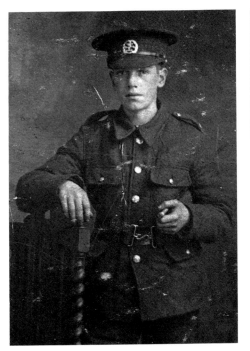

1. Jack's father, John Ashley, during National Service, 1914.

2. Jack's mother, Isobel Ashley, September 1945.

3. Jack (aged six) with sisters Helen (left, aged eight) and Mary (centre, aged four).

4. Jack aged eight.

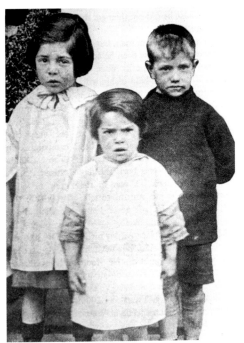

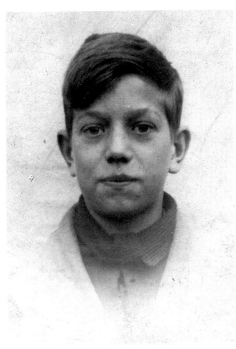

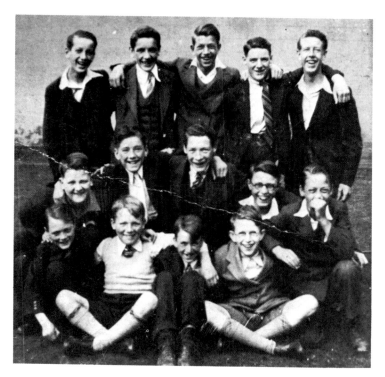

5. The last year of school (top row, centre, aged fourteen).

6. The young labourer (left) during a summer holiday from Ruskin College.

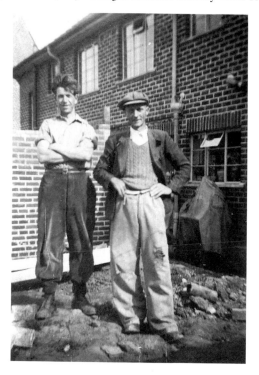

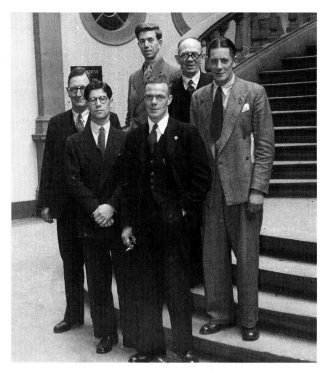

7. Shop steward (top, aged twenty-two) with fellow members of the National Executive of the Chemical Workers' Union.

8. Widnes at the turn of the century.

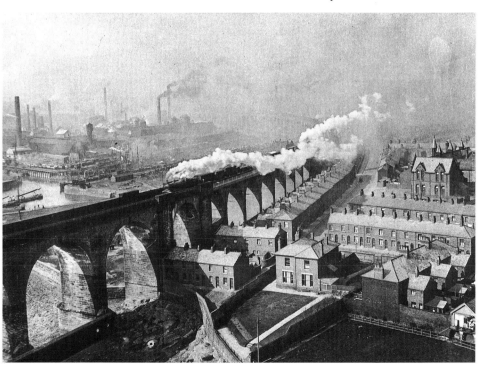

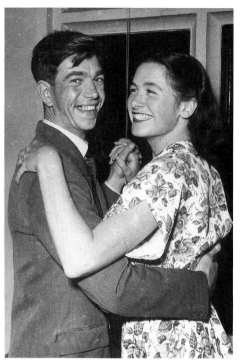

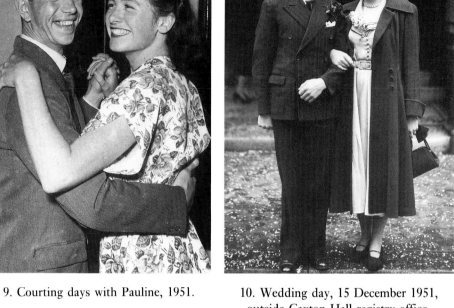

9. Courting days with Pauline, 1951.

10. Wedding day, 15 December 1951, outside Caxton Hall registry office.

11. President of the Cambridge Union, during a debate, January 1951.

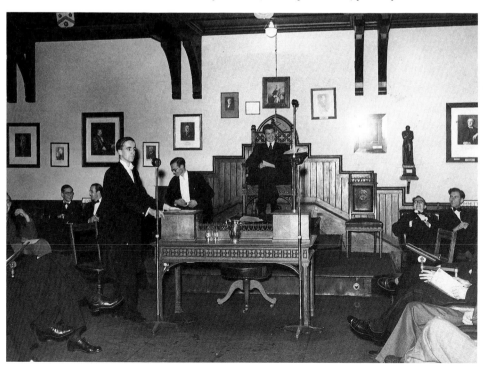

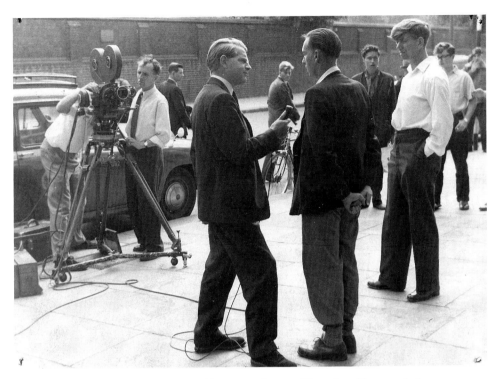

12. On location with Christopher Chataway, former Olympic athlete, and then current affairs commentator for the BBC's *Panorama*.

13. During time as a BBC radio producer, impersonating interviewees outside the Tower of London.

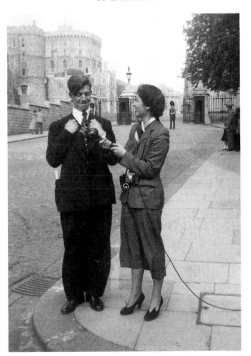

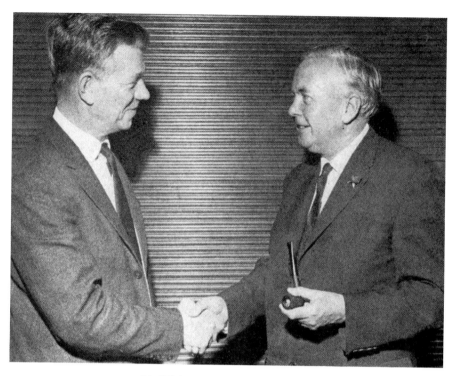

14. With Harold Wilson in 1966.

15. Opening of the Houses of Parliament, October 1974.

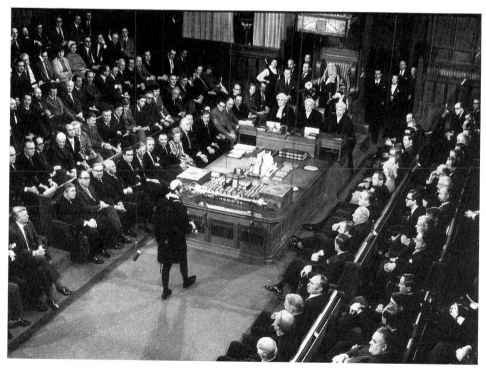

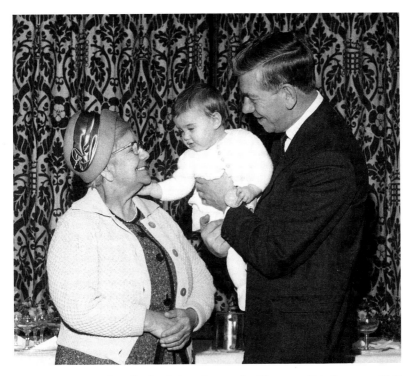

16. With Mam at Caroline's christening at the Houses of Parliament, 1966.

17. An election photograph of the family in the garden at Epsom, shortly after Jack became totally deaf.

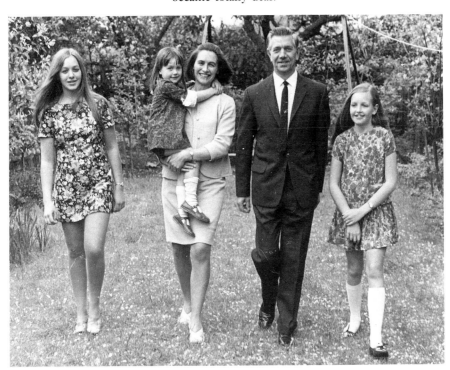

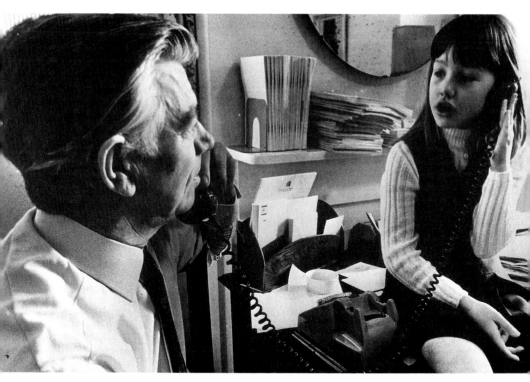

18. Caroline helps with a telephone call.

19. Caught by surprise on television for *This Is Your Life*, with Caroline and Jackie.

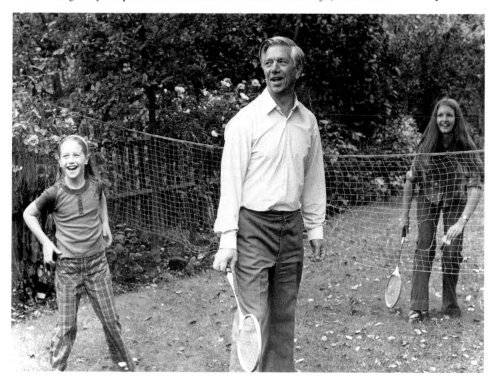

Balham, a local councillor, Martin Ennals, a vigorous campaigner, and Brian Stanley, a trade union leader. Just as in the Finchley selection conference fifteen years earlier, we chatted together in a small ante-room as each man took his turn to deliver a speech and answer questions. It was all so apparently easy-going, yet we knew that on the decision hung a Parliamentary career, for this was a safe Labour seat. Although my speech and answers to questions appeared to go well, it was disturbing to hear applause in the distance as other candidates spoke. We all pretended to ignore it as we indulged in small talk. When the votes had been counted the chairman came into the ante-room and told us that I had been selected. I was delighted; I was back in politics and assured of a seat in Parliament.

Pauline and all the family were as pleased as I was, but I wondered how the BBC would react to this news. Despite their earlier refusal to give me permission to apply for the seat, they accepted the information blandly, even casually. Arrangements were immediately made for me to move to *Tomorrow's World*, a programme which did not involve politics or current affairs. Until the General Election, I worked on scientific programmes, a gesture of goodwill from the BBC which I appreciated. Later they went further, and after the election Huw Wheldon and other executives gave a lunch in my honour. They and I knew that I was now on the other side of the political television fence.

8

Entering Parliament

Polling day in the 1966 General Election, 31 March, promised to be a memorable one for me. Defending a majority of 10,000 in Stoke-on-Trent South, with opinion polls favourable to the Labour Party, I looked forward to becoming a Member of Parliament. But first I had to win the votes. Although I had met party workers on many occasions since the selection conference the previous summer, the election campaign was my first close contact with them. They were led by Sir Albert Bennett, chairman of the party and Leader of the City Council. A dominant man, he could turn from banter to anger and back again within minutes. No one, especially his opponents, ever took Albert Bennett lightly. Befriending me from the first meeting, he was a benevolent chairman of my public meetings, a terror of hecklers and an astute political tactician.

The headquarters of our election campaign were an old, decrepit building tucked away in an alley. The Labour Hall, normally quiet, was transformed overnight, crowded with busy party workers. They sat on hard wooden chairs at long trestle tables, chatting to each other as they addressed thousands of envelopes for my election address and did all the assorted necessary jobs. I laughed and joked with them, especially the older ladies, many of whom had been party workers for years. I appreciated their dedicated efforts – and the endless cups of tea they prepared.

The party workers were mainly working-class trade unionists, retired workers and housewives, with a sprinkling of teachers, lecturers and other professionals. They were a hard-working, supportive group. During the day they helped me to canvass people in streets and shopping centres, or tour with a loudspeaker van. It all came naturally to me and was done with good humour. I mixed politics with jokes about preferring to kiss mothers rather than babies and, on the loudspeaker, I gave a running commentary about shoppers, traffic jams or the weather. It created a warm, friendly atmosphere that helped me to get over the serious political message.

As I had expected, I was indeed fortunate with my constituency. The 'Potteries' were the product of their unique history. The six towns of Stoke, Hanley, Burslem, Tunstall, Fenton and Longton, described inexplicably by Arnold Bennett as 'The Five Towns', were federated in 1910, but their history stretched back over centuries. Pottery had been made in Stoke since the Romano-British period. In this century, the names of Wedgwood, Royal Doulton, Spode, Minton and Crown Staffordshire have been famous throughout the world, and the industry had provided jobs for many women workers. In 1966, coal-mines and steelworks also employed many people in the city.

Inevitably, these industries scarred the environment. The extraction of marl for pottery manufacture left yawning holes in the ground; slag-heaps dotted the landscape, and coal workings honeycombed underground. Yet the warmth of the people shone through the dereliction. They were unpretentious and generous and had a fine community spirit. Although the industrial heritage denied them a city of idyllic beauty, the local authority had transformed derelict areas into splendid parks.

It was easy for Labour candidates to promote their party in 1966. Despite its short life and narrow majority since 1964, the Labour Government had a good record, having halved the inherited £750 million deficit on overseas payments and achieved record investment in schools, hospitals and houses. These were the basic issues of the campaign; the fun lay in tweaking the Tories when they offered alternatives. Why, if they were so good, had their panaceas not worked in the thirteen years they were in office?

Pauline wanted to play an active part in the election but she was pressed not to as she was shortly expecting our third child. She came up for the last few days of the campaign, and together we enjoyed the excitement and activity which went on feverishly until the booths closed on polling day. Because of an irritating convention in the city, votes were not counted until the following day. So when they were locked away, we went with friends to watch other results announced on television.

Next day, at the Town Hall, the count was almost a formality, though I felt oddly apprehensive just before my result was announced – as if the whole thing were too good to be true. My majority was the forecast 12,000. At last I was going to Westminster, and on the crest of a great Labour Party wave.

By coincidence, all three Stoke seats had new MPs. John Forrester, a warm and cheerful ex-teacher, represented the North, and Bob Cant, a serious, highly intelligent academic had the Central seat. Together we posed for the ritual photographs, then Pauline and I went with our loyal and delighted party workers for a celebratory drink. They left to resume their normal lives. For me it was different. I was to find a second home in Stoke and to begin a new career in London. My future promised to be as rewarding as it was exciting. The Labour Government had increased its majority from three to ninety-seven, and there seemed little to prevent the fulfilment of Labour's hopes.

The Queen opened the new Parliament on 21 April 1966, amid the traditional pomp and ceremony. Although I was more concerned with the serious business to follow, I had a special interest in the ritual. Watching the royal procession as it passed through the House of Lords was a small, white-haired old lady, utterly absorbed in the colourful pageantry. After all her years in Wellington Street, Mam had come to the Palace of Westminster to see the Queen. Still possessing that magical mixture of diffidence and personal warmth, she was aglow with excitement. She had been given a warm send-off in Widnes where Ken Merrifield drove her and my sister Helen to the station. The *Widnes Weekly News* photographed her departure and reported her visit under a front-page headline that was probably one of the longest in the history of journalism: 'Widow who was once an office cleaner gets a seat in the Royal Gallery and sees her son at Westminster'. It was an unforgettable day for her and for me.

Later that morning I went to my first meeting of the Parliamentary Labour Party in Church House, Westminster. At this crowded and enthusiastic gathering, Harold Wilson was given an ovation for leading a great victory. Jim Callaghan, the Chancellor of the Exchequer, said that while the Prime Minister had done his best for the party, loyalty was a two-way process and he was entitled to it in the years ahead. As he spoke, I wondered what the reaction of some Labour MPs would be when the euphoria had evaporated and the Prime Minister had to make difficult and unpopular decisions. I pondered, too, on how the Tory leader, Edward Heath, would fare at his meeting after electoral defeat; for it is not only Americans who admire success.

That afternoon I went to the Chamber in good time and took stock of my new surroundings. They were not wholly unfamiliar, because I had often watched debates from the gallery, but the angle was different; instead of being an onlooker I was now involved. When MPs crowded into the Chamber I realized how small it was. I was conscious of a sense of intimacy.

We crowded happily on the Government benches while our subdued opponents faced us. They were close – out of arm's reach, but not much more. The public gallery to our right seemed remote and irrelevant, while the press gallery on our left, high above the Speaker's chair, seemed much closer. In fact, it was roughly the same distance from our benches as the public gallery; the illusion was because the press, reporting and commenting on the proceedings, were intimately involved with the House.

In accordance with tradition, the new Speaker was selected, and the debate on the Queen's Speech began. However, I heard only the opening of the first speech before an urgent telephone message was passed along the crowded benches to me. Pauline had been taken to hospital and our baby was due any moment. I left the Chamber in an instant and rushed back to Epsom. Shortly afterwards our new baby daughter, Caroline, arrived. The twenty-first of April 1966 was a joyful day for Pauline and me. We now had three lovely daughters and a comfortable home in Epsom, near Pauline's mother; and I was on the threshold of an exciting Parliamentary career. We had no idea what the future might bring, but it seemed full of promise.

I had been so long on the sidelines that I was impatient to participate in the hurly-burly of Parliamentary life. But first I had to make my maiden speech. Some Members said the sooner the better; others suggested waiting some months until I was accustomed to the atmosphere. Most people counselled a non-controversial speech; a few felt this convention was outmoded. On 28 April, just a week after the opening of Parliament, I spoke defending the Government's prices and incomes policy which was being strongly criticized at that time. It was opposed not only by the Tories but by some MPs on our own side. The policy was to become one of the major issues of that Parliament.

I soon realized that while Parliamentary reputations could be made on the floor of the House, influence was exercised elsewhere. In committee and small subject groups, reason replaced rhetoric. There were also innumerable small cabals based on a mixture of common political outlook and personal friendship, and one often led to the other. New Labour Members were invited to meet Ministers, including the Prime Minister, in their private rooms for discussions. Sometimes there were further meetings and suggestions of alliances.

Party reputations were also affected by the meetings of the Parliamentary Labour Party. These were held in a large committee room in an atmosphere strikingly different from that of the Chamber. There was none of the formality of Parliamentary debates where we had to refer to Members by their constituencies and follow long-established conventions and procedures. Even though we were all in the same party, there were often strong differences of opinion. I had heard of rancorous clashes during the days of some early Labour leaders like Ramsay MacDonald. Older Members had vivid recollections of the debates between Hugh Gaitskell and Aneurin Bevan in the 1950s; these were so vindictive that some party Members stopped speaking to each other. We had no such scenes at the meetings I attended, though divisions existed, particularly between the critical left-wing Tribune group, who wanted faster progress towards an egalitarian society, and the majority of the party who recognized that no Labour Government could race too far ahead of the electorate.

Surprisingly enough, one of the most serious disputes in the Parliamentary party cut across those left–right lines. The Government's policy of maintaining military bases east of Suez was opposed by Christopher Mayhew, himself a right-winger, and the man I had worked with in television on programmes about class. At one of the most dramatic and crowded party meetings he proposed a motion critical of the Labour Government's policy. The Prime Minister, insisting that 'the Government must govern', seemed to imply that it would be an issue of confidence in him. Presiding over this vital debate was Emanuel Shinwell, one of the most fiery characters in Parliament. An authoritative chairman, he allowed no speaker from the floor to exceed five minutes, however famous or distinguished they might be. Anyone who attempted to do so was warned menacingly with a flourish of his gavel before he hammered them to order.

I opposed Mayhew's motion, although more on the question of timing rather than principle. I argued that divisions within the party delighted our enemies and dismayed our friends. Sometimes they could be irreparably damaging, and it would be wrong to cause a split merely on a question of timing. The debate was passionate. Mayhew's motion was defeated, and my speech was well received. But my pleasure at this was marred by sadness later that day when I attended the funeral of a man who had vigorously supported my early efforts to enter the House of Commons. Nat Birch, the kindly Jewish orator from Finchley, had died a few days earlier, and I left the exciting atmosphere of Westminster to go to Golders Green crematorium. For me it was a quick transition from delight to dejection.

Although I was a Parliamentary novice, my broadcasting experience enabled me to respond succinctly to journalists. Many of them started to telephone frequently for my opinions, and I was invited to take part in various television programmes. In the autumn of 1966, on 18 November, I appeared on radio's popular programme *Any*

Questions?, along with Margaret Thatcher, Jeremy Thorpe and the playwright Alan Melville. I travelled down to Paignton, Devon, in the same train as Jeremy Thorpe, who was brimming with bonhomie, confidence and humour. He had been President of the Oxford Union when I was President of the Cambridge Union and we already knew each other slightly. With incessant patter and humorous asides, he was an engaging personality and, of course, good value on the programme.

Margaret Thatcher, by comparison, was rather quiet, although she, too, was confident. At the dinner before the programme I found her fluent and friendly, although by no means as extrovert a personality as Jeremy Thorpe. On the programme, she was competent but not more than that, whereas Thorpe delighted the audience with his colourful antics, dramatic presentation and lively sense of humour. For me it was a particularly interesting evening, participating rather than producing, and enjoying the clash of debate.

On the train journey back to London the following morning, one of those arguments developed which tend to escalate when two people are obdurate, neither prepared to concede a point. Margaret Thatcher and I discussed racial issues, and before long the argument became overheated, to the discomfiture of Alan Melville. Had Jeremy Thorpe been with us, he would have punctured the atmosphere with a witticism. Melville hastily suggested that we should break for coffee, and that brought a truce. The conversation was then diverted to more acceptable channels. Margaret Thatcher and I parted amicably as we left the train, agreeing, as MPs tend to do, how busy and rushed our lives were. As she strode from the station platform, I thought she was an extremely capable and determined woman.

My first friends reflected my experience in both Widnes and Oxbridge. MPs with working-class backgrounds like my own, such as Bob Brown, a gas inspector from Newcastle upon Tyne, were natural allies. On the other hand, I became friends with three Labour MPs regarded as intellectuals: David Owen, David Marquand and John Mackintosh. The four of us met regularly for discussions in the smoking room or dining room or an outside restaurant. Sometimes we had dinner at Owen's house. He was the most critical of the Government's economic policy, although both Marquand and Mackintosh also had strong reservations.

Mackintosh, a professor of politics, had a keen, analytical mind. He saw most things in wide historical and political perspective. He was outspoken, partly because he was not excessively tactful, but mainly because he was politically courageous.

Marquand, who later became a professor, also had an academic approach to politics. Although he had encyclopaedic knowledge and a good grasp of the issues, he never made the mark in Parliament that many people expected. Eventually he resigned his safe seat because of disenchantment with Labour's attitude to Europe, and after a period in Brussels working for the European Commission he joined the Social Democratic Party. His constituents took a poor view of his resignation, and his very safe seat was lost in the ensuing by-election.

Owen was the most interesting of all. Attractive, intelligent and tougher than he looked, he was never afraid to hit hard. Far from attempting to disguise his criticism of the Prime Minister, he went out of his way to declare it to him. Even in those early days, Owen was a man with a mission.

At Westminster, I participated enthusiastically with speeches and questions on a whole range of subjects including prices and incomes policy, foreign affairs, social security and disablement. In Stoke-on-Trent, I campaigned forcefully on the many issues that arose – for an improved telephone service, for a medical school for Keele University and for the College of Technology to become a polytechnic. I spoke at schools, visited pottery factories and crowned carnival queens. At regular advice bureaux, I did all I could to help with constituents' personal problems, many of which were reminiscent of those I knew in Widnes. Not all my efforts were immediately successful, but I became increasingly aware of the value of publicity and sustained pressure in achieving results.

My activities were well reported in the local paper, the *Sentinel*, but only rarely in the national press. But then in February 1967, an incident occurred which pushed me into the national limelight overnight. A personal story that caught the public interest, it became a subject of articles and editorials as well as news reports.

One of my constituents was arrested as a deserter, even though he claimed he had been discharged from the Army. The man, Leslie Parkes, had been taken into custody by the local police, handed over to the Army and imprisoned in a military barracks in Surrey.

When I went to see him, he showed me the marks of handcuffs on his wrists, and said he had been manacled for a long time. Claiming that he had been discharged from the Army a few weeks earlier, he said that he had lost the discharge ticket but colleagues in his unit in Germany could vouch for it. He also complained that his cell was windowless and empty but for a bed. I asked the officer in charge if I could see the cell. Conditions in it were just as Parkes had described them. The Parkes case was fully reported on television and radio that night, and splashed on newspaper front pages the following day. It was my first experience of national publicity.

I asked the Ministry of Defence to inquire into Parkes's allegations and meanwhile release him. The Minister who replied, James Boyden, the Under-Secretary of State, ordered the inquiry, but he refused to release Parkes. Public opinion was aroused, and when the Chief Constable of Stoke-on-Trent admitted that the police had arrested Parkes under false pretences, a major Parliamentary row was inevitable.

The Speaker gave me permission to raise the issue immediately in the House with a Private Notice Question – a device which enables MPs to question Ministers on urgent matters. In a crowded House, I was careful to avoid a general attack on the police and the Army but criticized their handling of this individual case. Although Members on both sides supported me, the Defence Minister would not change his mind and release Parkes, so I decided to apply for a writ of habeas corpus. In view of the false arrest I felt certain that there was a strong case for releasing him pending the result of the inquiry.

Meanwhile some MPs were angry at what they regarded as an attack on the Army. The most upset was George Wigg, the Paymaster-General. Aggressive, conspiratorial and unpopular, he never doubted that the Army was right and he strongly objected to my handling of the case. When he met me in the Members' Lobby of the Commons we clashed angrily.

As I was discussing plans for the writ with Parkes's solicitor, I had an urgent telephone message from the Ministry of Defence that the Secretary of State, Denis Healey, would make an important statement in the House that afternoon. Hurrying back, I was just in time to hear Healey's statement; he said he had decided to free Parkes, and the Army had 'wiped the slate clean'. He generously said he could not imagine any Ombudsman performing his duty more effectively and more expeditiously than I had done. I was aware of pitfalls, and there was no danger of this praise going to my head, but just to make sure someone wrote to me asking, 'Who the bloody hell do you think you are to challenge the Army?' George Wigg was even more venomous when I met him in the lobbies. He told me that I was a fool, that Parkes was dishonest, and my antics were damaging the Army. All this was delivered with the considerable vindictiveness and malevolence of which Wigg was notoriously capable. The language I used in response about Wigg, his parentage and his judgement would have made sergeant-majors quail. Wigg did not respond, but as he stalked off I had no doubt that he was not deterred. Wigg meant business.

Days later I was forewarned by Gerry Reynolds, the MP who was second in command at the Ministry of Defence, that 'certain people are gunning for Parkes'. A critical article was published in the *People* newspaper; and when Parkes repeated his story on television, some relatives claimed he had been lying all the time. After a further inquiry he was accused of perjury and found guilty. Although I was disappointed, Parkes's perjury did not excuse his peremptory arrest. I was also relieved that the media attention had not beguiled me into making wild claims. I had stuck to a valid request for an inquiry, realizing that MPs could lose reputations as easily as they could get attention and that 'caution until certain' was a good maxim.

With my background, it was natural that domestic issues concerned me most when I first entered Parliament. But in August 1966 I was invited to be one of a four-man delegation to Zambia. The object was to meet President Kaunda and his officials and to acquaint ourselves with the country's economic problems. My first overseas Parliamentary visit, I found it enormously interesting and stimulating.

It was also my first visit to Africa and different from anything I had experienced before. The MPs' beautiful villas, with peacocks strutting on the lawns in hot sunshine, contrasted sharply with primitive villages we later visited. We flew to the Copper Belt, Ndola and Kicwee and talked to black and white employees at the mines. I was fascinated by the colour and the vivid scenery, so far removed from industrial Widnes. Yet, as we travelled over miles of bush, under a bright blue sky, I saw people grappling with great poverty with the same cheerful determination as in my own home town.

In Lusaka we discussed Zambia's problems with President Kaunda and his officials. The sombre Kaunda was angry with the British Government for what he saw as its failure to deal with Ian Smith's rebel regime in Rhodesia. We argued that sanctions were working, but Kaunda was unimpressed and told us he would boycott the Commonwealth Prime Ministers' Conference the following week. This visit stimulated my interest in the country and in foreign affairs generally. I became eager to visit other countries.

Back in London, I knew I needed to specialize but I wanted to feel my way before concentrating on a few major issues. I had little opportunity to do so, however, as the Government's prices and incomes policy soon became the dominant Parliamentary issue. Attempts by previous Governments to achieve steady economic growth had failed; for over a decade Britain had oscillated between bouts of inflation and deflation. The so-called stop–go cycle was inevitable with low unemployment, a fixed exchange rate, inadequate reserves and no policy on prices and incomes. In the previous year earnings had risen 9.5 per cent, prices 5 per cent. Economists were predicting that our exports would be priced out of world markets and the country would face bankruptcy.

In these circumstances I welcomed the Government's controversial Prices and Incomes Bill in July 1966. This put the Prices and Incomes Board on a permanent basis and gave the Government statutory powers to demand early warning of intended price or pay increases. The Government could impose a standstill for one month while it considered whether to refer any proposed increases to the board. If it did refer, it could impose a further standstill for three months. This was a portent of stiffer measures.

After the board had considered a claim, trade unions and employers were free to act on their own judgement, so there was not such a significant restriction as some opponents of the Bill claimed. Nevertheless in the second reading debate on 14 July, some of our Labour colleagues were as critical as the Conservatives in opposing them. They were even more incensed six days later when the Prime Minister announced emergency measures to deal with the economic crisis sparked off by a seven-week seamen's strike. This stoppage, coupled with steadily rising prices, led to overseas speculation, causing a heavy loss of sterling reserves. With a fixed exchange rate, the Government had to act, and it proposed a six-month freeze on prices and incomes. I knew this would intensify the fight with Conservative MPs and critics within our own party.

The Bill was piloted through the Commons by the Secretary of State for Economic Affairs, George Brown, one of the most ebullient and colourful characters in the House. Provocative, aggressive and sometimes overbearing, Brown tended to bulldoze his opponents and some of his colleagues. His explosive temperament resulted in rowdy outbursts which were often followed by great geniality. With his fine intellect, he could also be a powerful and persuasive advocate. I was appointed to the committee examining the Prices and Incomes Bill and I watched his handling of it with admiration. We sat throughout the night for many arduous and wearying debates which were frequently enlivened by powerful speeches by George.

Late one night, after he had slipped out, he returned to find that Tory MPs had vehemently attacked his junior Minister, Bill Rodgers. Rodgers was well able to look after himself, but when Brown heard of the incident he stormed into the committee room. Disregarding the contents of the Bill, he blasted those Tories present for daring to attack his number two – regardless of the fact that in his absence that was their job.

Brown was, however, far more upset by the opposition coming

from within the party. Frank Cousins, former General Secretary of the mammoth Transport and General Workers' Union, had recently resigned as Minister of Technology and soon became leader of the dissidents on our benches. It was no pleasure to be a loyal back-bencher on the Government side of this committee, because our votes were needed while our voices were not. Ministers put forward each section of the Bill and fought it with the Opposition – or Frank Cousins.

I had known Frank while I was a television producer, and he once came to dinner at my home. But our friendly relationship had changed; he despised my views. In turn, his continual sniping at our Government angered me. In a debate on the floor of the House, I accused him of confusing long-term solutions with short-term necessities and of being unable or unwilling to see the relationship between wage inflation and the balance of payments. I claimed he was peddling panaceas which were one-third argument and two-thirds hogwash. The following day when I walked into the committee meeting, an angry Cousins shouted to me caustically to ask if I was now satisfied. I brushed him aside, and he never spoke to me again. Looking back, I regret the incident. I wish I had dealt more with the issues and less with the man.

These remarkable committee sessions were presided over by a witty and diplomatic chairman, Harold Lever. A very wealthy Labour backbencher with a fine mind, he later held high office in the Treasury before going to the House of Lords. He was always even-handed and alert regardless of the hour, and gave the impression of enjoying the exchanges between 'Honourable Members deliberating in our proceedings'. If George Brown was going over the top or if disarray threatened, Lever would intervene as if speaking to a happy group of Boy Scouts: 'We are making excellent progress. I suggest, however, that we should break for refreshment and reflection.' That phrase always brought smiles from MPs on both sides of the committee room; and usually, after a discreet break, frayed tempers would be restored.

At this early stage of my Parliamentary career I was vigorous and enthusiastic, but also impetuous. On one occasion I attacked the

Prime Minister, Harold Wilson, without justification. During his clashes with left-wing Labour MPs over the prices and incomes policy, I had been a strong supporter. At the Labour Party Conference in 1967 I was attending a party when he entered. He came in my direction, then walked past, ignoring me, and chatted and joked with his left-wing critics. Although this was probably a sensible tactic from his point of view, it annoyed me. Later, I angrily told his Parliamentary Private Secretary, Harold Davies, that he was stupid to ignore his supporters and soft-soap his critics. Davies listened open-mouthed at my diatribe, after which I told him to tell the Prime Minister what I had said. He duly did so.

Before that incident I had been chosen by Wilson to second the Loyal Address to the Queen's Speech in the new Parliamentary session – a rare honour. I next met him on 30 October, a few weeks later, at the Downing Street party which traditionally precedes the Queen's Speech. All Ministers and the mover and seconder of the Loyal Address are invited. It was an embarrassing moment. When Wilson approached me I expressed regret, but he brushed it aside: 'Good luck, Jack. We will all be supporting you tomorrow.' Wilson was often accused of being devious or cynical or both. But his personal warmth to me despite my misjudgement showed consideration.

As a well-known supporter of Wilson I was a little surprised when I was invited to lunch by Cecil King, Chairman of the Mirror Group, in early 1967, because it was common knowledge that he was highly critical of the Prime Minister. The arrangements were made by John Beavan, a fine journalist then working for the Mirror Group and later to become a member of the House of Lords. The lunch was to be in Cecil King's private dining room in the Daily Mirror Building at 12.45 p.m. Caught in heavy traffic, I drove up after 1 p.m. An anxious Beavan was waiting and hurried me to the lift to King's flat. There the three of us talked about the Government's economic policies, and King did most of the talking. While he was implicitly critical of Harold Wilson's handling of affairs, he made no outright attack on him. I expressed my own views, although, as I was his guest, it was a friendly exchange rather than a debating one.

Some months afterwards I received another invitation to lunch with King. This time only the two of us were present. By now he was speaking of doom and gloom for the Labour Government, mainly because of what he regarded as Harold Wilson's personal failure; he seemed nonplussed by my support for Wilson's policies.

I did not disclose these discussions to anyone else and was uncertain whether to break this strange relationship with a powerful newspaper executive. The decision was made for me, because shortly afterwards King was ousted as Chairman of the Mirror Group and replaced by Hugh Cudlipp.

Mam was quietly thrilled that I was a Member of Parliament and she greatly enjoyed visiting Westminster. It was another world to her, and I took a special delight in showing her round. MPs and their families are regularly invited to one of the Buckingham Palace garden parties. In the first year I had taken Pauline and I asked Mam for the second. We walked through the Palace to the crowded lawn which looked rather like Ascot without the horses. Soon the Royal Family appeared on the terrace. After the national anthem, they slowly made their way through the guests. Three separate avenues were formed where the Queen, the Duke of Edinburgh and the Queen Mother met small groups of people.

Hovering, and escorting the Queen in a morning suit and tall hat, was Charlie Grey, an old miner from the Whips' office. Charlie was designated Comptroller of Her Majesty's Household, which meant that he had some responsibility for occasions like this. He caught my eye on the edge of the crowd, saw Mam, whom I had mentioned to him in the House, and gestured to us to come inside the avenue of people and await the Queen. When she came she chatted with us for a few minutes; it was simple chit-chat about Stoke and Widnes but it was a happy day for Mam. I knew that her health was failing, and my only worry was that the pressure might be too much for her. But she enjoyed every moment.

By this time my political career was flourishing. After just over a year in the House I was invited to become an assistant Government Whip. Although flattered by the invitation after so short a time, I rejected it. The job, which gives an insight into managing the party, is a customary stepping stone to office. Government Whips are responsible for discipline and ensuring that Members vote in divisions the right way and at the right time. But a condition of the job is that they do not participate in debates. After so many years of producing BBC programmes which expressed other people's opinions, I was anxious to voice my own. Another young MP, Eric Varley, was appointed instead. He subsequently became the Parliamentary Private Secretary to the Prime Minister, Secretary of State for Industry and in due course a Life Peer.

A few months later, Michael Stewart, Minister for Economic Affairs, invited me to be his Parliamentary Private Secretary. A PPS is the political link between a Minister and backbench members of the party. Some are merely messengers, conveying opinions from backbenchers and acting as assistants to the Minister. Others become their confidants, close and trusted friends whose views are taken into account. It is an excellent introduction to the machinery of government, providing experience without responsibility, and I accepted Michael's invitation with alacrity. A quiet and intelligent man, he had previously been Foreign Secretary but was now trying to get the economy right.

The newly created Department of Economic Affairs had been created by the abrasive George Brown as a counterweight to the power of the Treasury. Its massive task was to rejuvenate the economy, improve productivity in industry and engineer growth. The National Plan had been designed to fit the complex and sometimes chaotic arrangements of management and labour into a coherent framework. For this thankless task, one of the main instruments was a Declaration of Intent which Brown had secured from employers and trade unions. They had committed themselves to behaving moderately over wages, profits and prices. Their failure to do so led to the acrimonious Prices and Incomes Bill which gave the Government power to control these incomes. After this frustrating and exhausting process was completed, Brown persuaded Harold Wilson to make him Foreign Secretary and switch Michael Stewart to Economic Affairs. Thus Stewart was landed with one of the most unrewarding jobs in the Government.

I enjoyed working with him and improving his relationship with our backbenchers. I got on well with most MPs and, as an active member of the Parliamentary trade union group, I was close to nearly all its members. A fine Minister, Stewart was, nevertheless, a shy man and he was delighted when I offered to arrange social meetings with the group. The first one was a great success, although as he was so polite there was some danger that he would be trapped on a sofa with two or three opinionated members. My self-appointed function, as I poured the drinks, was to manage a discreet turnover of MPs so that during the evening he had met and talked to all of them.

Stewart gave me as much responsibility as he could. I became immersed in the work, and we developed an increasingly close relationship. When he subsequently became the Minister for the long-term development of social policy, I transferred with him. At that time there was press speculation about my possible promotion. Reports in the *Daily Telegraph* and the *Statist* suggested that a number of backbenchers should be made Ministers including Roy Hattersley, Eric Heffer, David Owen and myself. All the others became Ministers eventually, although not at the same time. When a Government reshuffle was announced, and two of the new Ministers' names were not disclosed, a press report speculated that I was one of them. I telephoned a friend, Gerald Kaufman, who was a member of the Prime Minister's staff at 10 Downing Street, asking him if the report was true. When he told me that it was not, I was disappointed but by no means disconsolate. I was content to wait, and everyone seemed certain that before long I would get office.

9

The Silence Falls

On the evening of 1 December 1967, I attended a splendid dinner party at No. 1 Carlton Gardens, the official residence of Michael Stewart. Behind the splendour lay an exercise in power; discussion at dinner could affect the lives of millions of people. As I listened intently to the experts planning radical changes in our social services, I felt that the evening signified a new era for those in need in Britain – little realizing that it was to mark the end of my normal life and the beginning of a remarkable new one.

One of the guests was G. D. N. Worswick, the Director of the National Institute of Economic and Social Research. Wearing the large and cumbersome National Health hearing aid in use at that time, he was able to discuss deafness without inhibition or embarrassment. I noticed with admiration, and some amusement, how he unclipped the microphone from his breast pocket during dinner and placed it prominently in the middle of the table to facilitate conversation with the people opposite. He told me that he had undergone an operation which had seriously damaged his hearing – though fortunately not destroyed it.

I was interested because the following day I was to enter hospital for an ear operation. My left ear-drum had a perforation, due to a childhood infection, and although this caused a partial loss of hearing it was not a significant one. But my right ear was failing despite three operations, known as stapedectomies. As the large rooms and halls of Parliament caused me slight hearing difficulties, I decided to

(133)

have a minor operation to repair the perforated left ear-drum. If successful, it would give me virtually perfect hearing in one ear.

The decision was not made lightly, because my hearing functioned reasonably well and I did not believe that slight deafness would be a major barrier to a political career. I deliberated for some time, but the surgeon's confident prediction of the outcome swayed me. It was a minor operation; improved hearing was virtually assured; and the risk of deterioration – even slight – was described as '1 per cent'.

The day before the operation I had a mild sore throat and because I was uneasy I told the surgeon and the anaesthetist. The surgeon's response was that he would make sure I had good antibiotic cover. The anaesthetist, who examined my throat, said: 'It's no reason why I shouldn't give you an anaesthetic.' I felt reassured, yet the precise nature of his reply raised a disturbing question. Was it a calculated evasion of comment on the desirability of an operation, or simply the straightforward response of a man who restricted himself to speaking within his own specialist field?

The following day I had the operation. Immediately afterwards my hearing was very low. I comforted myself with the thought that the dressings would be mainly responsible, but I was sufficiently disturbed to ask the surgeon if he had performed a more serious operation than the repair of the ear-drum; he told me he had not and that the dressing was reducing my hearing. His attitude was reassuring, yet I was vaguely aware for the first time that an event of profound significance in my life had occurred. I was not deeply worried, but a suspicion persisted in my mind.

During the evening I developed a heavy cold which seemed more feverish than any I had ever known. When the surgeon came the following day he told me that he was ordering more antibiotic injections. Although I was not disconsolate, I was uncomfortable with the cold, and tense because my hearing was so low. Michael Stewart kindly offered to visit me, but I declined because I felt the difficulties of understanding him might be embarrassing. Pauline had to speak slowly and clearly before I could follow her; she was very concerned about my deafness despite the confidence of the surgeon. He told me that there was nothing to worry about, my hearing would be all right and I could go home after a few days. When I went, it was with grave misgivings.

It was soon obvious that something had gone badly wrong. I was ill, weak and deaf, unable to hear without the help of an old bone conduction hearing aid of Mam's, which we happened to have in our house. Even then voices sounded like vague mumbles, limiting my comprehension of speech. Each time Pauline telephoned the surgeon he was reassuring, but he agreed to visit me. He diagnosed a new infection but took no further action since he thought the slow-acting antibiotics I had already been given would be sufficient. On our return visit a few days later he was obviously surprised that my hearing was still very low, and this time he prescribed new antibiotics. The infection would clear up, the surgeon assured us; he was going abroad for three weeks and he expected my hearing to be normal when he returned. In the meantime I was to take the antibiotics. It would be all right for me to travel to Widnes for Christmas, he said.

As I was still unwell, I travelled alone by train, Pauline and our three children following by car. My thirteen-year-old eldest daughter, Jackie, was disturbed by my deafness but assumed that it would be cured before Christmas. Jane, our nine-year-old, unquestioningly accepted our assurance that it was a temporary difficulty which would soon be resolved. Caroline, eighteen months old, was blissfully unaware of the problem. Despite the lurking doubts, we hoped to enjoy our usual family reunion with Mam, my sisters and their families – but my confidence had begun to waver. The operation had undoubtedly failed: was it to become a disaster? It bothered me that while the powerful hearing aid amplified the sound of voices, they were still incomprehensible. During the journey I switched off the hearing aid, trying to listen to the familiar clickety-click of the train speeding over the line. There was nothing but silence.

When I arrived, my mother and sisters were very worried. My mother had been deaf for many years and she managed only by using a powerful hearing aid. Now my hearing was worse than hers and we did not know whether it would deteriorate further. The infection showed no sign of clearing up, so a few days before Christ-

(135)

mas, with the London surgeon still abroad, Pauline and I visited a Liverpool hospital. I was examined by a young doctor of Chinese origin who was suffering from a heavy cold. I decided against joking with him about Asian flu and asked to see the head of the department – an ear, nose and throat consultant whom I had met some time ago. He was off duty but he kindly invited me to his home for an examination. For the first time since the operation my hearing was tested on an audiometer.

The results confirmed my worst fears. My right ear was dead, and only a flicker of life remained in the left one. The most powerful hearing aid was useless for the dead ear and of little help to the other because the vital nerves were damaged and were failing to transform noise into meaningful sound. It was a bleak diagnosis, and I felt the shadows falling on my life. But the consultant was cautiously hopeful that a little hearing might be restored, possibly just sufficient to enable me to continue as a Member of Parliament. He prescribed new treatment and made arrangements for me to contact him if necessary during the Christmas holiday. I hoped it would not be necessary, but took some telephone numbers as a precaution.

The next few festive days were not as happy as those I had regularly enjoyed with Mam and the Widnes family, but on Christmas Eve at our traditional gathering we carved a large turkey, distributed presents and sang Christmas carols. Christmas Day was charged with its own magic of happy children and a gay and intimate family. I was cheerful, for the new treatment was successfully bringing some hearing back, making speech comprehensible. As I was still convalescent I went to bed to rest after Christmas dinner. Caroline, sleeping in her cot nearby, roused me with her crying when she awoke shortly afterwards. I was elated at being able to hear some sounds again without a hearing aid. The whole family rejoiced. My eldest sister Helen said, 'Wouldn't it have been awful if your hearing hadn't come back?' My fears were proving unjustified and the threat of unmanageable deafness receded.

Our relief was short-lived. On the afternoon of Boxing Day, as I was watching rugby on television after lunch, the words of the commentator became blurred and indistinct. Afterwards the family had tea together, but as the strain of trying to understand the conversation became too great I went upstairs to rest. Shortly afterwards Pauline came to see me; when she spoke I could not hear her voice at all. My first reaction was that the borrowed hearing aid had failed, so she went downstairs and brought the powerful one my mother used. It was only when I tried it with the power full on and still could not hear Pauline's voice that the truth dawned on me. My hearing had completely gone.

I appreciated the potential consequences of the disaster immediately, yet I felt oddly cool and dispassionate about it. Perhaps it was due to the shock, or possibly I subconsciously assumed that my hearing would return. Yet I was aware of a growing, icy apprehension.

Pauline hurriedly telephoned the Liverpool consultant, arranging for me to enter hospital the following morning. The implications of deafness were ominous, as I reflected on them that night, but I refused to let my imagination roam too far; it may have been through fear or perhaps because I still had some hopes. Like a drowning man I clutched at an imaginary straw. I tried to invest medical science with an aura of infallibility I knew it did not possess.

It was a grim journey to Liverpool with Pauline. For the first time driving together, we were unable to communicate except when she made brief notes as we stopped at traffic lights or in queues of vehicles. At the hospital it was no longer a question of having difficulty in understanding some people; it was impossible to understand anyone. The formalities of answering questions for admission had to be conducted by Pauline. I was afraid, angry and frustrated – and I knew I was powerless to do anything about it.

I was taken to a small, soundproof cubicle where a solemn-faced technician clamped a pair of earphones over my head and indicated that I should signal when I heard anything. Watching him adjusting the controls, I recognized a contradiction in my attitude. I knew without doubt that my hearing had gone, yet I hoped that this complicated piece of machinery would magically produce some evidence to the contrary on which the doctors could build. The technician played his part perfectly. He was non-committally pleasant,

(137)

but I felt instinctively that he regarded my case as hopeless, my hope as forlorn.

The consultant began an intensive course of treatment in a desperate attempt to retrieve some hearing. He asked the advice of other specialists and eventually decided on a comprehensive approach. I was given antibiotics, cortisone, pills to reduce the water supply in my body, pills to increase the circulation of my blood, and even whisky. I wondered whether the whisky was administered for psychological purposes, but apparently it had medicinal value, helping to stimulate the circulation of blood to the ears. Most of the pills and potions were administered every four hours, and it was an odd experience to be wakened at 2 a.m. and 6 a.m. to be given a stiff dose of neat whisky. I came to hate it, but at that time I was prepared to swallow anything if it was going to help to restore my hearing.

Every morning the technician came to my bed with his mobile equipment, clipped earphones on my head and tested my hearing; it was practically non-existent. Three or four crosses on the audiogram formed a tiny curve which only just fitted on to the bottom of the paper. I was still unable to hear speech even with a hearing aid, but by banging a spoon on a table or a piece of china I could hear a vague blur of sound. I did this constantly, checking my hearing in the only way I could, until the nurses asked Pauline if there was anything wrong with me. I was making such a din that they probably thought my mind was affected.

The daily tests dominated my thoughts because the results were of crucial importance. Sometimes the crosses on the chart would rise a little, or occasionally another one would appear. These were occasions for rejoicing and soaring hopes. On other days, when the chart showed a loss, I was correspondingly gloomy. It was a desperate fight to retain normality, yet the whole procedure was conducted in a cool, clinical atmosphere, completely without obvious drama. Everything I did and all the actions of the doctors and nurses were conducted in a matter-of-fact way, but we all knew that success meant a return to an ordinary life and the resumption of my political career, while failure meant a lifetime of total silence.

Soon after entering hospital I heard the Liverpool trams clanking and roaring outside; but, remarkably enough, their screeching and shrieking sounds did not vary with the changes recorded on the technician's equipment. The first time I was allowed out of bed I went to the window and looked out at the street. To my astonishment, there were no trams or tramlines; the screeching and shrieking I could 'hear' were noises within my head. Known in the medical world as 'tinnitus', head noises are a profoundly distressing by-product of some forms of deafness and they are incurable. My experience then was the first dose of daily suffering which any victim endures throughout his life. Doctors and consultants are helpless, so I was faced with the prospect of living in the worst of both worlds, deprived of any meaningful sound yet denied the tranquillity which others imagine to be a tiny consolation of total deafness.

During those days of tension and anxiety Pauline sustained me. Two of our daughters, Jackie and Jane, had returned to Epsom to go back to school and were cared for by Pauline's mother and sister. Caroline, now twenty months old, stayed in Widnes. Every morning Pauline would dress and feed her, leave her with one of my sisters and drive the twelve miles from Widnes to Liverpool. She always entered the ward radiating infectious optimism. The dying days of 1967 were bitterly cold, and as she came in, rosy-cheeked and smiling, I always felt my spirits soar. She sat on my bed with pen and paper, conversing in this odd way as if it were the most natural thing in the world. She masked her misgivings with great courage, invariably interpreting the technician's results to my advantage. Thus my slender hopes were kept alive.

I knew that Mam and my sisters Helen, Mary and Margaret were deeply worried, anxiously awaiting news from Pauline every day. We were a close and loving family, and as I did not want to distress them I suggested they should not visit me for a little while until my hearing improved. But they came after a week, hiding their anxiety and affectionately lifting my spirits. I only learned years later from my sisters that on their sad bus journey home, for the first time in their lives, they saw Mam in tears.

My morale was boosted one day when the door was flung open

and the massive figure of Bessie Braddock, the local and legendary MP, burst in. She was a great Parliamentary warrior who fought many battles. When she heard I was in the Liverpool ear, nose and throat hospital she turned up at my bedside and wrote me confident, reassuring notes. Her attitude and spontaneous gesture were a tonic.

One cold morning, a few minutes after leaving with a cheerful wave, Pauline returned looking pale and shaken. She had slipped and fallen on the frozen snow outside and broken her wrist. While arrangements were being made to have it set and put in plaster, she rested in a room close to mine. While I was with her I tried to be as cheerful as she had been with me. A broken wrist was no lifelong tragedy, yet I felt more upset than at any time since I had entered hospital. When she went for treatment my spirits sank and I imagined all kinds of complications in her injury. But Pauline did not allow this setback to upset her. Although it meant that she was now unable to drive from Widnes to Liverpool and had to wait in the cold for an inadequate and slow bus service, she continued to spend every day with me.

When we were together, *she* looked like the invalid, with her arm in a sling. Gradually we began to notice that the nurses seemed more concerned about Pauline's injury than my deafness. One disability was visible, the other was not, and this affected their attitude. We were able to smile ruefully about this at the time, but it was a foretaste of the future when some people were to treat me with near condescension if I failed to understand what they said.

A few days after Pauline broke her wrist a bigger blow fell. As I was shaving, I noticed that the normal faint buzzing of my electric razor, which I felt rather than heard, had vanished. It was an ominous moment. When the technician arrived for his tests I did not mention it but waited for his reaction. He usually took about fifteen minutes, but after one or two tests lasting only a few minutes he left hurriedly, returning shortly afterwards with the consultant, who completed the tests himself. There had been a serious setback and the little hearing that had returned during my stay in hospital had almost completely gone. With only three crosses right at the bottom of the chart, my deafness was almost total. Every known method had been used, and now there was nothing left to try. The suspense had ended, but with disastrous results, despite the dedicated skill of the consultant. He advised me to go back to Widnes and to return periodically to the hospital for tests.

Before I left, he gave me new hope by explaining the possibilities of lip-reading; he said that in two or three months, speech could be understood quite well. Of course it was an overstatement, because mastering lip-reading takes years and even then it is a very poor and inadequate substitute for hearing. Yet without his encouragement, I would have despaired in the next few months. He made me feel that there was a mountain to be climbed and I resolved to climb it. Otherwise I might never have coped with what was to follow.

I left hospital in a car driven by one of my brothers-in-law, who chatted to Pauline on the journey. This apparently simple, natural scene caused one of the greatest shocks of my life. I was astounded to see them sharing a car with me yet having a conversation from which I was totally excluded. The hospital environment had insulated me against the reality which now had to be faced.

My spirits, already low, plummeted when I was unable to understand my mother and sisters at home. I was no longer the confident, jocular person they had always known; we all tried to pretend but we saw through each other's pretence. During the afternoon I went for a short walk with Pauline and it was the bleakest stroll of my life, for on that cold, gusty day in Widnes I was obsessed with the enshrouding silence now dominating my life. All rational thought was engulfed by powerful emotion and depression. The unthinkable was becoming a reality.

On one of my visits to hospital in Liverpool I was asked to try some powerful hearing equipment. This was the moment I had been waiting for, and I entered the room apprehensively, accompanied by Pauline. The consultant and a technician adjusted the apparatus; the large headphones were again gently clamped over my ears. Pauline was given a microphone and began to speak to me. Even with the help of this powerful machine I could hear only a few unintelligible scratches of sound. The consultant was delighted I could hear anything at all, but I was bitterly disappointed that I could hear so little

– although I tried to hide it to avoid hurting his feelings. I knew then that my tiny wisp of hearing was so slight that even with the most powerful hearing apparatus the human voice remained incomprehensible.

We stayed in Widnes for another few weeks, making frequent visits to the hospital, but there was no significant change in my hearing. Near the end of January we went back home to the children in London. Pauline's mother and sister, Barbara, had readily agreed to stay with Jackie and Jane while we were stranded in the north, and we appreciated their kindness. Barbara stayed with us for some months longer, giving us support and encouragement as well as unobtrusively taking over many household chores despite the pressure of her own demanding job. With remarkable understanding the family adapted to my deafness, speaking very slowly and clearly for me. Pauline constantly sought to instil a sense of proportion by emphasizing the faculties I had retained. Yet we were two baffled people groping in an eerie situation, endlessly searching for a solution to an insoluble problem.

The operation had been a terrible mistake, but the damage was done. My remaining option was to see if the London surgeon could repair it. The confident consultant I had seen before the operation now seemed nervous and very apprehensive. He did a hearing test on an old-fashioned machine lacking the precision of the Liverpool instruments. It failed entirely to register any wisp of sound, confirming once more that my hearing was almost certainly irretrievably damaged. But the consultant said he would prescribe a further course of treatment, which, I was to discover later, consisted simply of daily injections of vitamin B.

When I asked about the chances of recovery he was non-committal. He was shortly going to the United States and would discuss my case with two doctors – 'the best in the world at this kind of thing'. I was astonished at this sudden display of self-deprecation, since he had never taken pains to conceal the fact that he considered himself to be one of the leading ear, nose and throat consultants in Britain. In reply to my question 'Will I be able to hear sufficiently to remain a Member of Parliament?' he shook his head. Then he spoke one word. Of course I could not understand it, so he picked up a small pad and wrote, 'Journalism.' After showing it to me he pulled the pad out of its case and pushed it back so that the word was erased. I felt I ought to be impressed by the trick, and he obviously thought so too; but in fact I was amazed at the casual way he was dismissing the political career I valued so highly. He made it seem like his writing on the pad – now you see it, now you don't.

His discussions with the two leading doctors in the United States never took place. On his return he said that he had not seen them but would write. Later he told me that he had received replies and only one of them had heard of a similar case. The information was as useless as his vitamin injections. In a last desperate hope that my hearing could be restored I made the usual round of other ear specialists, but they were all as helpless as witch-doctors so far as I was concerned. Some simply shrugged and gave encouraging smiles; others treated me as if I were a congenital idiot and discussed my condition with Pauline.

'How old is he?' one inquired. He spoke without moving his lips, like a ventriloquist.

'Why don't you ask him?' Pauline replied. 'And try speaking a little more clearly.'

The consultants did their best, but their knowledge of deafness was limited and their knowledge of how to treat deaf people was lamentable. Pauline and I left every hospital with sinking hearts and a growing certainty that medical science had nothing to offer.

It was not in my nature to accept defeat, but resignation seemed inevitable. The idea of an MP who heard nothing seemed ludicrous – yet I wondered. Would it be possible, by a crash course in lip-reading and the minute help given by a hearing aid, to remain a Member of Parliament? Everything depended on my ability to communicate. The most powerful electronic aids were only of marginal value because the aural nerves were almost completely destroyed; nothing could magnify speech to more than a vague, indefinable blur to me. I had to learn to lip-read.

I was advised to go to the Institute of Further Education for the Deaf in London, then housed in a large, gloomy building. Although the teaching staff were helpful, many of the lessons were based on the presumed chit-chat of retired people – 'Would you like one lump of sugar or two?' Sometimes they took the form of soundless half-completed proverbs which individual members of the class had to lip-read and complete – 'A stitch in time . . .' When I moved to more advanced classes the material was less banal, but it was a desperately depressing experience.

Apart from one or two individuals, I felt no rapport with other people at the classes. Although they were pleasant enough, and some tried to be helpful, I had nothing in common with them. Many were old, with no interest in politics, seeking to overcome the slow erosion of their hearing by learning lip-reading. Yet we were thrust together through the shattering loss of our hearing, groping for understanding. For me, these lessons were overlaid by sadness, yet there was no alternative but to pursue them in the hope of acquiring some skill.

I read every available book on the subject and found many of them old-fashioned and inadequate. The surprisingly large number of people who speak without any clear movement of their lips underlined the limitations of lip-reading. Some consonants and vowels are scarcely visible, being formed by tongue movements often hidden by teeth and lips; beards and moustaches create more difficulties and so do regional accents. Groups of consonants like 'p', 'b' and 'm' or 'sh', 'ch' and 'j' are indistinguishable, while short vowels are extremely hard to identify. Lip-reading, I found, was infinitely more difficult than learning a foreign language; the Liverpool consultant had only been encouraging me when he said the skill could be achieved in a few months. Anyone trying to learn Chinese can at least theoretically master the language; but in lip-reading much of the 'language' is not available to be learned.

Lip-reading is an art based on recognizing slight visual clues and using them imaginatively. The mind has to register lip patterns while working like a computer to select the correct meaning from a vast number of possibilities. It is immensely difficult and a grossly inadequate substitute for hearing. The miracle is that, despite such tremendous limitations, it works at all.

Pauline thought I was good at interpreting clues but weak on identifying them. To help me to identify the slightest lip movement and match it with appropriate sound, she compiled a series of charts. I found these charts more helpful than the textbooks. Every morning and afternoon I visited the wives of some of our friends, who would repeat words and sentences from the charts while I vainly tried to understand them. It was a desperately fatiguing business for me, and they must have found it oddly trying. I wondered what the neighbours thought as they saw me regularly enter the houses of friendly wives, then depart weary and bleary-eyed after half an hour.

Some of our friends suggested I should have additional practice with them in the evenings. We would stand in front of a mirror, trying to identify and compare the lip movements of some elusive vowel or consonant. I have since learned that a half-hour intensive session of learning to lip-read is enough to cause eye strain and tax concentration, but at that time I was doing up to six half-hours a day. With the combination of eye strain, tinnitus and the battering of my nervous system, I could feel myself ageing day by day. The head noises were painful and sometimes agonizing. Their intensity varied from day to day, and even during the day, but I was never free from them. They created a ceaseless cacophony sometimes bordering on bedlam. I began to feel punch-drunk, sometimes despairing of ever understanding the silently moving lips, but with my hearing aid the minute whisper of sound made some of the lip movements more meaningful. Occasionally I practised lip-reading without the aid, hoping to improve more quickly, but it was extremely difficult; at that time only the scratches of sound made the near-impossible possible.

The sense of isolation was stunning. My inability to participate in conversation was the worst of all, but I was also acutely aware that others were participating in the now remote but wondrous activity of Parliament. My colleagues in the House of Commons were still debating all the exciting political issues of the day, while I was excluded. On the bleak train journeys to the Institute for the Deaf, I would read of the lively exchanges and see in my mind's eye all my friends, and my political opponents, arguing and clashing in the

Commons. I felt like an exile, deprived of a homeland, yet clinging to hope that one day I would return.

Meanwhile I resigned as Parliamentary Private Secretary to Michael Stewart. Shortly after the operation I had offered him my resignation, but he had refused to accept it. When in March 1968 he was suddenly reappointed Foreign Secretary, I knew I could never fulfil my responsibilities to him. Accompanied by Pauline, I went to No. 1 Carlton Gardens to hand in my resignation. It was our first meeting since the splendid dinner party; this time it was a quiet, personal occasion over a cup of tea. We were both sensitive to the drastically changed circumstances, and I shall never forget the immense depth of understanding and unspoken affection he showed. We seemed to have a tacit understanding that the words we spoke to each other bore little relation to our feelings. He was the first MP I had met since leaving hospital and he fully understood the significance of my resignation as his PPS, suggesting as it did a future resignation from the House of Commons. Whether it was our personal empathy, the peculiar circumstances or both I don't know, but our meeting was a source of solace and encouragement to me at that difficult time.

Although I was virtually totally deaf, my other faculties were unimpaired. Yet I did not know whether I should be able to use them effectively in Parliament. After Easter 1968, the final decision could no longer be delayed. I had been dealing with correspondence and my Parliamentary colleagues John Forrester and Bob Cant were helping out in my constituency, but it was time for me to return to the House to see whether I could continue or would have to resign.

The day I returned, Tuesday 23 April 1968 – just two years after I had entered Parliament – was one of the most testing and memorable of my life. For the past four months I had been fighting to preserve my political career, which hung precariously by the most slender thread. If I succeeded, all the work, concentration, eye strain and weariness would have been worthwhile. I left for the Commons exhausted, bewildered and apprehensive – but oddly hopeful.

As I walked through the Members' Lobby I was aware of curious eyes observing me. There was a warm welcome from many of my friends, who looked at the hearing aid, with its long cord, obviously wondering how I would manage. But I did not stop to talk to any of them; I waved, walked into the Chamber and sat down. Would I be able to understand the debate? I turned the powerful hearing aid to full volume. There were only vague and meaningless blurs of sound as each speaker made his point. I tried to lip-read, but the Government speakers were sitting with their backs towards me, and speakers from the Opposition side, whose lips I could see moving, were too far away for me to hear even the slightest sounds. I could follow very little indeed.

I left the Chamber, took a long, deep breath and walked into the bar. It was the most embarrassing experience of my life. Three or four Members converged on me at once, shaking hands, slapping my back and welcoming my return. Others waved, and somebody handed me a glass of beer. After the pleasantries, someone asked me a question. I could neither hear nor lip-read him so I asked him to repeat it. He willingly repeated it, but as I still could not understand I asked him to repeat it again. Then I saw an expression that was to haunt me endlessly in the years ahead. It was one of total perplexity and embarrassment – he did not know how to deal with the situation. When he repeated the question again he was probably shouting, because out of the corner of my eye I could see nearly everyone in the room turn and watch us; but I was still unable to understand.

Swift and meaningful glances were exchanged, and by this time I was perspiring. I muttered apologies and hurriedly tried to finish the glass of beer as one of our colleagues, who had evidently had a few drinks, decided he would clarify the situation. He joined us and obviously bellowed at the top of his voice, but to me it sounded like the rustle of a leaf – and I could not lip-read him. I finished the drink, smiled all round, thanked them and walked out.

By chance I met a colleague who was himself very hard of hearing. We went out on the terrace to talk, but I found it almost impossible to follow anything he said. The only message he conveyed to me was that he was a very clear speaker and that if I could not understand him he regretfully felt I would not understand anyone. 'But don't leave immediately,' he said. 'Give it a few months before you resign.'

When he left I sat alone on the terrace watching the Thames. It looked bleak and cold. It was early evening, and although I did not expect the river to be busy it seemed exceptionally still and silent. I thought I had known despair, but now I felt a chill and deeper sadness, as if a part of me was dead. After a while I went back to the Chamber, where the debate was continuing, but as speakers made their points there was for me total and unbelievable silence. Each Member on his feet appeared to be miming. My last support, that vague buzz of sound which had come to mean so much, had vanished – perhaps obliterated by the last desperate use of the hearing aid. At that moment I felt in my heart that I had begun a lifetime of tomb-like silence. I took a final look around the Chamber before leaving for home and my family, and to prepare for my resignation from the House of Commons.

10

Resignation?

I was shattered when I lost the crucial remnant of hearing on the day I returned to the House of Commons. My future was in ruins, and I was plunged into a new, blank world, isolated from all external sound. The odds against my remaining in Parliament had been heavy for months, but I had buoyed myself with hope while taking the crash course in lip-reading. Now the pressures had proved too great. I was mentally and physically exhausted from forcing myself so hard immediately after the illness, then failing the vital test. Success would have been a psychological boost – a springboard for further advance. But I could not build my life on what might have been; I had to live with the diametric difference between success and failure.

If only a job had been involved I would have been disappointed but not desperate. The problem was infinitely more complex and profound. Cut off from mankind, surrounded by an invisible, impenetrable barrier, I could see people clearly, but they belonged to a different world – a world of talk, of music and laughter. I could hardly believe I would never hear again. I tried pressing a radio to the side of my head in a vain attempt to make contact; when I turned the volume to full pitch I could only feel a delicate vibration as the set trembled. It was undeniable confirmation that although sound existed it was not for me.

That fragile wisp of hearing had maintained for me a slender contact with the ordinary world; it had given some sense of reality, a hint of that background of sound which, to a normal person, is so familiar as to be unnoticed. Without it, life was eerie. People appeared suddenly at my side; doors banged noiselessly; dogs barked soundlessly; and heavy traffic glided silently past me. Friends chatted gaily in total silence.

The greatest deprivation was being unable to hear the human voice. Casual conversation – the common currency of everyday life – and even a passing joke were things of the past. All I could manage to understand were simple messages spoken very slowly. Even talking to Pauline and the children had become almost impossible. This above all made me realize just how much was lost. Minute as it was, the residual hearing had been a vital adjunct to lip-reading; the vague sounds had helped to make lip movements comprehensible to some extent. Now, with total silence, they had become meaningless. The most experienced and skilful lip-readers invariably encounter difficulties, but I was new to the subject and found most people impossible to understand, even when they spoke clearly. I was struggling like a newly caught bird in a foolproof cage.

Had I been alone, I would almost certainly have despaired, because the exhaustion was exacerbated by unfathomable depths of depression. I felt isolated, but I was not alone, as throughout that time Pauline never left my side. She spoke clearly and, incredibly, optimistically about the future. There were many better jobs than being a Member of Parliament, she said, and I could do them better than anyone. She reminded me of the chance that some hearing might return; that was the faint hope we clung to. She telephoned the Liverpool surgeon, and although he was not optimistic he prescribed rest and further drugs. I swallowed them faithfully for a week, but this time they failed to restore the slightest hearing. As a final resort we went to see another consultant in a London hospital. He examined my ears, then simply looked at me and shook his head. It was the end of our hopes. Together we left with that odd mixture of despair tinged slightly with relief when one knows the worst, although the worst now had to be faced.

There was an atmosphere of quiet crisis at home, and all the family was aware of it. At the end of a traumatic week we knew that

I had to leave Parliament and pick up the threads of a new, silent world as best I could. I wrote to the chairman of my constituency party, Sir Albert Bennett, telling him that I had no alternative but to resign. It was a simple message. I added that although I was young for memories I would always remember with pleasure my time as the Member for Stoke-on-Trent South. Having written the letter I let it lie on my desk for the rest of the day. In the early evening I posted it with a sense of reluctant finality, feeling exhausted in a world of limitless despondency. In the House of Commons I had been supremely happy, working on issues of my choice, fighting for causes I believed in and facing a bright political future. Now I was looking for a job. None but the brave would employ a former politician who was totally deaf, and my family was obviously going to face serious economic problems. That night I wrote a batch of letters to people I knew, asking about jobs. I resolved the conflict between my wish to avoid asking favours and the need to provide for my family by saying in every letter that I would understand if they felt that in their particular field deafness was a major handicap.

The news of my resignation emerged in a strange way. The *Sentinel*, the local newspaper in Stoke-on-Trent, had always been scrupulously fair to me. It is a newspaper with high professional standards, always leavening its criticism with a touch of humanity; it could differ without damning. I appreciated this fairness and as a final gesture before leaving the constituency gave the *Sentinel* the news as an exclusive story. Pauline telephoned it to the paper's lobby correspondent, who thanked her and expressed his personal regret. Later in the morning the London editor of the newspaper group, Will Stewart, telephoned to say it was the saddest exclusive he had ever had for the paper. It was through him that I had first become interested in campaigning in Parliament for the disabled, and now I was resigning because I was disabled.

The story was published in Stoke-on-Trent in mid-afternoon, a few hours after Sir Albert Bennett should have received my letter. In fact, the letter was delayed, and he only learned of my decision when the *Sentinel* telephoned him for comment. He gave a non-committal statement. The news was now public, and Pauline discussed it on the telephone with a Press Association correspondent in the constituency, but somehow it did not reach the London office. It was only after nine o'clock that night that the London office of the agency telephoned to say they had just got the story from 'another source' and asked if we could confirm it.

The message went on the news tapes at 9.30 p.m. From 9.35 p.m. there was a stream of telephone calls from the House of Commons. Everyone wanted me to carry on. It was touching but futile. I assumed they thought I was merely hard of hearing and they did not realize the fundamental difference between that and total deafness. Their messages showed the quality of the friends and colleagues I was being forced to leave, but they did nothing for my peace of mind.

One of the letters I had written, attempting to explain that resignation was probably for the best, was to Mam. Neither she nor my sisters had telephones at that time. Unfortunately that letter was also delayed in the post, and the first she heard was a radio bulletin next morning announcing my decision to resign. It was a terrible blow to her.

Later that day there were more telephone calls, and two Members of Parliament, Eric Ogden and Michael McGuire, arranged to come and see me at my home in a few days' time. Although I appreciated the gesture, I felt that there could be only one conclusion. Continuing as a totally deaf MP was out of the question, despite the goodwill of my colleagues. Apart from the personal problems involved, I had been chosen as an MP with all his faculties and it would be presumptuous now to stay.

The Times carried a sympathetic story about my resignation, and reading the *Sentinel* editorial was like reading my obituary; the words were generous, but it was an unnerving experience. One of the telephone calls that morning was from a producer on the BBC's *World at One* programme. He wanted an interview, and after some hesitation I agreed, although I explained it would be necessary to let me have advance notice of the questions. I had frequently broadcast but I never arrived at a studio with such trepidation as I did that morning. Pauline came along to help if necessary. The interviewer, William Hardcastle, took it all in his stride, and in the programme I tried to explain as coolly as possible how I felt. His last question was interesting and significant: 'Even though you are totally deaf, would you stay on if you were pressed strongly enough?' I said I thought not. However, a seed had been planted in my mind; were all the messages I had received merely expressions of sympathy, or did people really believe I could stay on? I didn't really know, nor did Pauline, but as we walked out of Broadcasting House something had subtly changed – it was as if a nerve suddenly flickered slightly in an apparently dead body.

That night we had dinner at home with an old friend, Stephen Bonarjee, with whom I had worked at the BBC. He was our first visitor from outside the family and we welcomed the opportunity to discuss our problems with him. I had wondered whether to cancel the date, which had been made before my total deafness. Perhaps he too feared an embarrassing evening, but in the event it was pleasant and stimulating. Since we valued his judgement we told him of the tiny flicker of hope that had been revived; his reaction was interesting. He paused, thought for a moment and then said that it might well be possible to stay in the House of Commons. 'Yes,' he added after reflection, 'it might well work.'

When he had gone, Pauline and I talked long into the night. Although the hope of a miracle to save my hearing had vanished, there seemed now to be a slender chance that I could return to Parliament *despite* being totally deaf. We decided to see how things developed – and laughed at my suggestion that we should play it by ear.

Next day there was another flood of telephone calls and letters from constituents and Parliamentary colleagues. I knew that the Government was passing through an unpopular phase, and my electoral majority was not as safe as the figure of 12,000 suggested; but both Labour and Conservative MPs urged me to stay on. One of the kindest letters of all came from Tory MP Iain Macleod, then Shadow Chancellor.

Shortly afterwards the Government Chief Whip, John Silkin, wrote to say he had felt at first that I had no alternative to resigning but had changed his mind after careful consideration. He said that he had been approached by a large number of MPs who felt I should stay. His view was important, for he was ideally placed to judge the mood and feelings of Members.

We looked forward to hearing more from Eric Ogden and Michael McGuire, though not without some apprehension. Every encounter was a strain for me, and I felt strangely diminished when meeting people I had known before I was deaf. Fortunately the obviously sincere goodwill of the two MPs carried us over the initial difficulties on arrival; they said everyone agreed that deafness was no insuperable problem to remaining in the Commons.

A few days later my Parliamentary colleagues from Stoke-on-Trent, John Forrester and Bob Cant, came to see us. They confirmed what we had already been told about opinion in the House, and added that local people in my constituency were also anxious for me to stay. This was a crucial consideration; it was obviously time to visit Stoke-on-Trent.

Before I did so, I heard from an old Cambridge friend, Peter Townsend, who had become one of Britain's most distinguished professors of sociology. He and his wife, Ruth, told me they felt strongly that I should remain in Parliament, and they put forward a reason which had not been advanced before. They said that in addition to my being able to help disabled people, it would benefit Parliament to have in its midst a disabled person with practical and personal experience of disability. Sir Ian Fraser, who had served for years as a blind MP, was mentioned as a notable example of this.

Peter's reputation as a pioneer of sociological studies made his opinion an influential one. He wrote to *The Times* and the *Sentinel*, saying that despite my disability I could still make an effective contribution in Parliament. His intervention was significant because it authoritatively contradicted the widely held belief that disabled people were fit only for a few simple, specialized jobs. He made people think again, and I warmly appreciated his initiative.

A few days later we made an anxious journey to Stoke-on-Trent. The tidal wave of goodwill was fine, but we were now to meet leaders of the constituency party to discuss my future, and I would be unable to hear a word they said. When we arrived, there was a

(154)

heading in the local paper: '"Jack must stay" Chorus Swells'. The story quoted Professor Townsend and others who felt as he did. After a friendly welcome from an informal group of party workers, we went into a small office to talk with Sir Albert Bennett.

He explained, slowly and clearly, that though the decision rested not with him but with the local party, he personally felt that I was capable of representing the constituency in the House of Commons, and that I had a duty to stay on. He was eloquent, forceful and, at the same time, gentle and understanding. Eventually, after a slow and lengthy discussion, I agreed that if the party wanted me to stay I would reconsider my decision to resign.

Next day the *Sentinel* carried a photograph of Pauline and me among party workers and a guarded comment from Sir Albert saying that a statement would be made later. In Parliament, and in my constituency party, the omens were promising. But I wondered how the public of Stoke-on-Trent would feel about being represented by a totally deaf MP. We went to see Bernard Sandall, one of the best-informed men on the *Sentinel*. A reserved and intelligent man, his judgement commanded tremendous respect in the Potteries. He affirmed that I would have the support of my constituents if I carried on, though I felt he was painfully aware of my dilemma.

As we drove back to London we began to realize that the minor miracle was now a distinct possibility. Pauline drove most of the way as I was still exhausted, but instead of sitting in silence as before she fixed a mirror to the windscreen so that I could see to lip-read her. Although she had to speak very slowly and clearly, we were beginning to stumble back towards some kind of normality. We felt confused but hopeful.

I was under no illusion about the difficulties if I was to return to the House. I sensed that the problem would be even more intractable and complicated than anyone could visualize. Even conversation with Pauline, the most patient and clear speaker, was a strain. There were many busy people in Parliament, some of whom spoke like machine-guns; would they have the time or make the effort to accommodate me? Would I be able to follow the debates adequately? Would it be possible to understand my constituents as they explained their problems? How great a physical and nervous strain would it be? Could I justify the confidence placed in me? Above all, could I make a really useful contribution and maintain my self-respect, or would I be there on sufferance and sympathy? These were some of the questions which worried me as we travelled back to London to await the outcome of this extraordinary situation.

A few days later I was invited to discuss the problem with the Prime Minister at the House of Commons, another of what was becoming a series of ordeals. As Pauline and I drove into New Palace Yard, I felt bewildered because it was only a few weeks since I had decided never to enter the Commons again as it would evoke too many thoughts of what might have been. Yet there I was – neither a visitor nor a normal Member, for I had given public notice of my impending resignation.

We were escorted to Harold Wilson's room by his Parliamentary Private Secretary, Harold Davies, the genial, rotund Member for Leek, the constituency adjoining mine. I knew that the Prime Minister would be aware of my problem because Davies had been present at the informal meeting in Stoke-on-Trent, though he stayed discreetly in the background.

My political future was the subject of the discussion, but what was fascinating was the way it was discussed. Harold Wilson behaved as if it were an ordinary conversation. Instead of addressing Pauline and talking through her, as so many people had already begun to do, he spoke directly to me. Because he was not embarrassed I felt relatively at ease, although I could not understand what he said. After each comment or question Pauline, who was quite unflustered, repeated his words for me, and the conversation went relatively smoothly. Urging me to stay in Parliament, he said he would be glad to help in any way he could. He was warm, friendly and encouraging. I thanked him and said I would stay if the constituency party wanted me to.

In the meantime I began to see some of the people whom I had asked about jobs. Many of them, like Sir Hugh Greene, the Director-General of the BBC, Cecil King, Chairman of the International Printing Corporation, and Lord Cooper, General Secretary of my union, the General and Municipal Workers, had replied immediately asking me to go and talk with them or their senior staff. I had also received kind, spontaneous letters from organizations like Political and Economic Planning and the National Institute of Economic and Social Research. At the BBC, Kenneth Lamb, the Secretary, said they were anxious to find me a job I could not only do efficiently but would also enjoy doing. We discussed various possibilities to be pursued when my personal situation had clarified.

Cecil King had suggested that I should see Edward Pickering, his executive director. As we walked into his office in the Daily Mirror Building he was just finishing a meeting with Hugh Cudlipp and one or two other people. We met them briefly, then discussed my prospects with Mr, later Sir Edward, Pickering. A quiet, friendly man, he said he would be glad to employ me in labour relations because of my experience in that field. I arranged a further meeting with him, but shortly afterwards Cecil King was deposed from the chairmanship of IPC and Hugh Cudlipp took over. I did not know if this would affect the offer made to me, but Edward Pickering assured me that it remained open. It was a helpful insurance policy if I had to leave the House.

When we went to see Lord Cooper at the union's head office in Claygate, Surrey, we were kept waiting in an outer office for half an hour. As the minutes ticked by, I felt more like a supplicant than an applicant. I wondered if he might be reluctant to discuss the problem – and I could understand that – but when at last the door was flung open he breezed in and greeted me warmly. The reason for the delay was a sudden strike he was trying to settle. Without hesitation he offered me a job as soon as he had discussed it with his colleagues. So the economic threat receded, though I was still worried about my future. I knew the job offers had been prompted by generosity, but that could not be the basis for long-term employment.

The continuing flow of letters and messages of support influenced me greatly, strengthening the possibility of my staying in Parliament. I was under no illusion about the magnitude of the task, but knowing I had Pauline's support, I finally decided to continue in Parliament if invited by the local party.

The answer was to be given at a special meeting on 20 May at the old Labour Hall in Stoke-on-Trent. When Sir Albert Bennett came to see us before the meeting, he was properly non-committal about the likely outcome, but we knew that he was in favour of my staying. He felt it was better if the party made their decision in my absence and of course he was right. Pauline and I arranged to wait in the Working Men's Club nearby in case I was wanted for questioning.

The meeting began at 7.30 p.m. I ordered a drink for Pauline and myself and settled down for an anxious wait. Within five minutes some delegates came from the meeting to tell us that a unanimous resolution had been passed inviting me to stay as their Member of Parliament. It was one of the rare happy moments I had known since going deaf.

Pauline and I joined the meeting and were greeted enthusiastically, even emotionally, as we entered. Grateful for their support, I made a short speech of acceptance, a wholly inadequate expression of my feelings. Ahead lay a challenging, even intimidating, task. My Parliamentary career, to which I seemed temperamentally suited, was one I loved, and I was delighted. Yet the nagging reservation remained – that I might not be capable of doing the job and I was also imposing an unbearable strain on myself, on top of the crushing burden of deafness and tinnitus. But I was determined to try, hoping that, from the despair of the past and the exhaustion of the present, a more promising future would emerge.

The BBC TV programme *Twenty-Four Hours* expressed interest when they heard about the special meeting at Stoke-on-Trent and they asked to interview me. Michael Barratt, one of their reporters, came with a camera crew to my home. We were old friends, having worked together in television, but when he arrived he was obviously apprehensive about how to conduct the interview. After the handshake and welcome he seemed nonplussed. 'How do I talk to you?' he asked. Pauline and I laughed at this discomfiture, but he took it in good part. I was relieved to notice from these opening words that he was not too difficult to lip-read. We discussed the general line of questions together before recording the interview in our living room.

I was able to follow the series of questions, and Michael seemed satisfied with the interview. He asked me how I would cope in Parliament and I responded, 'You can either retire within yourself or say, "Hell. I'll fight."' I was displaying more confidence than I actually felt, and I suspect my voice sounded a bit strangled. Some months later, after I had again appeared on television, one of my colleagues said that my voice was 'better than on the *Twenty-Four Hours* programme'.

The transmission of the interview coincided with an important vote in the House. I did not want to meet colleagues on that occasion, and although I was in the precincts to register my vote, I was excused from the lobbies. While other members voted, I sat in the Chief Whip's office with Pauline and watched the *Twenty-Four Hours* programme. An official from the Whips' Office, Freddie Warren, who also watched, seemed touched by my perversity in staying on. Normally a cheerful person, he said nevertheless, 'I felt like crying.'

So was I right to reject well-meaning advice to take a quiet job and have an easier life? Was I being perverse? I didn't know. I was fighting back, but there was nothing noble about that. It was an instinctive reaction, influenced by my upbringing and my nature, and by the knowledge that the alternative of surrender would have been even less palatable than the struggle.

Whatever the reason, I was now staying in Parliament, albeit without the golden promise and soaring hopes. The first stages of the battle had been so intense and all-consuming that there had been little opportunity to think far ahead; the rest was to unfold in the coming years. That night, Pauline and I were content, for we had endured a deeply traumatic experience together and begun to emerge from the shadows. Without her, it would not have been possible to get so far. Now, back in Parliament, I had to face a unique journey into uncharted territory.

11

Would It Work?

The sudden onset of a devastating disability had transformed me from a confident Member of Parliament with a promising future into a totally deaf politician struggling to maintain a tenuous foothold in the Commons. Would it work? Although most people were encouraging, I sensed that some were very doubtful. They probably thought it was hopeless but that there would be no harm in my hanging on until the next election. My aim was different. The last thing I wanted, or would accept, was a charitable extension of time. I was fighting for a Parliamentary career – nothing less.

The main challenge was at Westminster. Inevitably, the difficulties of a totally deaf person are multiplied if his occupation involves much speech. In Parliament, the spoken word is paramount, and even simple and straightforward actions, such as talking to colleagues, would be difficult. It was with trepidation that I returned. If I was not afraid I was extremely anxious. On the last occasion, clinging to the wisp of hearing like someone hanging on a cliff face by his fingertips, I had held on for only a day. This time I was enveloped in an inescapable shroud of silence.

Since losing my hearing, I had relied heavily upon Pauline, but now I was going alone to the House of Commons. Arrangements could possibly have been made for her to accompany me, but I did not want that, partly on account of our three young daughters at home, but also because I wanted to be as independent as possible in the Commons.

If this gamble failed I would be forced out of Parliament. I needed time to improve my lip-reading; but however great the improvement, I knew I would always require the understanding and co-operation of colleagues, busy people involved in controversial matters which did nothing for their patience. If I was to be an active MP, I must engage in these controversies which could be as emotionally charged between party colleagues as between political opponents. Could I hope for understanding while speaking as frankly and vigorously as I had in the past? Being mealy-mouthed would be out of character, and would do less than justice to the issues.

At least this time Members would be aware of my disability. They knew I was totally deaf and dependent on lip-reading – yet they had urged me to return. Not all had, of course, and I doubted whether any fully appreciated the enormity of the problems. Despite their letters of encouragement, I wondered if they would be shocked when confronted with someone requiring immense patience before being able to understand a limping dialogue, and whether I would be able to establish any semblance of ordinary relationships with colleagues and officials of the House.

Understanding debates was important, but other occasions, previously taken for granted, would now be difficult. To check a point made in debates I could always read Hansard, the official report, but there is of course no report of informal discussions in corridors, cafeterias, libraries and smoking rooms which are a crucial part of the Westminster network. These exchanges enable MPs to comprehend, and react to, shifts of policy, positions and power. From now on I would be excluded from these unless I made exceptional efforts. Even conversation over a meal would be difficult, partly because of inadequate lip-reading but also because to eat I had to glance at my plate; either I lost the tenuous thread of comprehension, or people would have to pause.

After a few more weeks of intensive lip-reading work, the time came to take up the challenge of my next return to the House. As I left, on 10 July 1968, Pauline and I smiled reassurance to each other. We had discussed every detail of the problems, but now I was on my own. I drove through uncannily silent traffic in a subdued mood, as if reserving my energies for what lay ahead; I felt like a spring coiled for action, without the faintest idea of what the action might be. As I walked through the Members' entrance I was approached by a policeman with a thick, bushy moustache. Normally he would be difficult to lip-read, but he said slowly and clearly, 'Welcome back, sir.' They were the first words spoken to me on my return and, because he made a special effort, I understood them.

In the Members' Lobby, I was surrounded by friends and well-wishers. I did not pretend to understand all they said, and no one launched into a detailed conversation. It was a unique atmosphere compounded of extraordinary warmth, a little bewilderment and the faintest suggestion of embarrassment. Everyone wanted to welcome me, yet no one knew how to say it other than in the simplest terms. I dallied for only a few moments before going into the Chamber.

There is no ideal seat for a lip-reader in the House of Commons. Long benches divided by a gangway face each other in the Chamber across a central aisle – the front benches above the gangway are for Ministers on one side and Opposition leaders on the other. Benches behind, and the front benches below the gangway, are for backbenchers. I thought my best position would be at the end of our front bench below the gangway; I could then pivot round and see both sides. The redoubtable Bessie Braddock, who had visited me in the Liverpool hospital, always sat there, but when I wrote to ask her about it she assured me there would be no problem.

When I walked in, it was Question Time. The front bench was full, so I stood undecided at the Bar of the House. Until a Member crosses this line near the end of the Chamber he is technically not in the House and unable, therefore, to take part in the proceedings. The usual fusillade of questions was being fired at Ministers, and I was anxious to avoid interrupting by trying to squeeze on to the crowded bench.

I was uncomfortably aware that many Members from both sides were beginning to look at me, but the moment Bessie Braddock spotted me she turned to the crowded bench and called 'Push up!' She gave them a friendly shove as she spoke, and as she weighed at least fifteen stone the effect was dramatic. A space was provided where she had been sitting a moment before. She patted it in welcome, and I thankfully slid into it, shielded to some extent by her massive frame from the full gaze of the House.

After a few moments I tried to lip-read. I had not expected to understand much, but the reality was chilling. I understood practically nothing. To add to my discomfort, I had no idea where to look. By the time I had swivelled round to locate a speaker he would be halfway through his question; a brief question would be finished before I could start to make any sense of it.

This did not seem like the Chamber where I had vigorously interrupted other speakers and impatiently waited my turn to speak. It was transformed into a mysterious, menacing arena where I could be trapped into misunderstanding the arguments and passions which swiftly ebbed and flowed. It would be all too easy to make a fool of myself; somehow I would have to make sense out of this silence. As I sat there uneasily I reflected on this daunting prospect.

I became conscious for the first time of the shifting patterns of light in the Chamber. The high windows above the Distinguished Strangers' Gallery caught and reflected the slightest change of sunlight on this fitfully cloudy day. As shadows flitted across the faces I was trying to lip-read, they made a difficult task nearly impossible. I thought they seemed symbolic of the sun setting on my political career.

Soon my spirits drooped and my eyes grew tired. I left the Chamber and went into the tea room. There, touched by warmth and friendship, I felt my depression lifting. Conversation was not easy but it was not impossible. Colleagues mainly inquired about my health, and if they had to repeat themselves they were ready to do so. The House of Commons is a remarkable institution; its Members are individually diverse but collectively they act in subtle unity. Crushing to anyone who offends their canons, they can sometimes lavish affection which is powerful and moving. I was the fortunate recipient of this immense goodwill at a time when I needed it most.

Later, at a meeting of the Parliamentary Labour Party, the main item on the agenda was a proposal to rebuke a group who had refused to accept a majority decision. I decided to see if valour was

(163)

the better part of discretion and I intervened in the debate. Although I grasped only a little of the opening speech, I used that fragment as a peg on which to hang a speech of my own. I regretted the group's action but supported a proposal that the issue be dropped. The speech was well received, but I knew that the applause was more in the nature of a welcome back. Douglas Houghton, the Chairman of the Parliamentary Labour Party, added generously to the welcome in a press statement: 'One must state amazement at Mr Ashley . . . entering into the debate.'

That evening I went home weary but cautiously optimistic. My welcome in the House had been encouraging, and Pauline typically focused on this in our discussions that night. Yet the problems ahead seemed to stretch to infinity. The strains since becoming deaf had exhausted me. My eyes were permanently shadowed, and the psychological pressure of my return was intense. Added to this, and the difficulties of lip-reading, was the perpetual roaring and shrieking of tinnitus. During the past few months I had not been able to keep up with fast-moving political events, but now I had returned I could not operate in a political vacuum. I had to begin reading and acquaint myself with current controversies. Although drained, I had to press on, pick up the threads, continue my constituency work, participate in the House of Commons and simultaneously try to improve my lip-reading.

I was invited to present a Ten-Minute-Rule Bill on disablement. These Bills enable backbenchers to present in ten minutes a case for changing the law, and although they are not allocated further Parliamentary time as Private Members' Bills are, and are not enacted, they enable an MP to focus attention on a subject. If it is a good issue, it can be taken up by MPs who are successful in the ballot for Private Members' Bills and then it stands a good chance of becoming law. This Bill proposed a commission to investigate the problems of disabled people. It had been prepared by David Owen, but he had just been appointed Minister for the Navy and, knowing of my interest in disability, he suggested that I should present it.

Delighted as I was with the opportunity, I was conscious of the hazards. Being totally deaf, I was unable to hear my own voice and it was sometimes difficult to control the volume. The tendency was to shout – perhaps a subconscious effort to hear what I was saying – and when I did so the modulation and pitch could go awry. But lowering my voice could make it inaudible. I could sometimes tell if I was speaking too loudly in conversation because people from beyond my own circle would look across. But I often couldn't tell when my voice was too quiet unless colleagues told me; and sometimes they just pretended to understand me.

These were my anxieties as I prepared the speech about disabled people. I had long taken an interest in their problems and now by an odd irony of fate I was one of them. The weekend before I was to present the Bill, there was a rally of disabled people in Trafalgar Square. Hundreds of people in wheelchairs or on stretchers made it a moving demonstration. Travelling from all parts of Britain, some of their journeys had been ordeals, with relations and friends having to wheel or carry them to the rally. Yet, in the bright sunshine of Trafalgar Square, the atmosphere was cheerful as they supported reasoned demands for a disability income.

I was struck by the spirited way they coped with their handicaps. Even simple actions, which most people take for granted, like drinking a cup of tea, required an elaborate and contorted performance from some of them. As I was leaving after the rally, I saw a paralysed old man on a stretcher being lifted by two friends into an old van. Helpless, he joked as they carried him. The plight of these people, so totally dependent on others, gave me a new perspective. I had been feeling anxious about my own performance in the House of Commons a day or two later, but it was clearly time to forget my problems and state an effective and persuasive case.

The day I was to present the Bill, 16 July 1968, I arranged to meet a colleague, Eric Ogden, Labour MP for Liverpool Derby West, in the empty Chamber before proceedings started at 2.30 p.m. He sat within my range of vision and we arranged and practised a series of unostentatious signals about my voice level. If it was satisfactory, he would sit still and upright with his hands on his lap. If I spoke too loudly, he would raise his hand to his face and rest his chin on it, whereas if my voice was too quiet he would lean forward

as if straining to listen. No one would notice these natural movements, but for this first speech in the Chamber I needed the guidance. When we had completed and rehearsed these arrangements I
waited with mounting anxiety for the summons to speak. Pauline
went to the visitors' gallery with two good friends, Jean and Peter
Thorpe, who had helped me to learn lip-reading.

The House was full for Prime Minister's Questions, but when
they ended, at precisely 3.30 p.m., the usual exodus did not take
place. MPs normally leave at this time if they have no interest in a
particular Ten-Minute-Rule Bill or have other engagements. But on
this occasion, as I rose to speak, nearly everyone remained in their
seats, including the Prime Minister and the Leader of the Opposition.

As the minutes ticked by I felt I was winning the House. I told
them of the Trafalgar Square demonstration and what it meant to
disabled people. The bleak, impersonal word 'disablement' was a
synonym for personal and family tragedy, and I explained the need
for assistance, pointing out that disabled people had no powerful
trade union or pressure group to fight for them. As I moved from
specific examples to the national problems and on to international
comparisons, I occasionally glanced at Eric Ogden. Hands in his
lap, he sat like a statue. Harold Wilson looked up at Pauline in the
gallery and smiled his approval at her. Well before the end I knew
that the House was with me and I lost my fears. As I sat down I
could sense the cheers although I could not hear them; then the
Speaker rose to ask for the names of the sponsors of the Bill, which
I read aloud before moving to the Bar of the House. From there, I
walked in the traditional manner through the Chamber to present
my Bill to the Speaker. On my way I passed the Prime Minister
sitting near the dispatch box. He touched my arm and I lip-read,
'Well done, Jack.'

Pauline and I went out into the sunshine on the terrace with our
friends. As we enjoyed a celebration drink, Members from all parties
crowded over, offering congratulations. In the excitement, I found it
difficult to lip-read, but it did not matter. I had returned to the
House of Commons without any hearing and my first speech in the

Chamber had been warmly accepted. It was a memorable day shared with Pauline, who had accompanied me through a tunnel of despair and helped me to emerge, and friends who had helped when needed. I noticed that the Thames no longer looked bleak and cold but seemed to reflect a new sparkle in the air.

The first major hurdle in my new Parliamentary career had been overcome, but others lay ahead. If I was to stay in Parliament, I had to keep the support of my constituency. Fortunately I found that deafness affected my work much less than I had feared. At my regular advice bureaux people were willing to speak clearly and some even came with explanatory notes. I could usually understand them by lip-reading, supplemented by glancing at Pauline's notes.

My local party was warm and understanding. Sir Albert Bennett, the dominant leader and chairman, was succeeded on his death in 1972 by Arthur Cholerton, who with his wife Ethel became close friends. After a working-class childhood similar to my own, he became a long-distance train driver. Like many intelligent working-class people, he found an outlet for his talents in local politics. Active on both the City and County Councils, he subsequently became Lord Mayor of the city, Chairman of the County Council and an effective campaigner for development throughout Stafford-shire. For me, he was a rock-like supportive figure. I was extremely fortunate in having him as my chairman from 1973 to 1990 apart from a brief interlude.

With Arthur as chairman, I was not pressed to attend meetings other than those that were essential. At those I did attend, I had very few problems, although at first people were reluctant to ask questions. This was soon overcome when they found I could follow them. I rarely missed a question or failed to answer immediately but, when this did happen, I would jocularly blame Pauline's writing for the delay. Once people laughed, the difficulties were over.

Pauline's signals at meetings became so subtle that they were imperceptible to others. An apparently natural inclination of her head indicated where I should look when a question was asked. When I had difficulty lip-reading I would glance at her writing pad and the words would be written for me. If I was concentrating on

(167)

lip-reading someone as she got to the end of a page, she would keep it in a convenient position until I acknowledged it. I also refined return signals. At first I would mutter to her; this developed into a nod; then a single blink meant I had read the note or did not need it. The notes and signals were invaluable aids which helped me to cope with total deafness.

However understanding my constituents were, I had to be able to fight for them as vigorously as any hearing MP if I was to justify my role. The first test came a few weeks after I lost my hearing. The Coal Board was rejecting many subsidence compensation claims made by people living in one small locality. Visiting their damaged homes, I met another problem imposed by deafness; I could follow their explanations until they turned to the cracked foundations or broken walls they were describing. Then, if I looked from their lips to where they were pointing, I lost touch with their train of thought. On the other hand, if I did not look where they pointed, they waited till I did and then they again spoke as they pointed. Nevertheless with Pauline's help I managed.

Subsidence was a serious problem in Stoke-on-Trent because the city was honeycombed with coal seams. On the estate I visited, I found some striking examples of damage. An 82-year-old widow had badly cracked walls, and her stairs were so seriously affected that when I put my foot on the staircase the whole thing moved. She was unable to get to her bedroom and had to sleep in her living room despite its cracked walls. It was the only moving staircase I had seen outside a fairground.

Nearby, a married couple lived in a relatively modern house in which every wall and ceiling was cracked. The gable end was so badly fractured that I could put my hand between this and the floor on which it was supposed to rest. It was reminiscent of my old home in Wellington Street.

Although the Coal Board had in the past carried out repairs, they were now denying further liability, claiming that the present damage was not due to subsidence. I got in touch with the chairman, Lord Robens. After much local publicity and many brisk exchanges, he agreed to my demand for an independent investigation; he even said that I could choose the independent investigator.

This was a happy outcome to a vigorous battle. Yet I was none too sanguine because I feared it might indicate not generosity by Lord Robens but his confidence in the Board's own case. I checked the reputations of mining engineers and chose Professor Potts of the Department of Mining Engineering at Newcastle upon Tyne University. Robens agreed.

Professor Potts made a careful study of the houses, land and mining plans while the homeowners and I waited expectantly. When his report was issued it was unequivocal; the damage was not caused by mining subsidence but had arisen because the houses were built on inadequately compacted 'fill'. To describe this, as I did at the time, as a harsh blow and a severe setback was an understatement. All I could salvage from the wreckage was the consolation that few other MPs could have fought harder or persuaded the Coal Board to go as far as they did in trying to prove their case.

People were usually appreciative of any help I could give, but there were exceptions. One angry old man wanted the bus stop outside his house moved. At my request, the City Council investigated his problem and calculated the cost of moving the stop and the trouble it would cause others; they decided against any action. When I told the irascible old man his retort was, 'Bloody fine MP you are. Can't even get a little bus stop moved.'

As the months passed, I was gradually compelled to acknowledge that the major problem of coping with deafness was in the House of Commons. Making contact with other Members proved to be remarkably difficult because an invisible, impenetrable barrier lay between us. They could feel all the goodwill in the world, but if they were unable to talk to me, I was left out in the cold. Conversations usually began agreeably but ended in confusion and sometimes embarrassment. Sometimes I was tempted to pretend that I had followed and nod acknowledgement, but this created a sense of mutual uncertainty, no better than a simple acknowledgement of my failure to understand. Occasionally they would jot notes for me but there was an obvious limit to that method of conversation. It was disconcerting to see such affection yet be unable to make meaningful contacts with the people who displayed it.

The problems I had foreseen became daily realities. After a few difficult encounters, many Members whom I had difficulty in lip-reading were still pleasantly disposed but they made no further attempt at conversation. This was partly to avoid embarrassing me but mainly because they themselves were embarrassed.

On one occasion in the tea room I took my cup of tea to a table to join four MPs. When one of them asked me a question which I could not understand, he and the others repeated it for me but I was still unable to follow. They paused while one of them wrote it down and I was aware that the easy-going conversation they had been enjoying before my arrival was now disrupted. When I answered the written question it was understandable that none of them should risk a repeat performance by asking another. Within a few minutes two of them left, and after a brief pause the others explained that they had to go because of pressing engagements. They were genuinely sorry and I understood, but it was small solace as I sat drinking my tea alone.

Human nature being what it is, even relationships with close friends were eroded by deafness. The first indication came when suggestions that we should have a drink, or dinner during the long evenings at the Commons, were no longer forthcoming. Some MPs shied away from formerly close contact. They smiled and nodded when passing me in the House – but the rapport had vanished. I missed it more than I cared to show.

The drastic change in my life was shown most vividly one evening as I sat alone at a table in the Commons library. David Owen passed by and returned a few moments later with David Marquand. As they approached I hoped they would ask me to join them for dinner as in the old days. They nodded, smiled affably and walked past. I turned to look at the retreating figures of my two friends, feeling unbearably isolated, and went to eat alone in the cafeteria.

The loneliness could not be eased simply by mixing in a crowd. During important votes I would walk slowly with other Members as they drifted through the packed lobbies, but few came to talk to me. People were aware of the inadequacy of my lip-reading and, as it was noisy, I had difficulty adjusting the level of my voice. Their attitude was understandable, but there can be no more demoralizing sense of isolation than to be alone in a crowd.

These experiences desolated me in the months after my return to the House. There were others which under normal circumstances I could have brushed aside as of no consequence. Some MPs, or their wives, amended their guest lists. Invitations to their homes for formal and informal lunches, dinners and parties become notably scarce. I consoled myself that the quality of friendships was more important than the quantity, but I was trying to rationalize.

Another reason for the isolation was that at first deafness pushed me out of the mainstream of politics. The lip-reading difficulties were compounded by my having less to talk about with my colleagues. There was little point in them asking me what I thought of a speech they knew I had not heard and they were probably reluctant to ask if I had lip-read it. This was in marked contrast to my experience before I was deaf. Then my judgement was respected, and although my views were not always accepted, they were often sought. Now I could only wait and try to improve my communication skills. The difficulty, if not impossibility, of doing this added to my frustration. No one in the House of Commons could understand sign language, so there was no point in learning it for Parliament. And as hearing aids were useless to me, I had to rely on the imprecise art of lip-reading.

The simplest jobs became difficult. If I went to ask a clerk about procedure for Motions, and could not understand him, he had to speak slowly and sometimes write out part of the explanation. Officials were invariably helpful, but I found these encounters embarrassing. Yet there was no escape if I was to resist the temptation to opt out.

A few minor problems were more easily solved than I anticipated. I had expected to miss important Divisions because of being unable to hear the bell, but this never happened. I could detect a surge of movement in any part of the Palace of Westminster. As soon as three or four Members moved briskly in the direction of the Division lobbies I would check the television monitors and confirm there was a Division. Very occasionally I would be reading or writing and fail to notice the movement. Colleagues working nearby would let me know, and Conservative Members smiled as they nudged me to go and vote against them.

Parliamentary questions posed particular problems, since a failure to lip-read replies could result in asking an inappropriate supplementary question. I arranged to receive from Ministers a draft of their initial answer, though this still meant I had to lip-read the reply to my supplementary. It was more difficult when I intervened in other Members' questions. If I missed the answer or following question I could easily misconstrue or be repetitious. I occasionally asked colleagues to make a note for me before I intervened, but this created as many difficulties as it solved. Question Time requires speedy reflexes, as a dozen Members may jump up the moment a Minister sits down. While I was reading a colleague's note of the Minister's reply, other MPs would be on their feet and the Speaker would have called one by the time I looked up. I had to choose between glancing at the notes and swift lip-reading; I generally chose the latter and hoped to manage.

The Speaker's attitude was important; my difficulties would have been immeasurably greater if he had been indifferent or lacked understanding. Speaker Horace King was a firm and sometimes impatient man who normally allowed no one to delay Parliamentary business. The first time I met him after my return was at a formal reception in his palatial apartments. I joined the queue to be received and when I reached him he dropped protocol and substituted for the formal handshake a warm and long embrace. He took great trouble to ease my way back, promising to let me know in advance whether I was to be called in debates, so that I could avoid the eye strain of sitting, watching and waiting from mid-afternoon until late at night.

I was fortunate also in having two supportive colleagues representing the other Stoke-on-Trent constituencies. Bob Cant, the ex-university lecturer, could hold his own in economic debate with the best in the House of Commons. John Forrester, the ex-teacher, always spoke with balanced common sense. With me they were very helpful, invariably taking the trouble to bring me into the conversation and explain anything I missed. John made notes at many meetings and on other occasions when it was needed. I was aware that making notes made it less easy for him to contribute, and I was fortunate that he was so willing to assist me as he did. Few other MPs were so generous.

Worst of all were those acquaintances who, although civil, showed by their demeanour that they wanted no part of the problem. They were always careful to keep their distance and they soon got the message from me that I would do the same. There were not many people like that, but they existed, and their attitude could be hurtful. Embarrassment could be overcome, but coldness never. No matter how politely people displayed this, they wanted to close the door, and my natural reaction was to keep it closed with pressure from both sides.

In sharp contrast was an MP who was unstinting in his kindness – Michael Stewart, who was now Foreign Secretary again. Despite the pressure of his office, soon after my disastrous first return to the Commons he invited Pauline and me down for the day to his official weekend residence at Dorneywood. When we arrived at this beautiful house, deep in the Buckinghamshire countryside, I wondered how deafness would affect our relationship. When I had been his Parliamentary Private Secretary he tolerated my exuberance, allowing me to run affairs at social functions while he talked to the guests. Despite the loss of some of my vitality, our conversation went well, with pauses for him to repeat only a few sentences that I found difficult. One of the most thoughtful men, he was sensitive, gentle and kind, wanting to help in any way possible. We had a rare rapport. He was, I think, rather amused at my rumbustiousness when I first became his PPS; and even on this occasion, rather sadder and quieter than our earlier meetings, my jocularity kept breaking through. Michael accepted it with good humour.

After lunch we went for a walk which developed into a procession, with Michael and me together, followed by Pauline and Michael's wife, Mary, and the personal detective trailing discreetly behind. I had to understand the conversation without prompting from Pauline. Walking and talking while lip-reading can obviously be hazardous.

When we stopped to clarify a sentence, the detective would pause about ten yards behind us; I wondered what he thought of the Foreign Secretary and his guest making slow, stumbling progress through the woods. It was an odd experience and it sadly reminded me of what I had lost, but I was encouraged by it. It helped to rebuild my flagging self-confidence.

I badly needed gestures of support and friendship because the shock of total deafness still reverberated daily and shook me every time I entered the House. Whenever I walked into the Chamber I was struck by the absolute silence of this noisy debating forum. I joined in as best I could, though for many months I felt that I was only on the periphery of Parliament.

The transformation in my life was still difficult to comprehend. Without Pauline it would have been impossible to carry on. She provided the practical help and the moral support that were so vital. Her invaluable notes, clarity of speech, unlimited patience in dealing with the difficulties, and practical assistance enabled me to cope. For example, television is largely meaningless to a totally deaf person except for purely visual programmes such as those featuring sport or wildlife. In those early days no programmes were subtitled, so Pauline took notes of the political ones to help me follow current affairs. On social occasions she would discreetly observe my conversations and if they were proving difficult – perhaps if someone had a beard or moustache, or spoke quickly – she appeared at my side, explaining the points I had missed. When Pauline was around, the problems of total deafness were never insuperable.

I had worried, for example, about the telephone. It was essential for busy, active MPs, and as I was totally deaf it seemed beyond my reach. But checking with the telephone authorities, she found that they could provide an ear-piece extension which enabled her to listen and repeat simultaneously the words of a caller; I lip-read her and answered accordingly. With practice, the system became near word perfect. With the help of Pauline and my secretary I have used the telephone without difficulty over the years, including doing many live national radio interviews.

Pauline's understanding, based on an appreciation of the brutal buffeting of deafness and tinnitus, meant a great deal. In addition, I was strengthened by the affection of our three daughters. Jackie and Jane were full of warmth and kindness. Aged fourteen and ten respectively, they appreciated the devastating effects of deafness and did all they could to help. They quickly learned to speak clearly and to help on any social occasion. As she was only two, Caroline was unaware of my deafness, but when she was a little older her delightful sense of humour caused total confusion until I discovered her game. She would say something I could not understand, so I would ask her to repeat it. Smilingly, she would do so and, if I still could not understand, she again repeated it, but to no avail. When this had happened a few times I called Jackie or Jane to interpret; they told me she was talking gobbledegook, and was greatly amused by my attempts to lip-read. We all shared her joke, but I quickly learned to keep a sharp eye open for repeat performances.

Caroline grew up with my deafness from early childhood and accepted it as natural. I learned that it was a mistake to try bluffing her, because when I failed to lip-read her and pretended to understand she would ask with impish innocence, 'What did I say?' It is not often one can learn from a child, but she taught me that it was dangerous pretending to understand because it could be exposed so easily.

Another sanctuary of love and generosity was Widnes, where I visited Mam and my sisters Helen, Mary and Margaret as often as I could. They were as affectionately anxious and helpful as it was possible to be, and I did my best to show them that I was coping, although not always successfully. The moment I entered Widnes I felt at home, and physical and mental pressures fell away. No doubt it was because Mam, my sisters and friends, and my roots were all there. The refreshment from these relationships in that industrial environment was better than I could get at the finest and most luxurious seaside resort.

It was predictable that the deaf organizations would contact me as a deaf MP, and an approach was not long in coming. Just a few weeks after my return to the House I was asked by Air Vice-Marshal Dickson, Chairman of the Royal National Institute for the Deaf, to give the opening address at their biennial conference to be held in October. The invitation posed an interesting question. Was I to begin campaigning for deaf people now that I was myself deaf, and would this be seen as special pleading? Although my first speech in Parliament had been on disability and I intended to continue pressing that, I was anxious not to be seen as pursuing a subject to help myself.

Rejecting the invitation, however, would be churlish. I thought that the best thing would be to try to help deaf people in much the same way as I would aim to help all others who were disabled.

The conference was in Edinburgh, and my most striking recollection of that fair city is of being driven to distraction by tinnitus. Pauline suggested that we should walk around the castle and shops, hoping no doubt that my mind would be diverted. However, the shrieking and roaring in my head dominated that stroll, as they have on so many occasions since.

In the Assembly Rooms, where the conference was held, there were hundreds of people, some with hearing aids, others intently watching the sign language interpreters standing on the platform, as well as doctors, audiologists and sociologists. It was a very different audience from Parliament and I felt no rapport with them until I rose to speak. Then the warmth of the reception showed how welcome I was. Their disability was often neglected and sometimes derided. They obviously hoped that I would be their champion and speak for them in Parliament. A substantial press corps awaited my speech, and I made a forceful and wide-ranging one. My anger at the public attitude to deaf people came through, and I attacked the discrimination they suffered. Explaining that there was no proper provision for rehabilitation centres or training lip-reading teachers, I said that if the blind were deprived of sticks and guide dogs, or the crippled denied crutches, there would be an outcry; but the deaf were denied the strong support of lip-reading.

I had some harsh words for those people who laughed at deaf people: 'Braying donkeys who mock the deaf should be treated by society for the asses that they are.' Attitudes were a major problem, and I suggested a planned and professional approach through the mass media to change the public mind; this should be an organized and sustained campaign. The audience responded generously, and the media coverage was extensive. At Edinburgh, I struck a small blow for deaf people and passed another landmark in my own rehabilitation.

It was reassuring to find that I could still campaign and be listened to despite my deafness. Now that Ministerial office was out of the question, I felt I could only achieve something worthwhile by campaigning in Parliament. I knew I needed a new role.

During the next Parliamentary year, 1968–9, I took up several issues. I pursued my interest in industrial relations by supporting Barbara Castle's controversial policy *In Place of Strife*. I called for a minimum wage to help low-paid workers. And I pressed constituency concerns such as the availability of flu vaccine.

But the many letters I received following my speech on disablement helped to determine my main interest. In Parliament I took up the concerns of these disabled people. The result was remarkable. I found that disability was for the disabled; MPs were not interested, and Ministers were disinclined to commit resources. They knew there was little political pressure to do so. The polite but consistent rejection made me even more determined to change the dismissive and complacent attitude.

All kinds of pressure groups are active in the House. MPs at or near the top of the ballot for Private Members' Bills are inundated with scores of pre-packed Bills, complete with briefs and even speeches, because they are allocated Parliamentary time, and a Bill chosen by them has a real chance of being enacted. Parliamentary interest in disability increased dramatically when Alf Morris, MP for Manchester Wythenshawe, won the ballot in November 1969. Members are tempted to take an easy, straightforward, already prepared Bill, but Alf Morris selected this then obscure subject. He was an MP whom I could lip-read without difficulty, and together we discussed the general lines of a comprehensive Bill to help disabled people. Beginning with a few notes on the back of an envelope, the Bill expanded rapidly as MPs from all parties suggested clauses on subjects which particularly interested them.

(177)

The battle for the Chronically Sick and Disabled Persons Bill turned out to be a lively one. MPs on the committee for the Bill became increasingly aware of the problems facing disabled people, and no one tried to make political capital. It soon became clear that disabled people were neglected, depressed by disability, oppressed by poverty and hidden behind closed doors. Small wonder that their desperate needs were largely ignored by local authorities; even their numbers could only be guessed at.

The most important provision of this Bill was to impose an obligation on local authorities to discover the disabled people living in their area. If the authorities had no information, they could neglect people with impunity; once disabled people were discovered, evasion would be difficult. The Bill was based on one of the first principles of politics: make it visible.

As the Bill passed through Parliament, my political reflexes returned. I argued, bulldozed and encouraged people so as to get the vital provisions. Throughout our private discussions, civil servants, understandably cautious about the imposition of expensive commitments on local authorities, kept trying to insert the phrase 'as far as is practicable'. Ministers parroted it in the Chamber and in committee. I knew it would create gaping loopholes which would undoubtedly be exploited by reactionary local authorities who had neglected disabled people. On financial grounds, they could argue that it was impracticable to build a new rehabilitation centre or even to provide a white stick for a blind man. Perhaps I was sometimes rather too aggressive about these points, but whenever the phrase was left in, and it was in some clauses, it was only after bitter opposition.

While working on the Bill, I found that my views were wanted again, and to get them people were willing to make the effort to communicate. But the familiar problems of deafness could never be totally brushed aside. At one stage we wanted the Government to acknowledge the mobility problems of haemophiliacs. The Secretary of State for Health, Dick Crossman, was procrastinating, and Alf Morris asked me if I would press the Prime Minister. It was my second meeting with Harold Wilson since I had become deaf. This time I was alone, and it was in striking contrast to the first when Pauline was present and everything went smoothly.

Wilson greeted me cordially as I entered. I said I would try to lip-read him, but if I couldn't could he make a note for me. He nodded and replied, but I could not understand him. I asked him to repeat, but he merely gestured as if to say, 'Don't worry', and wrote down a friendly comment. Thus encouraged, I told him of the special problems of haemophiliacs, explaining why we needed recognition of them as a group requiring special help. In response, he wrote another note. Halfway through the conversation – if it could be called that – I asked him to leave the notepaper alone and I would try to lip-read him. He said that what he was explaining was difficult to lip-read – which I lip-read! – and went on writing. He was motivated by kindness and consideration, but for me it was a depressing experience. He was unable to offer any assurances about helping haemophiliacs, although I heard later that he urged Ministers to try and help.

By coincidence I met his wife, Mary, a few days later at a reception. I was able to lip-read her relatively easily and I told her about my abortive attempt to talk with Harold. She was very understanding. When I met him some time afterwards for a further conversation he did not touch pencil or paper, speaking so clearly that I could understand him almost as well as I could his wife.

The final stages of the Bill were rushed through Parliament because of the imminence of a General Election; if it was called before enactment, the Bill would fall. The pressure of work was so great that I had little time to reflect on personal difficulties. The Bill became law on 29 May 1970, just before the dissolution of the House for the June General Election. It was an important Act creating many new rights for disabled people over a wide field and elevating the subject of disability in Parliament. My involvement, entailing more work than I had expected, pulled me out of the isolation of deafness. It was a psychological tonic which helped me to cope with a silent Parliament. I was at last certain that despite total deafness, and the cacophony of tinnitus, I could continue as an MP.

One of my greatest regrets was that Mam did not live to see the re-emergence of my political vitality. Despite being unwell for some years, she gave me tremendous encouragement and affection. On 25 July 1969, I had an unexpected, anxious telephone call from my sister, Mary, in Widnes. Mam was very ill, and Mary asked if I could go at once. The last time I had seen this wonderful, affectionate, gentle woman had been a few months earlier when she came to stay with us in Epsom. Her heart was already weak and she had difficulty walking any distance. At Euston Station it had been hard for her to walk from the ticket barrier to the train, so I went to collect a baggage truck on which I could pull her. She was rather embarrassed about this but accepted without demur, knowing that the alternative would be more painful effort. As soon as I received Mary's telephone call I rushed to start the drive to Widnes. A few minutes later, when I was about to leave, the telephone rang again. Mam had just died. I had no opportunity to say goodbye; a great, loving light of my life had suddenly been extinguished.

In the early months of 1970, there was much speculation about the date of the next General Election. Just as we had our own bookmaker in the Wellington Street of my Widnes boyhood, so at Westminster we had Ian Mikardo, the MP for Poplar, taking bets on the election date. There were over 600 well-informed tipsters in the House of Commons and their advice was supplemented by newspaper opinion. The only man who refused to comment was the Prime Minister, Harold Wilson, though it was obvious that his choice really lay between June and October. It turned out to be 18 June. As the election approached, there was no sign of any change in the warm support the constituency had given me when I lost my hearing. I wondered, nevertheless, if there were some who, although they had not wanted me to resign earlier and so cause a troublesome by-election, would perhaps feel I ought to be replaced at the General Election by a hearing person. My fears were misplaced. I was both encouraged and touched by the universal confidence shown in me, and I was unanimously adopted as the Parliamentary candidate.

Coping in Parliament was one thing, but how would I manage an

election campaign? I had more difficulty than I expected but it was
not due to deafness. My majority of 12,000 was comfortable –
providing the electors could vote – but Stoke-on-Trent came to a
virtual standstill for two weeks every year when thousands of families
deserted the city as all the factories, mines and schools closed down
for the Wakes Weeks holidays. Postal votes were not allowed to
holiday-makers. To make matters worse, many professional people,
generally regarded as Conservative supporters, took their holidays
later in the year. In 1970, the Wakes holiday fell in the last two
weeks of June, and polling day was 18 June. It was an unfortunate
coincidence.

My political opponents were a lively Tory schoolteacher, eager to
score political points, and a dour Communist bricklayer who was
less than formidable in debate. The days of well-attended public
meetings were already over; my job was to make personal contact
with the electorate and focus on issues of special interest to Stoke-
on-Trent. I aimed to visit every street in the constituency to meet
people, or address them through the loudspeaker. I thought that the
best tactics were to fight on the Labour Government's record, attack
the Conservative Party and ignore the Communists. As my opponents were unknown, I tried to give them the minimum of publicity.

During the campaign I met and talked to hundreds of people and
found they were mainly concerned about the cost of living. It was
obvious that the result would hinge on their interpretation of the
'bread-and-butter' issues. It was an enjoyable campaign with long,
sunny days and people giving us a good-humoured, lively welcome.
The local children added to the gaiety and excitement of the electioneering.

However, on the Saturday before polling day, Pauline and I drove
round the city and our spirits sagged. The Wakes Week holiday had
begun, and the place seemed deserted. Who was listening to my
carefully prepared political comments or reading the elaborate
manifestos in a city from which life appeared to have fled?

It was hard to calculate how many people were at home, and
there were many different views. Someone suggested counting the
houses with windows closed, because women who were shopping

(181)

would leave bedroom windows open on a hot day, whereas those on holiday would have locked them. This method showed that over 60 per cent of people in my strongest area had gone away. It was not encouraging.

On Thursday, polling day, Jackie, Jane and my sister Mary joined the party members who were working exceptionally vigorously because no one knew how close the votes would be. At 9.30 p.m., after touring the polling booths, my agent estimated that there was a 50 per cent poll – on our calculation this meant I had won. Nevertheless we kept at it until the polls closed at 10 p.m., before joining a group of helpers for a cautiously optimistic drink.

Before the count, the family went to our bungalow for baths and a quick meal. Although tired, we were in good spirits which were not affected by the radio news, just before we left. The first result showed a swing against Labour, but we assumed this was a freak and set off cheerfully for the count. There we found an astonishing scene. In the Town Hall, where the votes of all three Stoke-on-Trent constituencies were being counted, crowds of people milled around excitedly; but the local results were a side-show. Everyone was shouting about the national news coming over portable radios. Conservatives were celebrating, yelling the latest results to their friends, while our supporters were despondent. We were dumbfounded to learn that the Labour Government was tumbling to a disastrous defeat. It took the edge off my personal victory in Stoke-on-Trent South. My family and I had to be content that I had become the first totally deaf person to be elected to any legislature in the world – an achievement that had seemed unattainable just two years earlier.

Next day BBC television invited me to go to Birmingham to appear on their special election programme. There I sat in the same chair as a despondent Edward Heath had done a few days earlier. Now he was Prime Minister. My old friend Robin Day interviewed me and he gave me prior notice of the questions in case I had difficulty lip-reading him on the screen. They were mainly about my own campaign and the way I had handled the problems of deafness. On the air he made no attempt to obscure the difficulties he was expecting. He told viewers he intended to signal the number of each question to me and he did so, jabbing the air with his fingers. No danger of misunderstanding there!

When Parliament reassembled after the election, we knew, of course, that we would be occupying the Opposition benches while our opponents sat on what we had come to regard as 'our' side – the Government side. We had to accept it, but it was with a sense of unreality that we saw Edward Heath at the Prime Minister's dispatch box, accompanied by his newly appointed Cabinet and supported by jubilant backbenchers. They would make the decisions now; we could merely question and criticize. Only then did I appreciate the famous comment by Sir Hartley Shawcross from the Labour benches after the 1945 landslide victory: 'We are the masters now.' No doubt the thought was in the minds of our opponents. As for us, we had to pretend stoically that this was all part and parcel of a politician's life.

On 29 June 1970, the first business of the new House of Commons was to appoint a Speaker. The longest-serving Member on the Government benches, the 'Father of the House', Robin Turton, spoke for his side and I was chosen to represent the Opposition. It was a rare honour, and I recognized that it indicated my full accept-ance by the House of Commons. The atmosphere was unusual, since there was no Speaker in the chair to control a packed House. In accordance with tradition, the Chief Clerk stood and pointed to the Member selected to speak to the Motion. In a graceful speech, Robin Turton proposed the re-election of Dr Horace King.

When my turn came, I spoke of the character of Dr King and the combination of strength and humanity he had displayed in office. But there was also a political message I wanted to convey, because I was sure that immigration and the Irish question would become important topics in this new Parliament. I warned that if the witches' brew of racial hatred or religious bigotry was poured into the political cauldron the House could explode with feeling which could rock it to its foundations. There were formal congratulations from Tory Ministers and some warm compliments from backbenchers on both sides, but the comment I valued most came from Norman Shrapnel, the Parliamentary sketch-writer of the *Guardian*, who said it was an unusually meaningful speech for such a formal occasion.

The next few weeks were a period of readjustment for both sides of the House. It must have been particularly traumatic for Harold Wilson, the more so because it was unexpected. One moment he had all the Government resources at his disposal, the next he was practically on his own. I saw an example of this one night when I left the Members' entrance to drive home. No longer chauffeured in his official car, he was standing in a queue waiting for a taxi. I would have been delighted to help, especially as he was so considerate to others, but it seemed presumptuous to offer a lift to the man who had been Prime Minister a week before.

It was now part of my job to attack the Conservative Government, but I was faced with a unique difficulty. When the Labour Government had been in office, Ministers did what they could to meet my demands although they were naturally restricted by shortage of funds. But a Tory Government would have different, and sometimes opposing, priorities. To succeed in campaigning I knew I had to hit hard and ignore the consideration given to me because of deafness. The dilemma was underlined by a Labour MP after I had attacked Edward Heath during Question Time. Shaking his head, he said that if I persisted the Government might withdraw its co-operation. The real issue was more subtle than that because the Government was offering me no co-operation, merely the courtesy of Ministers speaking clearly when they addressed me. What my colleague had in mind, consciously or subconsciously, was that, as a disabled person, I should keep my place and not get above it by attacking the Prime Minister. It was a revealing comment, unthinkingly illuminating an attitude often taken by the general public towards disabled people as a whole, and deaf people in particular.

The last thing I wanted was to be all things to all men because I was coping with a disability – I expected, indeed preferred, to attack and be attacked, although I required consideration for my need to lip-read. Edward Heath got the balance exactly right. When I criticized him, he answered just as strongly, but looked straight at me and spoke clearly. His attitude was increasingly typical of many

Members in the House. At first, they must have been discomfited at my presence, but my disability was steadily and quietly accepted. While I was grappling with coming to terms with deafness, the House of Commons unostentatiously came to terms with me.

12

Thalidomide

On 24 September 1972, the *Sunday Times* ran a dramatic front-page headline: 'Our Thalidomide Children: A Cause for National Shame'. Beneath this emotional lead was a cool analysis of the plight of 450 children born in the early 1960s with dreadful deformities. After ten weary years the families were still struggling for adequate compensation from the mighty whisky company, Distillers, which had ventured into pharmaceuticals. The moment I finished reading I decided to help.

Thalidomide, a sedative, had been blamed for the deformities as early as 1961. Mothers who had taken it early in pregnancy gave birth to children with no arms, no legs, flippers instead of either, or limbless trunks. Others were deaf, blind, autistic or brain-damaged or had internal injuries. Worst of all were those with a combination of disabilities. One child, for example, was brain-damaged, deaf, dumb and visually impaired in one eye, had one hand without a thumb and the other with an extra finger, a large hole in his palate, one ear missing, the other deformed and his face paralysed down one side.

Thalidomide, advertised as completely safe for pregnant women, was alleged to have produced these appalling results. But little publicity followed because some parents issued writs in August 1962 and the case became *sub judice*. Despite the children's plight, and the anguish of their parents, virtually no progress was made throughout the decade as opposing lawyers wrangled about compensation.

At the first sign of public protest, when the *Daily Mail* boldly published three articles about thalidomide in December 1971, the Attorney-General, Sir Peter Rawlinson, warned of contempt of court, and the paper had to cease publication. Televised interviews with parents, planned by the BBC, were withdrawn when Distillers threatened legal action.

Thus Distillers and the Attorney-General, the twin warders of silence, were able to hide the scandal in the legal shadows for a decade. Fear of prosecution prevented publicity until Harold Evans, editor of the *Sunday Times*, forced his way through. Evans knew the risks but was determined to take them. That decision, and the assiduous work of his team of journalists, led to the shock headline and detailed story on 24 September 1972.

I telephoned Evans after reading the article, and we agreed to meet at his office the following Tuesday. When Pauline and I arrived, he had assembled his full team to answer questions and provide information. They included Philip Knightley, who had worked on the project for over three years; Bruce Page, head of the special projects unit; and Elaine Potter and Marjorie Wallace, two of their most experienced journalists.

I wanted to check the authenticity of their case, so I pressed them as a devil's advocate. Where was the evidence that thalidomide was the cause? How had the company been negligent? Why was the *Sunday Times* apparently flouting the law of contempt? Were they being wise after the event? Why had they decided to publish now? What discussions had taken place with the families? How about the reactions of Distillers? How valid was Distillers' defence? What were their proposed next steps? What sums did they have in mind?

Evans and his team fielded these and many more questions, painstakingly, patiently and in detail. I was told that the beleaguered families were being fobbed off with staggeringly inadequate compensation. After years of argument, sixty-two families had reluctantly agreed in 1968 to accept only 40 per cent of a hypothetical court award. They did so on the advice of their lawyers who believed they had a less than fifty-fifty chance of a successful court action because of the difficulty of proving negligence by Distillers.

No figure could be put on the 40 per cent award until the amount, resulting from a hypothetical victory, was known. To decide this, Mr Justice Hinchcliffe adjudicated on two representative cases. For each one, he had to decide the effect of the disabilities on a lifetime's earnings, the cost of special care and appropriate compensation for suffering.

Actuaries use sophisticated statistical techniques on behalf of insurance companies to assess likely life-span and appropriate pensions. The children's lawyer argued, reasonably enough, that actuarial evidence should be considered and allowance should be made for inflation. Opposing this, Distillers' lawyers claimed that actuarial evidence was for average cases, not for two specific individuals. Even more remarkably they claimed that inflation should be disregarded on the grounds that the Government had undertaken to control it, so that to allow for its effects would be to ignore Government policy. They also said that it was not legal custom to take note of inflation.

These arguments impressed the judge. Rejecting actuarial evidence and making no allowance for inflation, he decided that just £24,000 would be appropriate to cover loss of income and a lifetime of special care for a totally limbless boy. This compared with an actuarial calculation of £106,000. John Prevett, the actuary, estimated that £24,000 would last the limbless boy until he was only twenty-seven – and only 40 per cent of this amount, a mere £9,600, was to be paid. In addition, the judge decided that £28,000 was appropriate to compensate for pain, suffering and loss of amenities of life, and once again only 40 per cent was to be paid. The other child, a boy with missing arms, received 40 per cent of just £14,000 and £18,000 – minuscule amounts for major disabilities. The adjudication dispensed a curious kind of justice.

The 1968 settlement of £1 million for sixty-two families abysmally failed to meet their requirements. So it was not surprising that Evans and his team were disturbed to find that a further settlement of approximately half of that was being offered to the remaining 389 families who had sued later. Following secret negotiations, Distillers were proposing to establish a trust fund of £3.25 million spread over ten years. The families were warned that if any information leaked to the newspapers, or if any family refused to sign, the deal was off. Prevett, the actuary, estimated that a fair and realistic settlement for the second group of 389 families would be £20 million rather than £3.25 million.

At the end of the discussion with Evans and his team, I promised to raise the issue in Parliament and do what I could to help, although I was under no illusion about the difficulties. The Speaker would not allow discussion of any matter that was *sub judice*. Quite correctly, evidence on legal matters had to be weighed in the law courts not in the Chamber of the House of Commons. So my attack had to be carefully angled.

At the beginning of a Parliamentary campaign I would normally seek action first from the Minister concerned, in this case Sir Keith Joseph, Secretary of State for Social Services. But special cases require special measures, and I wrote directly to the Prime Minister. Edward Heath would have to consult with Joseph, but even if this led to a negative reply, my letter and Heath's response would generate helpful publicity.

I suggested that Heath should ask Joseph to convene and chair a conference between the children's parents and Distillers, so that the Government could assess the problems and allay widespread fears that the children were being left in a legal quagmire. I told him that the need was urgent.

My representations heartened the *Sunday Times*, whose dramatic story had been almost ignored by the rest of the media. I was the only Member of Parliament who had contacted them. Harold Evans commented later in his book *Good Times, Bad Times*: 'The first noticeable sequel to the launch of our campaign was the silence. Apart from a BBC radio interview with me ... every newspaper and television news programme ignored it ... There was still not a line in any other newspaper and nothing on television; there were no more radio invitations. It was demoralizing.'

Presumably in the hope of demoralizing him further, Distillers immediately complained about the *Sunday Times* article to the Attorney-General, who warned Evans of contempt. Evans nevertheless published a second powerful article the next Sunday. It was a high-risk strategy, and with a heavy immediate cost for the paper. Distillers were their largest single advertisers, spending £600,000 per annum before the campaign began, and nothing from the moment it started. Had Evans wavered because of the risk and the cost, the thalidomide tragedy would probably have been hidden in legal thickets for ever.

The first stirring of interest in the rest of the media came two weeks later when, on 8 October, I was asked to discuss thalidomide in a television programme, *Weekend World*. There I met David Mason, the father of a thalidomide child. Knowledgeable and amiable, he did not strike me as a tough campaigner; I could not have been more wrong. His daughter, Louise, had been born with no arms or legs. It had been his rejection of Distillers' meagre offer of £3.25 million to the second group of families that alerted the *Sunday Times*. Because of his rejection, he and five other families had been taken to a court which transferred their parental right to decide for their children to the Treasury solicitor. This outrageous decision was overturned on appeal by Lord Denning. Mason fought Distillers throughout the whole campaign with ferocity and relentless aggression. Determined to reject unreasonable offers, he played an outstanding role, and his persistent challenges and frequent television appearances were crucial.

Soon afterwards, *Weekend World* was in court for contempt, and proceedings were also taken against the *Sunday Times*. The Attorney-General had issued a warning after the first articles but he now told Evans that Distillers must see further articles before publication. This was like inviting one man to show another the size of his knuckleduster before a fight. Inevitably, when they saw the draft of the next article, Distillers cried 'foul'. The Attorney-General brought an action against the *Sunday Times*, and three senior judges banned the proposed next article.

Despite Evans's efforts, the gag was on again, even more securely than before. A specific ruling by the Lord Chief Justice and two senior colleagues put any further public comment out of the question. The *Sunday Times* could continue descriptive reporting but it was prohibited from attacking Distillers. I began to understand how Distillers had so effectively silenced the media for so long.

The media gag meant that a Parliamentary campaign was crucial. If I could attack Distillers in the House of Commons, the media would be free to report because Parliamentary comment is 'privileged'. Neither I nor those who reported my Parliamentary speeches could be sued. But I still had to contend with the Speaker of the Commons, who would not allow comment or debate on an issue which was *sub judice*.

As I expected, the Prime Minister's reply to me was negative. He and Keith Joseph were 'deeply sympathetic' – the deadly phrase so often a prelude to a dismissal – but he rejected the idea of a special conference because 'it would interfere with the legal process'.

Heath claimed that my letter did not give sufficient credit to the work his Government had put in hand on compensation and damages. This was merely a committee on safety and health at work. He seemed to fear that I would make party political capital out of thalidomide children. I had no intention of doing that. As Chairman of the Parliamentary All-Party Disablement Group, I was careful to invite the support of Tory MPs. The Secretary, Tory MP John Astor, lent his support throughout, aided by his Parliamentary colleagues, notably Dr Gerard Vaughan and Dr Tom Stuttaford.

A wild campaign would have alienated these MPs, whereas a mild one would have had not the slightest effect. A dexterous balance between hitting the company hard and winning widespread Parliamentary support was required. My next step was to table an Early Day Motion (EDM). This is a Parliamentary device for expressing opinion; it appears on the Order Paper, and can be signed by supporting MPs. If Parliamentary support is extensive, a debate can sometimes follow. My thalidomide EDM criticized the settlement proposed by Distillers and demanded adequate compensation for the children.

I handed the text to the clerks at the Table Office, hoping for the best but fearing the worst. As they read and re-read it, my fears were realized. They ruled that it was unacceptable to attack Distillers and demand compensation because the case was *sub judice*. My Motion was out of order.

The clerks in the Table Office are invariably helpful and sometimes suggest ways of amending Parliamentary Questions or Motions to put them in order. This time there were no offers. They could see no way of amending my Motion to permit it to go on the Order Paper.

Although the natural response would have been to go immediately to see the Speaker, the final adjudicator, I calculated that he would simply endorse the views of his experts. So I decided to kick up a public fuss in the Chamber to win support, and then go and see him.

It is rare to get a ruling of the Table Office changed, but there were three advantages in this approach. It would indicate a strong challenge to the ruling, and the Speaker himself would be obliged to consider the Motion; it would attract the attention and perhaps the support of other MPs; and it would enable me to make a strong attack on Distillers.

Next day, on a point of order, I asked the Speaker to reconsider the ruling on my EDM. In the well-attended Chamber I told him that it 'called for moral justice', that this was not a question of law and therefore could not be *sub judice*. Moral justice was a subjective concept beyond the jurisdiction of the most knowledgeable lawyer. I also urged him to allow the House to condemn the 'contemptible' offer by Distillers. The Speaker promised to consider my submission and rule upon it the following day. I was in with a fighting chance.

It was thanks to Harold Evans that I emphasized the moral aspect. Just before speaking in the House I had telephoned him. He told me that the Attorney-General had accepted the *Sunday Times* article of 24 September and he had accepted that there was a distinction between a moral and a legal argument.

I asked to see the Speaker personally the following day before he made his ruling, knowing that all was lost if he supported his officials. Selwyn Lloyd was perhaps best known as Foreign Secretary at the time of Suez, although he had held other Ministerial offices. He was depicted by cartoonists as a reactionary Tory with flared nostrils and bumbling arrogance. But when I went to see him on 20 October in the Speaker's rooms I found him considerate and concise.

He began by reiterating the difficulties about the *sub judice* rule, and defended his officials. He also expressed concern about my condemnation of Distillers. This was no surprise; my request for him to accept this was more in the nature of a negotiating ploy. I was willing to surrender the condemnation, which I had in any case already expressed in the House, but anxious to retain the basic message of the original – that Distillers had a responsibility for adequate compensation.

To get the Speaker's approval, I focused on the moral issue, amending the Motion to read: 'That this House, deeply disturbed about the plight of thalidomide children, calls upon Distillers (Biochemicals) Ltd, in dealing with these cases, to face up to their moral responsibilities.' Soon I was to add proposals that the Government should amend the law of damages to take account of actuarial considerations and set up a state insurance scheme to compensate for personal injury. But that was for the future. The vital need then was to get the Speaker's approval for the Motion as amended.

There was no rhetoric in our discussion; it was a quiet, constructive exchange in which we seemed to be trying to help each other. It ended as he looked at me sternly and said, 'Right, I'll accept your amended Motion. I can't comment either way on it but . . .' Then he smiled with an outstretched hand. Our warm handshake sealed a crucial advance in the campaign.

I was delighted. I now had a base in Parliament for an attack to outflank Distillers' legal defence. Thalidomide was firmly placed on the Parliamentary agenda. I immediately sought signatures from MPs of all parties, and there was virtually no resistance. It was like plucking ripe blackberries. Within a few days I got 266 signatures, an extremely powerful expression of widespread Parliamentary support.

This level of support from all sides of the House, and particularly from Tory MPs, must have disturbed Heath and Joseph; 266 signatures left no room for doubt. Over 100 signatures on a Motion is usually regarded as significant. Meanwhile, a Labour MP, Ray Carter, was successful in the annual ballot for Private Members' Bills, and he used his invaluable Parliamentary time to introduce a

Bill redefining the legal liabilities of drug companies. No one had any doubts about which particular company stimulated his interest. Another MP, Lewis Carter-Jones, introduced a Bill to speed up research and development for thalidomide children.

As I had expected, the Speaker's acceptance of the Motion was a crucial breakthrough. The general media, silenced by Distillers' fierce legal threats, could now freely report my increasingly strong attacks on the company. As interest grew, so did the media's confidence.

This change was steady but by no means complete. Arriving at the BBC Television Centre where I was to be interviewed about the Motion, I was told that the item was cancelled on the instructions of BBC lawyers. I demanded a word with them, knowing from my experience in television that they were cautious but amenable to argument. After a forceful, lively discussion, I persuaded them that as my Motion was subject to Parliamentary privilege, I could legitimately explain it and comment in a current affairs programme.

I took every opportunity to attack Distillers and challenge the Prime Minister. Pauline drafted numerous Parliamentary Questions demanding information on every related aspect we could think of; these continuously harassed him. At one stage, when he insisted that he would not intervene or set up a special fund, I responded that I was sick of expressions of sympathy, and the London *Evening Standard* led with a front-page headline 'Thalidomide: Heath's Letter "Sickens" MP'. It was reported, accurately as it turned out, that Heath was furious at this comment and the coverage it received.

A few days after this headline, I told Heath in the House that if he waited for the 'crafty lawyers of Distillers' to end their work, the matter might drag on for another ten years. He revealed his anger but expressed it in his usual polite and restrained terms: 'I cannot accept the Honourable Gentleman's view. I am sorry he has made comments in such an extreme form about the letter which I wrote to him.' The shafts were getting home, and I was delighted when Harold Wilson drove in a vital one of his own. He told Heath that he had studied his letter to me and that the Opposition intended to table an official Motion on the lines of my Early Day Motion – he wanted an early debate. We were on our way.

The pace was becoming frantic, and Pauline and I began to feel that thalidomide was taking over our lives. After eight weeks of continuous campaigning, we were talking about it non-stop every day, planning our moves and attending meetings with colleagues. Hundreds of letters poured in: some from anguished parents; others from the general public expressing support. Together we spent weary and exhausting hours on the telephone.

In 1972, MPs received only up to £1,000 for secretarial help. Pauline's research work was unpaid, and we could afford only minimal extra provision. My secretary typed my dictated letters in her own home, coming to my study only for filing, so it was left to Pauline to research and help with all the telephone calls in addition to her other responsibilities. Our youngest daughter, Caroline, was only six at the time. My study was upstairs; constant telephone calls meant that Pauline had to go up and down the stairs continually. Our fragile system of coping with deafness was bordering on collapse, so we turned the dining room into the study and installed extra telephones in every room. This gave Pauline more time and energy to help with the campaign. With her logical mind, she helped me to clarify issues and keep a clear line of argument in public.

The *Sunday Times* continued its comprehensive coverage, reporting human stories of thalidomide victims every week, detailing their injuries and explaining the struggles of the families. Patrick Pope had one kidney, no control of his bowels, thumbs without muscles, an abnormal penis and defective sight. He had endured forty-two operations by the time he was ten years old. In a letter published in the *Sunday Times* his mother explained that she did all the nursing for him at home before and after the operations. The strain must have been phenomenal. Pat Luce had an exceptionally difficult birth because of her limbless daughter's splayed-out feet. The *Sunday Times* referred to the agony suffered by parents having to steel themselves to the stares and comments of strangers. Anne Luce was accepted at school only if her mother also went to carry her around and care for her personal needs. Under the emotional, physical and financial strain, the Luce marriage collapsed, and Mrs Luce was admitted to hospital with mental strain and partial paralysis.

The *Sunday Times* did not place legal blame on Distillers for ruining people's lives, but the moral point was made in every article. It was a delicate, skilful balancing act, for who is to define the point at which publicity or moral questions will not affect juries deciding legal issues? Judging from the reaction, public opinion was moving strongly in our favour. How would Distillers react?

The All-Party Disablement Group invited the company to come and discuss compensation. But the chairman, Sir Alexander McDonald, refused. Distillers were remaining silent; it did not mean they were inactive. Not content with dragging the *Sunday Times* before the courts, they told one of their shareholders that in view of the continuing campaign by that newspaper they would consider ending negotiations with the parents and take a 'stand on the legal issues'.

This was a threat to withdraw the miserable offer of £3.25 million and an attempt to reinforce the gag on the *Sunday Times*; it required a strong counter-attack. In the House of Commons I sought an emergency debate on Distillers' action, which, I said, was a threat to parents seeking to protect their children. I made the emotional claim that 'For them, the Sword of Damocles has been replaced by the jagged edge of a broken whisky bottle.' The Speaker intoned his traditional rejection of my application, but the objective had been achieved. Harold Evans described it as 'rich stuff', and it was duly reported by the press. Although Distillers made no public response, nothing more was heard of their threat.

In the fog of war, military men may not know the strength of the enemy nor how a battle is progressing. They have to guess as much as calculate. I felt much the same at this stage of the campaign. Distillers, if anything, seemed more aggressive with legal threats than before. Yet their failure to pursue the threat of withdrawing the £3.25 million offer was a clue. Were they bluffing? Perhaps they were not as sure of their ground now as they appeared. I decided to try another public attack on them.

On 16 November 1972, I secured an Adjournment debate. These

are thirty-minute debates, which take place at the end of the day's business. They enable a backbencher to make a case, and a Minister is required to respond. Apart from helping to maintain momentum, the Adjournment debate could lead to a full-scale debate, which would transform the campaign. This was my first opportunity to speak at some length on the issue, and I made the most of it. I vigorously condemned Distillers for their outrageous advertising claim that thalidomide 'can be given with complete safety, and no adverse effect on mother or child', and for their subsequent attempts to gag Parliament, the press and television.

Labour MPs unanimously supported me, but it was Harold Wilson who gave most practical help. He had kept in touch with me informally, and it was no surprise when he called a special meeting in his room at the House to discuss the full-scale debate on thalidomide. This was to come out of the limited amount of Parliamentary time controlled by the Opposition, something I particularly appreciated. It was in marked contrast to the stony attitude of Heath. To this meeting Wilson invited Harold Evans, Sir Elwyn Jones, Labour's legal spokesman, Alf Morris, the Shadow Minister for the Disabled, and myself. They approved a Motion I had drafted, based upon the original one which had caused such a furore at the beginning of the campaign. Wilson invited me to open the debate from the front bench.

This was a unique honour, because traditionally only Ministers or Shadow Ministers speak from the front bench; all other MPs speak from the back benches. Wilson asked me to keep it brief because many MPs were anxious to speak. I aimed at ten minutes. By now I could have spoken for hours about thalidomide children but, after talking with Pauline, I decided on the main points to make. The challenge was to find the words that would illuminate and do justice to the children's remarkable plight.

Just before the debate, Distillers made their first gesture since the campaign began, increasing their offer from £3.25 million to £5 million. But they had fallen into the oldest negotiating trap in the world, offering too little too late.

It was a crowded House on 28 November 1972 when I rose to

speak at the dispatch box. Because of my deafness, I knew that other MPs would be uncertain whether to intervene because I might not be able to follow interruptions or questions. Pauline and I had agreed from the beginning that I should and could manage in the Chamber without her assistance even though at that time I had to rely solely on lip-reading.

Anxious that MPs should not feel inhibited from criticizing me if they wished, I had arranged for Alf Morris to write a quick note if there were any interruptions. Opening my speech, and asking to be forgiven a personal note, I said it was important for MPs to feel free to intervene. I would try to lip-read them but, if I couldn't, I would get a note from a colleague which would take about five seconds – a small price to pay for the cut-and-thrust of debate.

This was well received by both sides, which encouraged me as I tried to put the debate in context. I told the House:

> We are debating a great national tragedy, none the less poignant because it happened ten years ago. This is one tragedy in which the passage of time instead of healing the suffering actually heightens it, for children who were robbed of the magic of their childhood by a man-made disaster are now approaching the highly sensitive and emotional years of adolescence without arms, without legs, and in some cases without organs.

The House was silent and thoughtful. Harold Wilson sat at my side, the Prime Minister and Sir Keith Joseph opposite. Pauline was in the public gallery and Harold Evans in the press gallery. Then I described the youngsters' plight in words which were carried on all the television and radio bulletins that night, and on the front pages of most newspapers the following day:

> Adolescence is a time for living and laughing, for learning and loving. But what kind of an adolescence will a ten-year-old boy look forward to when he has no arms, no legs, one eye, no pelvic girdle and is only two feet tall? That is the height of two whisky bottles placed one on top of the other. How can an

eleven-year-old girl look forward to laughing and loving when she has no hand to be held and no legs to dance on?

It was not enough, however, to describe the ordeal of the children in emotive terms. The company which had fought them for a decade, using every possible manoeuvre to avoid paying compensation, had to be attacked with at least the same toughness as they had shown to thalidomide children: 'We are witnessing not only a shabby spectacle but a grave national scandal, a display of moral irresponsibility which has seldom if ever been surpassed. There are a thousand excuses why these children should receive no money and every excuse has been scavenged by the company throughout the last decade.'

There was only one interruption as I spoke, and thanks to a quick note from Alf Morris, I was able to deal with it reasonably well. The House listened carefully to my speech, and I was given a warm reception when I finished. Sir Keith Joseph replied for the Government, supporting an anaemic Amendment to our Motion. Expressing concern at the plight of the children and the delay in reaching a settlement, it merely welcomed the Government undertaking to investigate any thalidomide children's needs which were not met by the services available and offered to consider whether a trust fund for them would be needed later. He announced that £3 million was to be set aside for improving services for congenitally disabled children, but there was nothing specifically for thalidomide children. This money, financing what became known as the Family Fund, has helped thousands of children and still does so today, but in the debate on thalidomide children, the announcement seemed an irrelevance. Nothing could obscure the central demand of justice for them and the Government's refusal to help to provide it.

The debate had a passionate ring to it, with striking contributions from both sides. Dr Gerard Vaughan spoke from personal knowledge about the children, many of whom he had examined in his professional capacity. Barbara Castle, a former Minister, revealed threats to a mother that her legal aid could be withdrawn if she persisted in trying to publicize the evidence.

Gerard Vaughan's contribution, together with those of other Tory MPs such as John Astor, William Shelton and Dr Tom Stuttaford, put some Government backbenchers in a quandary. These MPs had spoken with such obvious knowledge and sincerity, yet their Government would not accept the Motion. In the division, party loyalties triumphed as usual; the vast majority of Tory backbenchers supported the Government's amendment, which was carried by 291 votes to 260.

The vote itself was of minimal importance compared with the tremendous public interest aroused by the debate. Suddenly, it seemed that everyone in Britain was talking about thalidomide – and people were practically all on our side. As Harold Evans said, the debate was the turning point.

Distillers responded by increasing the £5 million offer. In a long public statement, they offered an £11.9 million trust fund to compensate the 342 children. As they no doubt calculated, this won favourable headlines. One, which was typical, ran: 'Distillers Say: We'll Double It'.

The company was proposing a trust fund into which it would make ten annual payments of £1,185,000. But this was only the equivalent of a capital sum of £5 million from the company because the method of payment made it deductible from taxable profit. So the additional money was to come from the taxpayer.

Next day, in the House of Commons, I condemned Distillers. It was 14 December, and I called for an emergency debate 'to show that Distillers is still acting as Scrooge, but now in the guise of Santa Claus'. Although I knew my call would be rejected, it was calculated to hearten the families and dishearten the company – and the enormous press coverage ensured that both got the message.

A further blow to Distillers came from the Chancellor of the Exchequer, Anthony Barber. No doubt needled by the company's presumption, he told Sir Alex McDonald that there was 'no authority' for Distillers' suggestion that the Government might agree to a tax concession. Shaken by this, the company withdrew the offer and, as a spokesman said, went 'back to the drawing board'. No longer was it the arrogant and dogmatic company it had been for the past decade.

By now the thalidomide story was an international one, but it was the British public who would influence the outcome. Seeking to extend our support, I asked Vic Feather, General Secretary of the Trades Union Congress, for help. He contacted the General and Municipal Workers' Union, which had the largest number of members among Distillers' employees. The General Secretary, David Basnett, pressed for a meeting with Distillers. Other unions as well as local authorities, student bodies and voluntary organizations expressed their support.

A boycott of Distillers' alcoholic products was an obvious tool in the campaign. One of the keenest supporters of this tactic was David Mason, the thalidomide child's father whom I had met on the television programme. Ebullient as ever, he took off to the USA to persuade Ralph Nader, the famous American consumer campaigner, to intervene. After their meeting they warned Distillers that a boycott would soon be organized. Increasing numbers of organizations and political groups, including Conservatives, were now writing to tell me that they were no longer buying Distillers' products.

Mason's visit to the USA generated tremendous interest on both sides of the Atlantic, and he brilliantly exploited every opportunity of enlisting support. Even on his journeys he acquainted fellow passengers with the scandal of thalidomide and won their backing. His appearances on television were impressive, because he was fighting with feeling and tenacity for his own limbless daughter as well as for other thalidomide children.

The fuse of another explosive attack on the company was lit by a quiet, bearded, studious man to whom 'moral obligation' was a binding imperative. Tony Lynes was a social policy analyst whom I had met on a few occasions at the House of Commons when he was the Director of the Child Poverty Action Group. He would arrive on a bicycle, clips around his trouser legs, ready with erudite arguments and masses of statistics about poor families. He was a shy but persuasive advocate.

Lynes held just six hundred of Distillers' 300 million shares. Using his position as a bona fide shareholder, he had been an active supporter of the thalidomide children for some time. He had earlier

written to Sir Alex McDonald arguing that even from the narrow
commercial point of view the company ought to be doing what was
morally right. He was quite correct. The reputation of Distillers was
sliding and with it the value of its shares.

McDonald had brusquely rejected Lynes's proposals. It was in
this reply that McDonald said he would consider taking a stand on
the legal issues, widely interpreted as a threat to withdraw the
inadequate offer of £3.25 million. Incensed by this, Lynes contacted
other shareholders, and together they formed a shareholders' committee. Distillers were now to be attacked by some of the most influential
people of all.

The original small group beavered away to find other shareholders
and seek their support. Then came the priceless discovery that some
shares were owned by local councils and big insurance companies.
Ever helpful, Harold Evans got the *Sunday Times* to buy the thirty-
two volumes of shareholders' names from Distillers. He published
hundreds of names of the bigger shareholders, and stood back to
await the bang.

It was not long coming. Local authorities, trade unions and
churches holding shares were inundated with telephone calls from
the press. Where did they stand on thalidomide? Many swung in
favour of the campaign, agreeing to support a call for an extraordinary general meeting. But the most damaging move of all was
made by one of the largest life insurance companies in Britain, the
Legal & General Assurance Society, which held 3½ million shares.
Announcing its support for the shareholders' committee and the
moral claim of thalidomide parents, the company not only shook
Distillers but it stimulated other big shareholders, insurance companies, banks and local authorities to follow.

This turned out to be the final onslaught. Wobbling already from
the combined pressures of Parliament, the *Sunday Times*, David
Mason and other parents, Ralph Nader and a growing boycott,
Distillers were shattered by escalating action from their own shareholders. On 5 January 1973, I was suddenly invited to go to the
BBC television studios to comment on an announcement expected
from Distillers.

In the studio, waiting tensely and seemingly interminably for the announcement, I wondered if Distillers would attempt another manoeuvre. The news came a few minutes before going on the air; Distillers had capitulated and offered the £20 million we had demanded all along. This was a marvellous moment. After ten years of legal battles and making derisory offers to the parents, Distillers were willing to pay in full; the company would make ten annual payments of £2 million a year into a charitable trust. All the campaigning, the passion, the fighting and the tactics had been justified. For the first time in months there was no need to hit back and plan the next moves, or indeed to receive worried messages from desperately anxious parents. It was total surrender by a powerful corporation, and a victory of crucial benefit to the children and their families. All that remained were negotiations about payments rather than argument about principle.

Harold Evans and his colleagues set up a liaison committee, with me as chairman, to examine the offer in detail. An impressive committee, it included thalidomide parents, distinguished doctors, lawyers and financial experts. Among these was Lord Goodman, one of the greatest advocates of his day, Sir Gordon Newton, former editor of the *Financial Times*, and Dr Gerard Vaughan MP.

All their great expertise was needed, especially when they discovered that many thalidomide children had not been systematically medically examined. Until this was done, it would be impossible to allocate comparable and fair compensation to children relative to their different disabilities. In addition to the outstanding cases, the families who had settled for an unsatisfactory sum in 1968 had to be considered so that parity could be established between the two groups.

Negotiations with Distillers, lasting six months, were intensive and remarkably successful. The scheme which emerged was, in the opinion of the original questioning actuary, John Prevett, even better than any 100 per cent award the children might have won in court for negligence. A sum of £6 million was to be paid to the 340 outstanding cases to give them the same award as that secured by those who had settled in 1968. In addition, there were to be payments of £2 million a year for seven years to a charitable trust for the benefit of both groups; and £20,000 a year for ten years was given to help operate the trust. Inflation, which had been disregarded by the first judge, was acknowledged, and the annual payments were to increase by up to 10 per cent if prices rose, as of course they did.

The total liability to Distillers was £28.4 million. The firm recovered only £3 million from their insurers, Lloyd's of London, a higher payment being refused on the grounds that Distillers had failed to carry out adequate tests and research on thalidomide.

The war was over, or so it seemed. Then to my dismay I discovered on 19 October 1974 that the Treasury was going to tax the investment income the children would receive. This meant that £5 million would be claimed back, and all the allocations would have to be reassessed. The parents were deeply upset, and David Mason said he was 'back in the fight'.

By this time Edward Heath had been replaced as Prime Minister by Harold Wilson, following the 1974 General Election, and Denis Healey was Chancellor of the Exchequer. I knew that both of them were favourably disposed towards the thalidomide children, and of course it had been Wilson's decision to hold a full Parliamentary debate that had facilitated the eventual victory. However, a Treasury ruling is usually one of those immutable things – especially when officials argue, as they did on this occasion, that tax relief would create an anomaly because other handicapped people were not being similarly helped. What was to be done?

The first thing was to make strong public protests to prepare the ground for future discussions with Treasury Ministers. Within minutes of hearing the news I discussed it with Harold Evans, who acted immediately. He wrote a powerful editorial for the next day's *Sunday Times*, attacking the move and demanding concessions for the families. I asked the Treasury to provide £5 million to offset the tax demand. After all, Labour MPs had supported the Parliamentary campaign when we were in opposition, so Labour Ministers should give practical support in office. However, this was rejected by the Financial Secretary to the Treasury, John Gilbert, acting in Denis Healey's absence while he was abroad. I was furious at this refusal and publicly attacked the Treasury's decision. I arranged to meet Denis Healey on his return and urged other MPs to press the Government.

Before the weekend was over, Harold Wilson indicated that he was intervening and intended to help. So far as I was concerned, his statement meant that we had won, but when I met Healey in his office in the House of Commons I found him in a sombre mood. I had always liked and admired this brilliant and tough politician who would have made a great leader of the party. He was outstanding as Minister of Defence and Chancellor of the Exchequer; but it was his very toughness, and consequent outspokenness, which upset some of his colleagues and tipped the scales against him in the leadership stakes.

He had always been difficult to lip-read, and his first words to me, which I had to ask him to write as I couldn't follow him, were: 'You should have come to me in the first place.' He was annoyed at my attacks on the Treasury, but it had not been for me to decide which Minister would answer my questions earlier. That was a Treasury decision, and I told him so.

However, Healey was genuinely sympathetic. Once he had delivered his mild rebuke he softened and told me in confidence that the Government was to give the £5 million. He stressed the need to keep this private until the technicalities had been worked out and a Ministerial announcement was made in about a week's time. I was naturally delighted and of course I respected his confidence, but this meant I could not disclose the news to the parents or the press. Later, when David Mason telephoned wanting to know the outcome of my meeting, he was clearly suspicious. As I was unable to reassure him, because of my promise to Denis Healey, he wanted to resume the campaign; but I asked him to trust me and to take no action. Reluctantly, in view of my mysterious silence, he agreed despite his misgivings.

Some days later, on Friday 25 October 1974, two years and one month since that first article in the *Sunday Times*, the official announcement was made. It said that there had been 'genuine misunderstanding' and the Government would pay £5 million into the thalidomide children's trust fund. That marked the end of the re-markable battle for compensation to the families. It had been dramatic, complex and exhausting. The main objective, to secure the financial future of the children, had been achieved, and the victory had also set an important precedent for the future.

Harold Evans and his *Sunday Times* team continued the other aspect of their campaign, the fight for freedom of the press. They took their case against the banning of a draft article not only to the House of Lords but to the European Court of Human Rights. Following a protracted legal battle, they were ultimately vindicated.

The victory was marred only by the dispute that arose over which children should be compensated. Many of the deformities caused by thalidomide could occur naturally, and the children damaged by the drug were not easily or precisely distinguishable. Those whose mothers could prove that they had taken the drug were placed on an 'X' list of those to be paid. But if there was no proof, the child went on a 'Y' list, which meant no payment unless new evidence led to a transfer to the 'X' list. It was hard to argue against a severely handicapped child receiving compensation, and some people felt Distillers should compensate them all. However, although I was passionately opposed to Distillers, I could not accept that the company should be obliged to pay children for whose injuries they were not responsible.

It was the first time in Britain that compensation for injury had been won in the public domain. A few people subsequently argued that this was wrong because only the law courts should decide such issues. But the law had shown itself inadequate to secure justice; and because of the stranglehold on the media which Distillers maintained for a decade, there was no pressure for reform. Too much suffering had been caused and too much damage inflicted on families to allow continued prevarication. The special circumstances of thalidomide justified special measures.

The deformed children rightly won their compensation, but there was no cause for celebration because they still had to face life with dreadful disabilities. At least the compensation helped them to cope with some of the problems.

In an entirely different way, the campaign had a profound effect on my own life. My first major campaign since I had lost my hearing, it proved that I could fight in Parliament with success. The enormous press, radio and television coverage made me a national figure. To those who believed that total deafness was a disqualification for Parliament, and there were still some, it proved that the disability could be overcome. Thalidomide, a disaster for the children, unexpectedly helped me to cope with a disaster in my own life.

It also illustrated a subtle but powerful function of the House of Commons which is not widely understood. Although not a legal court of last resort, as is the House of Lords, in this instance it operated parallel to the legal system and, without interfering directly, significantly influenced the outcome. Without the Commons' intervention the families would almost certainly have been denied the justice eventually accorded to them.

The outcome of the thalidomide battle also showed something else. This was that when public opinion is aroused, by Parliament, the press or individuals – and in this case it was all of them – even the most powerful and obdurate multinational company must accept values which are demonstrably fair and just.

13

Campaigning for Women: Battered Wives and Rape

In November 1972, Pauline and I visited a decrepit house in Chiswick, West London. Although it appeared to be an ordinary terraced home in an undistinguished area, 130 women and children lived there, crushed into every inch, with makeshift beds lying side by side. They were refugees from violent husbands. By any normal standards, conditions were intolerable; yet, bleak as their environment was, the women shared a curious mixture of cheerfulness and comradeship, albeit laced with fear. The atmosphere was akin to the aftermath of a natural disaster when everyone tries to make the best of things.

In the Chiswick Women's Aid refuge, the first of its kind in Britain, were women who had been bruised, cut and even scalded; some were nervous wrecks. We could see the results of violence and sense the underlying fear. The combination of physical attacks, mental cruelty and insecurity had shattered their lives. But this unlikely, overcrowded terraced house offered security and hope.

. A large, confident woman with striking features dominated the scene. Erin Pizzey, supremely serene, was the driving force behind the refuge, reigning like a strong but gentle matriarch. All the women, especially the terrified ones, looked to her for comfort, guidance and advice. Her natural authority gave confidence to the women, with whom she was endlessly patient and helpful.

In 1970, Hounslow Council had allowed her, as a voluntary worker, to convert a derelict house into a place for mothers and children simply to meet and talk. Some of the mothers did not want to go home. They stayed, and Chiswick Women's Aid was born.

Erin's own troubled childhood, with a mother who beat her and a father she disliked, helped her to understand the women's fears. She was to make the cause of battered wives her own. A highly controversial one, it naturally enraged violent husbands; and, when Erin refused to comply with the safety by-laws, she angered the local authority. They wanted to limit numbers because of fire regulations. She refused to turn anyone away.

This courageous stand put her at risk of prison, but she was totally unyielding, insisting that no woman would be forced to return to a violent husband, by-law or no by-law. The Council's dilemma was that if they did not act they were condoning law breaking; if they did, they would put women at risk of serious injury. This conflict between legality and morality – between the anxious Council and the stubborn woman – attracted public interest and widespread support for her. The Council shrank from taking legal action against her, but they continued to insist that she should change her policy.

We talked to the women as Erin showed us round. Then she outlined the requirements: more financial help for the families, better accommodation and more sympathetic police attitudes. These were the immediate necessities; the further aim was to establish a national network of sanctuaries.

I was moved by the evidence of violence, the fear of the women and the insecurity of the children at Chiswick. Providing adequate housing and financial support would not be simple or easy, but something had to be done, and I resolved to press the case in Parliament. I expected to face some prejudice. Some of the male journalists I met when visiting the refuge, while welcoming the story, commented to me, 'They enjoy it' or 'They probably deserved it.' Such chauvinism in the face of brutality disturbed me.

My immediate response was to push Ministers into action. I asked the Home Secretary, Robert Carr, to make domestic violence a criminal offence and to discuss with Chief Constables how the police could help. To the Attorney-General, Sir Peter Rawlinson, I suggested that injunctions against violent men should be heard without delay. And I asked the Social Services Minister, Sir Keith Joseph, to collate information and create a network of sanctuaries. Their replies were placatory – the Home Office was consulting with police, the Attorney-General was giving publicity to legal aid and assistance schemes, and Social Services were exploring the problems. The answers were pat, more like easy responses than constructive involvement. I was far from reassured.

At Prime Minister's Question Time, I asked Edward Heath to make one Minister responsible for co-ordinating Government policies for advice and assistance to battered women. Although Heath refused – he said that the Departments concerned were working closely together – he did recognize that there was a 'grave and complex problem' and promised to investigate any evidence.

Domestic violence was not new in Britain. In 1878, an article in the *Contemporary Review* described wife beating as a mere preface to torture, maiming, blinding and murder. The author, Frances Cobbe, described the suffering of poor women who were blinded with acid, set upon by dogs, trampled by hobnailed boots, roasted before an open fire, stabbed and strangled as well as suffering the most vicious beatings.

Cobbe claimed that wife beating belonged almost exclusively to the artisan and labouring class. This was not the case in 1973, when, as the result of the publicity, battered women started writing to me. One, the wife of a senior civil servant, said she was constantly beaten and lost her sight after a haemorrhage of the retina. The ex-wife of an executive in Berkshire wrote:

> In the summers I couldn't swim or wear summer dresses because I was so covered with bruises. When I was eight months pregnant with twins I was knocked down and kicked repeatedly in the stomach and kidneys; the babies were born prematurely and although they had both been apparently healthy inside me at the time of my 'accident', one of them

(who had stopped moving inside me after the 'accident') was born dead.

Often the women had to endure the violence because there was nowhere to go. The terror of violent husbands and the shame of their plight demoralized them. They felt isolated and helpless. Many had a great sense of relief when the publicity showed they were no longer alone. With domestic violence out in the open, women began to talk of their ordeal and seek an end to it.

As the Department of Health had refused an inquiry into the prevalence of domestic violence, Pauline and I tried to collate a national picture from other sources. In Stoke-on-Trent, a city of 250,000 people, 80 women suffering habitual cruelty had asked the Social Services Department for help in the past year. In the county of Staffordshire, with a total population of just over a million, 320 assaulted women complained to the police in the year. Assuming those figures were typical, both gave an approximate figure for the country as a whole of 16,000 women being so severely beaten that they went to the police or local authority for help.

It was a crude way of estimating a national figure, and undoubtedly underestimated the true one. Fear, despair and maternal anxiety deter battered women from reporting assaults or seeking help. But these figures indicated that there was at the very least a significant amount of mindless cruelty and needless suffering.

There was little help available to prevent the cruelty or treat the suffering. Lawyers were often inadequate, the legal system cumbersome, and social services unable to cope. Police attitudes revealed 'an understandable but unacceptable schizophrenia in their approach to violence', as Erin Pizzey pointed out. A man found attacking a woman in the street would be immediately arrested and charged; but the same man could inflict violence on his wife in their home with impunity. The views of MPs were even more disturbing. 'Battering? It's a perk of marriage,' said one flippantly. He had a half-smile, but he was only half-joking. 'You must know,' said another, 'that some women ask for it.' I was by no means surprised by these attitudes, because they reflected to some extent the chauvinistic ethos of the factories and the Army, with which I was familiar. They were the adult equivalent of adolescent wolf-whistles, yet when they were articulated by MPs they angered me. Bloodied women were not a joke.

Nearly a century ago, an MP felt as angry as I did about battered wives. On 18 May 1874, Colonel Egerton Leigh MP appealed to the House of Commons for increased punishment for assaults on women. He wanted the men to be flogged. But he accepted an assurance that the Government would bear this in mind and withdrew his proposal. Disraeli subsequently set up an inquiry into wife torturing.

In an Adjournment debate on 16 July 1973, I pressed for strong but more civilized action than that demanded by Colonel Leigh. I sought a radical change in police attitudes so that they treated seriously criminal assaults on married women and common-law wives. I wanted more solicitors with expertise in domestic violence, and I called for immediate legal aid for wives taking action against husbands.

I instinctively felt about battered women as I would about someone in a burning house – get them out. But I knew that these women, especially those with children, would only leave their homes if they had somewhere to go. The priority was to persuade the Government to establish a network of refuges. In addition I suspected that if the men knew there was a certain escape route there would be less brutality. Refuges would be the first haven, but I also called for local councils to give women tenancy temporarily if there was evidence of brutality and permanently after the breakdown of a relationship due to violence.

During 1973, the campaign became increasingly effective. Some of the popular newspapers took it up with prurient relish, but the publicity was nevertheless helpful. It became a topical issue, discussed frequently in articles and on radio and television. Organizations like Chiswick Women's Aid, the National Citizens' Advice Bureaux and the National Council of Women vigorously pressed for action. Academics joined in, researching and writing reports. From every source it was clear that domestic violence was widespread and action was required.

Governments respond slowly on such issues, and Heath's Government was defeated in February 1974 before it had made any changes. But the new Labour Ministers acted without delay. I had a hand in this because Barbara Castle replaced Sir Keith Joseph at the Department of Health and Social Security, and as I became her Parliamentary Private Secretary, I made sure that she was fully briefed. She listened carefully to my suggestions and deputed one of her Ministers, Alec Jones, to deal with the subject. A few months later, on 12 November 1974, he opened a seminar which covered the whole spectrum of domestic violence. The recommendations included a national network of refuges, a 24-hour telephone advice service, information to doctors and social workers, and changes in police procedures.

While warmly welcoming these recommendations, I felt the main need was to focus on the home and move the balance of advantage towards the women. Why should a brutal man retain the comfort of the home while the woman and children had to scrabble around for makeshift accommodation? If he was the aggressor, why should not he be expelled from the home and have to find a refuge for himself?

There could be no doubt about a husband's violence if he was convicted of it; and for those cases I proposed a simple but drastic solution. Possession of the matrimonial home should go to the wife. Although I had strong support in the House, some MPs had reservations. The Government Chief Whip, Bob Mellish, wrote to me guardedly saying that my proposal would probably be discussed by a Select Committee looking into the subject, which was to be set up by Barbara Castle. Mellish asked me to have a word with the Lord Chancellor.

I did so, but Lord Elwyn Jones, ever the cautious lawyer, had strong reservations. 'I am sure you will not mind if I mention one point,' he wrote. 'On the one hand the court would be required to turn the husband out after any conviction, even if it was only an isolated minor assault. ... On the other hand [the proposed Bill] would not deal with the situation where no conviction has been secured.' He added that wives were often reluctant to give evidence. I was well aware of the reluctance of women to give evidence, and I was sure that it was only in the serious assault cases that a conviction was obtained. So I found his response unconvincing.

The simple solution of transferring the matrimonial home to the wife, because of a conviction for an act of violence, was regarded as impracticable by more people than the Lord Chancellor. The House of Commons Library, ever helpful on every subject, sent me a pained letter hinting at incredulity that I should press this case. A legal adviser to the Women's Aid Federation was concerned about the legal implications. I was not deterred and on 14 January 1975 I presented my proposal in a Ten-Minute-Rule Bill. I told the Commons that I was concerned not with normal domestic disputes or even serious rows, but with brutality – pregnant women kicked, women being beaten or even burned, the breaking of bones and the crushing of spirits – the kind of cruelty that would cause a mass outcry and marches on Parliament if inflicted on dogs. Yet in such cases the women had either to endure it or to get out.

If violence meant homelessness – as it often ultimately did – Parliament should decide which one was to go. Was it to be the attacker or the attacked? The man with good earning power or the woman with very little? My Bill provided that if there was proof of violence – and a conviction would be the proof – then the man must go. It was given an unopposed first reading with all-party support. Normally Ten-Minute-Rule Bills make no further progress, but I was fortunate in securing a second reading debate for my Bill the following July. In the weeks before, many of the women's organizations lobbied strongly in support; letters were sent to all MPs; and on the day of the debate, women gathered outside the House, while many more were in the gallery.

In my speech I welcomed the progress made in the two years since the issue was first raised in Parliament. Thirty more refuges had been set up. National and local government were now concerned, and a Select Committee had been established to consider the problems.

Attacking the complacency of MPs and the public in general, I made my call for the victim of battering to be given possession of the home. When I sat down, the political lawyers moved in. A Tory

MP, Ronald Bell, criticized the use of the word 'battered', describing it as a political cliché. He claimed that women had their own ways of wounding men, and Parliament had treated women gently on this matter. Other lawyers complained that the loss of home was too severe a punishment for a violent husband. Only Christopher Price, a Labour MP, gave the Bill whole-hearted support, suggesting to the nit-picking lawyers, as he called them, that if they did not know what a battered wife was, they should visit the refuge in his constituency. The Bill was talked out, but the debate had been valuable. Virtually every MP had been made aware of the issue, and they all knew it would not be dropped.

In the autumn of the same year, I was delighted when Jo Richardson, who had worked on women's rights for many years, chose this subject when she was successful in the ballot for Private Members' Bills. Her luck meant valuable Parliamentary time was available. She took up some of the important recommendations of the Select Committee on Violence in Marriage and against Children. In particular, her Bill enabled a wife to obtain an injunction against the husband without having to initiate divorce or separation proceedings. It also provided that the judge could attach power of arrest to the injunction order, so the police could immediately arrest the offender if it was breached. A further clause amended the Matrimonial Homes Act of 1967, so that a wife could obtain an order making a husband leave the home. This was a modified version of the proposal I had pressed for for so long.

Despite the opposition to the Bill, some of which was serious, some flippant and most chauvinistic, it was enacted in October 1976. This was the first legislation to help battered wives for nearly one hundred years. The 1878 Matrimonial Causes Act, which followed the inquiry set up by Disraeli into wife torturing, had provided for husbands to give some financial support to the wives they had assaulted.

Jo Richardson's Domestic Violence Act was later criticized in an article in the *New Law Journal* in 1980 as falling far short of providing a significant solution to the problem because of the limited ability of the law in solving intricate social and psychological problems. It is true that the law cannot alone resolve the problem of domestic violence, and the Act was debilitated by its weak implementation. The number of injunctions rose, but few of those who ignored them were sent to prison. Even more frustrating was that getting an injunction sometimes itself provoked violence. Nevertheless it was a useful and welcome step forward on the legal front.

Police attitudes and behaviour were more difficult to change. In the early 1970s, it was clear that change would be a long time coming. When I had suggested in the House of Commons that the police should treat assaults on wives the same way as those on MPs or the Royal Family, it merely raised a few chuckles. The replies to Parliamentary Questions and letters to Home Secretaries were perfunctory to the point of indifference, offering the feeble excuse that these matters were being considered.

A significant change did take place but not until fifteen years later. It resulted from the pressure exerted by the many organizations outside Parliament that were now concerned with domestic violence. The new police policy was spelt out in August 1990 by the Home Office Minister of State, John Patten, who said that 'brutality in the home is just as much a crime as any other sort of violence. The victims of this hidden crime must be helped and offenders must be punished.'

The police were urged to keep registers of victims 'at risk', to set up units with specially trained officers and to give more consideration to arresting and charging offenders. Patten rightly warned the police against attempting reconciliation as a substitute for arrest and charge, and against assuming that the victim's complaint would later be withdrawn. This is a common assumption by the police, because many women who complain withdraw the charge before it goes to court. The underlying reason of course is fear. Because women are afraid of more violence, they do not make use of legal protection, but that protection should nevertheless always be available.

The fear is often justified. When women go to refuges, some psychopathic husbands try to seek them out. If they succeed, the results can be catastrophic. For example, in 1986, one husband murdered his wife in the kitchen of a refuge in front of the children.

In 1991, a woman was stabbed to death in the domestic violence unit of a North London police station while she and her husband were supposed to be discussing the marital rift.

Although it is mainly men who kill in domestic disputes, some women kill the men, often as a result of provocation. When they do so they find that the legal defence of provocation is curiously inadequate. This was highlighted in 1990 by the case of Sara Thornton, who, after suffering great brutality, killed her husband. She took a knife, sharpened it and stabbed him once. After his death she was found guilty of murder – her plea of provocation was rejected.

According to English law it is wrong to kill in retaliation for brutality, however extreme. Otherwise people could take the law into their own hands. A plea of provocation can be accepted only if it can be established that the brutality led to a loss of self-control. In such cases a killing becomes the less serious crime of manslaughter rather than murder. This is particularly important, because a murder conviction results in automatic life imprisonment, whereas a manslaughter sentence is at the discretion of the judge – and can sometimes merely be probation.

Sara Thornton's plea of provocation was rejected because some time had elapsed between the provocation and the killing. Back in 1949, Mr Justice Devlin had ruled that, to be successful in a court of law, provocation had to cause a *sudden* and temporary loss of control. If there was a time gap, he said, there was time for reason to be restored. If reason was restored, the act was deliberate, and was murder.

I thought the Devlin dictum was flawed by its emphasis on 'sudden', and asked the Home Secretary, Kenneth Baker, to introduce legislation to change it. He declined to do so as he was satisfied with existing case law based on the Devlin judgement.

Given the Ministerial intransigence, a Ten-Minute-Rule Bill seemed to be the best way of pressing the need for change in the House, and I was lucky with the timing. I proposed my Bill on 18 December 1991, which was the opening day of a major debate on Britain's role in Europe following the Maastricht Treaty. When I rose to speak, it was to a packed Chamber, with the Prime Minister, John Major, waiting to open the debate after my speech.

I told the Commons that Mr Justice Devlin's view, that reason could quickly be restored after great brutality, was acceptable once. It was acceptable in the 1914–18 war when we shot shell-shocked young men. It may have been acceptable in 1949, when we did not really appreciate the effect of violence upon the human mind. But it bore no relation to what we knew in 1991 about the effects of violence.

I claimed that the fallacy at the heart of the judge's ruling was that it failed to appreciate that many people do not regain normal self-control soon after brutality. We recognized this with American troops in Vietnam, with British troops who fought in the Gulf and with British hostages in the Middle East. I felt we should give the same consideration to battered and brutalized women as we gave to soldiers and captives.

Although my Bill received an unopposed first reading, it did not become law because there was no Parliamentary time. Nevertheless the debate and the consequent publicity stimulated great interest. I subsequently went to see the Home Secretary, Kenneth Baker, to discuss the issue. As is common with Ministers, he made no commitment, but it was clear that he appreciated the nature of the problem.

The original Parliamentary campaign on battered wives was a good example of the limitations and strengths of backbenchers' activity. It stimulated and complemented other work: sociological analysis, feminist argument, legal debate and activities of women's groups. The issue was put back on the Parliamentary agenda after a hundred-year gap – and it will certainly not be forgotten again for so long. The publicity generated led to public interest, some action and a slight shift in attitude.

Women themselves have a vital role in trying to change the attitudes of society. The Women's Aid movement emerged with the growth in the number of refuges, but it was split by Erin Pizzey's later view that some battered wives were prone to violence. In her book *Prone to Violence*, published in 1982 with Jeff Shapiro, her second husband, she said that some women colluded with, and became addicted to, violence. Rejecting criticism that she was blaming women for being beaten up, she said that it was an attempt to show that women who had had violent childhoods, and knew nothing else, accepted and even became addicted to violence because it was the kind of communication they understood. But her views were rejected by many of her previous supporters, and the Women's Aid Federation denounced her theories.

No doubt psychologists will endlessly debate the reasons for domestic violence; sociologists will explore the relationship between women's role in society and battering; lawyers will argue about the effectiveness of law in deterring violence; and the police will discuss the difficulty of applying the law to close and violent relationships. These discussions are necessary for long-term solutions, but the vital short-term measure is to provide a haven for desperate women and children trapped with violent men. Until brutality can be prevented, a means of escape from it is essential.

By 1991, 279 refuges had been set up, providing over 25,000 places of sanctuary for women and children each year. This provision falls short of that recommended by the 1975 report of the Select Committee on Violence in Marriage – one refuge place per 10,000 head of population, indicating some 50,000 places. But it is still substantial progress in the twenty years since the Chiswick refuge pioneered the way. The finances of many refuges, however, remain precarious, based on limited Government grants, restricted local authority support, board and lodging payments, fund-raising and donations. Although the problems of battered wives have been recognized, they will not be solved until much more is allocated; and this is still not a high priority for many men.

In Parliament in the 1970s, what are customarily known as women's issues were either ignored or promoted by women MPs. I became involved because I was indignant about the general injustice of the indifference to battered wives and the absence of adequate help. Subconsciously, no doubt, and to some extent directly, I was affected by having three daughters and a wife, all of them with a lively concern for justice for women. It was a standard family joke that if, when we were together, I mentioned 'girls', Caroline would correct me by interjecting 'women'.

*

The next women's issue that concerned me was rape. On 30 April 1975, the highest legal body in the land, the Law Lords, although rejecting an appeal on a bizarre rape case, made a ruling which aroused heated controversy throughout the country. The appeal was by three airmen who had been convicted of raping the wife of a senior NCO named Morgan – at his invitation. He took the men to his home one night, told them to expect a show of resistance from his wife, but not to take this seriously because it was a mere pretext which stimulated her sexual excitement. The wife, awakened from sleep, was attacked and held down by the men while each took it in turns to rape her as she screamed and struggled.

Their conviction was influenced by the judge's summing up, which went to the heart of English legal principles. Mr Justice Kenneth Jones said that the airmen would only be innocent of rape if they honestly believed that the woman was consenting to sexual intercourse and if their belief was reasonable. The Court of Appeal, led by the Lord Chief Justice, Lord Widgery, endorsed this ruling but granted leave of appeal to the House of Lords.

But the full ruling of the judge was unacceptable to the Law Lords. By a majority decision, and after complex, erudite legal argument, they ruled in principle that the reasonableness of the belief was irrelevant. All that mattered if a man was accused of rape was whether he genuinely believed that the woman consented. They did not, however, free the three airmen, because they felt the men did not genuinely believe that the woman was consenting. The key to the Law Lords' argument was the legal principle of *mens rea* – the guilty intent – which is the basis of all English criminal law. Only if there was a guilty intent could a man be found guilty of rape.

My objection to the elevation of this sound legal principle was that it obscured an equally valid one, that people should be responsible for the result of their actions. It was surely wrong that a woman should suffer a sexual assault without penalty to her assailant because of an unfounded assumption by him. Arid legalism denied justice if one principle was elevated to the detriment of others. If the Law Lords' judgement remained unchanged, the strength of women's legal protection from sexual attack from men could be undermined.

I considered the Law Lords' ruling as bizarre as the rape itself. So I wrote to the Home Secretary, Roy Jenkins, telling him that if the law was really the ass that the judgement made it appear, it must be changed. It was the craziest situation since Al Capone's heyday. I went on to argue that 'Every vicious sexual attack can now be excused on the grounds that the aggressor claims to believe that his victim's protests were not sincere. A flimsy Shakespeare line that the "lady doth protest too much" has now become the rapist's cast-iron alibi.' His response was, however, disappointingly negative. So within days, on 6 May, I gathered a group of MPs from both sides of the House and went to see him. Although expressing sympathy, Jenkins was not convinced that the judgement would have much, if any, effect on rapes. Even if he had been, he said, emergency legislation was out of the question. He intended to wait and see if I was right that the judgement could become a rapist's charter; meanwhile he would consider the issues.

This response puzzled me. How could a compassionate and en-lightened Home Secretary sit back and wait? I told him that this was like waiting for a bank to be continually robbed before defending it. But he was adamant; he would wait and see. I thought not. Jenkins had to be propelled to act. His stand would discourage more women from reporting rape; and if women were unwilling to report rape to the police, how could rapists be caught? A rape victim already had to endure police interrogation, medical examination and a defence counsel's clever questioning in addition to the original assault. She would now have to listen to the rapist proclaiming his 'belief', however unreasonable, that she was willing to accept what was forced on her.

As I studied the subject, I began to realize that not requiring reasonable grounds for a man's belief in the woman's consent was only one factor deterring raped women from turning to the law. Rape cases in general, and sensational ones in particular, were widely publicized. A rape victim had to suffer, as well as the assault, the exposure of the lurid details.

In addition, court procedures made no allowances for the sensi-tivities of raped women. Legally, they were but witnesses while their assailants were innocent until proved guilty. Inevitably the defence counsels' normal tactic was to exploit the women's sexual history to demean them. Exposing women to this public ordeal and permitting their sexual character assassination could not be justified, and I set about changing it.

I drew up a Bill requiring that a man's belief that a woman consented must be based on reasonable grounds. It also provided that the Criminal Law Revision Committee should consider a guarantee of anonymity to rape victims, and it prohibited the disclosure of a woman's sexual history in court.

On 21 May 1975, I presented it as a Ten-Minute-Rule Bill. The issue had aroused much interest, and the Chamber was well attended when I put forward my arguments that the Law Lords' judgement was more likely to protect criminals than to prevent crime. I began by saying that rape was often seen by men with Tarzan minds and Tom Thumb imaginations as a bit of a game, but it was a vicious and degrading crime – far more important and evil than crime against property. In the absence of statute law for rape we had to depend on common law, now unhappily and unfortunately interpreted by the Law Lords. I then called for the three changes outlined in the Bill.

Fortunately, at the end of my speech, one MP, John Lee, rose to speak against my proposals. Had he not done so, we would never have known how many MPs supported my Bill. The Division that followed resulted in a vote of 228 for and 17 against. It was a massive majority. Among my supporters were influential MPs including three members of the Cabinet, Michael Stewart, Bob Mellish and Tony Benn, and four members of the Shadow Cabinet, Jim Prior, Norman St John Stevas, Michael Jopling and Willie Whitelaw.

My natural pleasure at the size of the vote changed to indignation the next day when I read the *Guardian* headline 'Government to oppose new rape law bill'. The journalist had obviously been briefed by the Home Office.

Just two days later, a convicted rapist, John Cogan, walked free having won his appeal against a two-year sentence for raping his friend's wife. The jury had originally decided he genuinely believed that the woman consented but that the grounds for doing so were unreasonable. In view of the Appeal Court's ruling in the Morgan case, he won his appeal after a one-minute hearing.

I promptly called on Roy Jenkins for an immediate statement on his attitude to the Bill and threatened a 'major row' if he flouted the known will of the House of Commons. If the Home Office sets itself up as a last bastion of defence of this outrageous law, I said, a long siege lies ahead. For good measure, I asked him to receive another deputation. I was intent on pressing the advantage accruing from the large Parliamentary majority.

Just over a week later, Jenkins sent me a written assurance that he had not yet come to any decision and that his attitude 'as reinforced by my abstention in the vote on your Bill' remained unchanged; he also said he would be glad to receive my deputation. So either the journalist had got it wrong or the pressures were forcing the Home Office to back off from total opposition to my Bill. Meanwhile, I was bombarded with letters and messages of support, including nineteen petitions containing 4,200 signatures which I sent to Jenkins.

The deputation's discussion with him was amicable. Far from opposing my Bill, he said, he welcomed it as a valuable test of Parliamentary and public opinion and would certainly not oppose it. Not only that, but the Home Office was willing to have detailed discussion with me about it and, as far as practicable, even provide me with assistance.

Jenkins acknowledged that the House of Lords judgement should be viewed not solely as a legal issue but in a wider context. As a matter of urgency, he was appointing an independent group, of both sexes and of legal and lay opinion, to advise him. This was a major step forward. As I pressed for women to be represented on this body, I was pleased to find, in due course, that the majority were women and Mrs Justice Heilbron was chairman.

While this group was examining the issues relating to rape, there was little to do except wait. But in June 1975, a month later, a separate but related issue arose. An eighteen-year-old man raped

two women in particularly brutal attacks. Forcing his way into the
home of the first one, he threatened her with a knife saying that she
had a nice face and he didn't want to spoil it; then he raped her.
Similarly with the second woman, he held a knife and threatened
that if she screamed it would go straight through her heart; then he
raped her. In court, after he pleaded guilty to these two vicious and
degrading crimes, Mr Justice Christmas Humphreys let him go free.

Sentencing him to a mere six months, which was suspended, the
judge said: 'The evidence against you is overwhelming. You lied to
the police to begin with and then confessed.' He added: 'Because of
your age and character and your shame and the fact that you have
parents who are going to keep an eye on you it is not necessary to
send you to prison.'

The rapist celebrated; the victims expressed their deep distress;
and I was outraged by this eccentric decision. I tabled a Motion
which deplored the judgement, described rape as 'a vicious and
degrading crime which should not be dismissed lightly' and called
upon Mr Justice Humphreys to resign or be removed forthwith.

The reaction from the legal establishment was to close ranks and
counter-attack. Mr Justice Humphreys countered by saying: 'Mr
Ashley probably knows only about 25 per cent of the background
and what goes on in a judge's mind. Don't forget I've been judging
and sentencing for twenty-five years. I do know what I'm doing.'
He betrayed his uncertainty, however, when he said: 'I may be
wrong – but my decision was right. I think I'm right.'

Lord Hailsham, a former Lord Chancellor, was far more vitupera-
tive in his counter-attack against me. Warning against encroachment
on the independence of the judiciary 'implicit in some recent actions
by some Members of Parliament', he said that demands for the
removal of a Crown Court judge by bringing political pressure to
bear on a Lord Chancellor began to constitute a serious danger to
judicial independence. Warming to his theme, though getting a bit
overheated, Hailsham went on: 'But to substitute for a judicial
process political pressures taking the form of savage denunciation of
individual judges . . . is indeed nothing but a modified and updated
form of mob rule.'

I could not take these words seriously. Hailsham's characteristic extravagance, however, did not obscure the serious point he was trying to make, which was that I was trying to substitute political pressures for a judicial process. Of course I was not. I was well aware of the need for an independent judicial system, but that did not mean abrogating all rights to criticize judges, or their sentencing policy. They were independent but not immune.

The issue was now attracting much media interest. Most comments were favourable, but there were some critics. The *Daily Telegraph* condemned my 'absurd' demand for the removal of Judge Humphreys and called it a petulant gesture. Lawyers were reported to be concerned, arguing that it was a basic rule of British justice that judges, like jurors, could not be punished for their verdicts.

A few days later, I took a deputation of MPs to the Lord Chancellor, Lord Elwyn Jones. He was friendly and placatory. While explaining that he had no powers to remove a judge, or to interfere in his decisions, he promised to discuss sentencing policy in rape cases with the Lord Chief Justice and, if necessary, issue special advice to judges. In addition, he was calling for a report on the Justice Humphreys case. Welcome as these developments were, I was surprised by his claim that he had no power to remove a judge so I checked with the Clerk of the House of Commons. Sir David Lidderdale, Counsel for the Speaker, said that the Lord Chancellor could remove a circuit judge on the grounds of incapacity or misbehaviour. Mr Justice Humphreys was a circuit judge.

I put this to Elwyn Jones and suggested that he could dismiss the judge, or ensure he was not allowed to hear further rape cases. Alternatively he could say that this dangerous precedent should not be followed by other judges, and lay down specific guidelines for sentences of rape. But when I took the deputation back to him just over a week later, he was much less amenable. The highly respected judge Lord Devlin had criticized him for agreeing to call for a report of the Justice Humphreys case. Elwyn Jones said that while he did not accept Devlin's criticism, it was important that he should not be seen to be telling judges how to do their job. Then he produced figures intended to prove that judges were not soft on rape. This was clearly a tougher line than at our first meeting, and we were more abrasive with each other.

Pauline analysed his figures, which proved to be unsatisfactory, and I told the Lord Chancellor so. I had frequently been told that the provision of a life sentence for rape meant that it was indeed taken seriously. But the figures showed that, of the 314 men convicted in 1973, only two got life sentences. Another 34 got over five years. The bulk of the sentences, 235, were for two to five years, while at the other end of the scale 43 got less than one year, a suspended sentence, a fine or probation. These were neither adequate nor consistent. I told the Lord Chancellor that legal bingo would do more damage to the judiciary than any criticism from MPs.

I aroused the ire of the legal establishment. The Lord Chief Justice, Lord Widgery, in a well-publicized speech, rejected my criticism of inconsistent sentencing for rape and condemned my call for the Lord Chancellor's intervention. The obvious unity between the Lord Chancellor and Lord Chief Justice was a clear indication of their opposition to change. Yet there were signs of movement. Sentences imposed by other judges for rape were becoming more realistic, and their comments were showing how seriously they took the crime.

In December 1975, the Heilbron Committee issued their report. While they were sitting, Mrs Justice Heilbron had invited me to give evidence and answer questions from her committee. I attended, accompanied by Pauline, and we found a friendly, intelligent, sensitive woman. She and her colleagues wanted to hear my views. Pauline, who had initiated many ideas throughout the campaign, left the talking to me. But on that occasion, as on so many others, she peppered her notes with suggestions which I could pick up when appropriate as the discussion proceeded. She put her own views in parentheses so that I knew how to differentiate between the notes she was making to supplement my lip-reading and her own comments. We left that meeting feeling that Mrs Justice Heilbron and her colleagues had listened carefully and taken account of our views, without necessarily accepting all of them.

In their report, the committee accepted many of my suggestions but they did not concede that an alleged rapist should have reasonable grounds for his view that a woman had consented. They supported the Law Lords' view that if *mens rea*, the intent to rape, was absent, it was irrelevant whether the belief that the woman consented was reasonable or not. They made the crucial point, however, that the absence of reasonable grounds for a man's claim of consent should be taken into account by juries when assessing the genuineness of his claim. In this way they were preserving the basic tenets of English law, yet ensuring that lack of reasonable grounds would be fully considered.

I was delighted that they accepted the proposal that publication of a raped woman's name should be forbidden. They also recommended that breach of anonymity should be a criminal offence. In addition they suggested that the cross-examination of private sex lives of rape victims should be banned, except in exceptional cases where judges felt this was necessary. A further recommendation was that of the twelve jury members in rape cases, no more than eight should be of the same sex.

These were major proposals of immense benefit to women which I warmly welcomed. But I knew that such reports are easily pigeon-holed in Whitehall, so I immediately drew up another Bill embodying most of the recommendations. The problem was how to get it implemented. Although the Home Secretary was now sympathetic, he had made it clear that the Government was short of Parliamentary time for legislation. Unless I could persuade an MP who had been successful in the ballot for Private Members' Bills to take on my Bill, the campaign objectives, and the Heilbron Committee recommendations, would dribble into the sand.

One of the six MPs who had won Parliamentary time in the recent ballot was Robin Corbett, a shrewd and compassionate MP whose judgement I respected. He did not have vast Parliamentary experience and had tentatively decided to take on another subject, but I put my Bill to him and he agreed to consider it. As the deadline grew closer I became a little anxious.

One afternoon, when he was on the back benches in the Chamber and Roy Jenkins was on the front bench, I engineered a meeting between them. I told Corbett that Jenkins was anxious that he

ACTS OF DEFIANCE

should take on my Bill and wanted to discuss it with him. He immediately agreed to talk with the Home Secretary, and I asked him to go to the Members' Lobby. Then I went to Jenkins and told him that Corbett was anxious to discuss my Bill with him and wanted to see him immediately in the Members' Lobby. He agreed to accompany me to the lobby, and the three of us discussed how best to proceed with the Bill. From there on it was relatively plain sailing!

Jenkins was supportive, and his civil servants helped in redrafting the Bill. Corbett piloted it through the Commons with great skill and dedication. There were one or two differences from the Heilbron Committee recommendations such as the proposal that a man accused of rape should also be given anonymity. The Heilbron Committee were opposed to this because they felt that an acquittal would give him full public vindication. I didn't think so because of the unique nature of rape and the public abhorrence of it. I felt that few men could ever really escape from this charge regardless of the courts' decision. I argued in the House that as 'the blaze of press publicity scorches anyone named in a rape case, guilty or innocent, naming them is wrong unless they are convicted'.

I claimed in addition that, if men charged with rape were to be named, women could damage a man's reputation by making a reck-less charge, secure in the knowledge that they would remain anony-mous while he would not. This would not help the cause of women. It was on these grounds that I supported the anonymity of men as well as women, and this was included in the eventual 1976 Act. To my regret, this decision was subsequently reversed by a Conservative Government in the Criminal Justice Act 1988.

However, the few differences with Heilbron did not obscure the important advances that had been made. The campaign resulted in the Sexual Offences (Amendment) Act 1976, which removed some of the advantages enjoyed by rapists in our courts of law and pro-tected victims from the ravages of damaging publicity. These changes would deter some rapists, and ease the public ordeal of rape victims.

14

Labour Government Backbencher 1974–9

In September 1974, I received a telephone call from a friend who was a press officer with the Labour Party. Would I take part in a party political television programme? I readily agreed, and she suggested that we use the natural setting of the garden of our home in Epsom. We arranged that I should be filmed playing badminton with my daughters before the interview. The film crew arrived. I began playing with Jackie and Jane as Pauline watched from the sidelines, when suddenly Caroline appeared hand in hand with Eamonn Andrews holding his famous red book *This Is Your Life*.

I was taken totally by surprise, and the cameras caught my expression. What they did not catch was my puzzled look at Pauline and her amused answering smile. Some years earlier she told me she had been approached by the producers who wanted to feature me but she declined. I was glad about this, so I had confidently assumed she would decline any further invitations.

When approached a second time she felt the time to be right and, using her own good judgement, accepted and kept it secret from me. I feared that the programme would be sentimental and embarrassing – but it turned out to be a happy occasion with my family and friends from all periods of my life. All my family were there and close friends came from Widnes. Norman St John Stevas spoke of my Cambridge days, the Cohelans flew in from the United States, and Barbara Castle and Michael Stewart talked about my Parliamentary career. It was also humorous. Michael Barratt got the biggest laugh of the evening when he recalled the time when as a television producer I sent him to Sweden to do a story on their shipyards: 'Well, would you believe, in one week in a year, the shipyards are locked, shut – everyone's gone off to the islands . . . that's the week he sent me to Sweden.' He also said I sent him with just £56 and booked him into the most expensive hotel in Europe so he could not afford food. 'I desperately wanted money, rang him up at the BBC, and of course he wasn't there. Where was he? In Widnes.'

The programme was transmitted on the night of the October 1974 General Election, a pleasant ending to electioneering. Since February 1974, when Heath's Government was defeated and Labour took office with a tiny majority of just four, the political temperature had remained high. No one doubted that another election would be held before the year was out. However, neither election was as tense for me as the one in 1970. There was no Wakes Weeks crisis, and I had an excellent agent in John Wallis. A railway signalman, he was a warm, caring but determined man. He and his wife Jean were to become close friends. In later years he stood for the City Council in the ward in which he lived. Although opposed by a popular and well-entrenched Tory councillor, he kept fighting despite successive defeats; after four losing campaigns, he eventually won his Council seat and went on to become Lord Mayor of Stoke-on-Trent.

An election agent is responsible for the whole complex organization of a campaign and he or she controls the constituency party. A good agent can win an election and a bad one lose it. John pitched into the election campaigns with characteristic energy. In the first one, he was conscious of his responsibilities and aware of his inexperience. He worried about every aspect, yet he was effective, winning co-operation from people because of his good nature and obvious concern to get things right. If he had a fault it was that he was too kind to wind up conversations either on the telephone or face to face, and consequently worked very long hours. I was fortunate to have him.

There was a striking contrast between the two election campaigns. In February, everyone was enthusiastic because Ted Heath was unpopular and they worked hard to get rid of him. The great objective was the return of a Labour Government. But in October, Heath was a figure of the past, a comfortable Labour majority was likely, and party workers did not welcome a re-run of their efforts so soon after the previous election. Many of them were busy councillors, but we managed to conduct a workmanlike campaign.

In that October election, the Labour Government achieved a satisfactory majority of forty-two. My own majority was 16,495, which was the highest of the three Stoke constituencies, and I was delighted with the result.

The 1974 elections brought a change in my Parliamentary role. The Labour Party was again the Government, and that February Barbara Castle was appointed Secretary of State for Health and Social Services. Soon afterwards she asked me to go to see her and invited me to become her Parliamentary Private Secretary. I was uncertain how to respond. As Michael Stewart's PPS, in my early years, I had been very active attending numerous meetings on his behalf. But the loss of my hearing had forced a reassessment of my Parliamentary priorities: I was now a campaigner rather than a committee man. Constant lengthy meetings were exhausting, but I was able to campaign against injustice. I knew how to present a case and, equally important, persist against strong opposition. Campaigning needed a high profile, however, and this would not be possible on health and social security issues if I became her PPS. On the other hand, I would be able to exercise influence inside the Department. I was interested in drug safety and disablement, as well as health, all relevant to Barbara's responsibilities. Would I achieve more by campaigning outside her department or by operating within it? Weighing up the advantages and disadvantages, I decided to accept.

Barbara had given me staunch support during the thalidomide campaign, and I knew that I could work happily with her. I was also close to other Ministers in the Department. They included one of my early Parliamentary friends, David Owen, who became Minister of State for Health, and Alf Morris, from the disability field, who was made a Parliamentary Under-Secretary. Barbara's specialist adviser, Professor Brian Abel-Smith, was an old friend from our Cambridge days when we were both active in the Labour Club and

Union Society. I did not know then that although Barbara called my appointment one of her 'inspirations', her husband, Ted, was opposed because it was 'sentimental'; she said in her diaries that her instinct told her he was wrong. She also said that the Prime Minister, Harold Wilson, 'warmed to the idea'. My acceptance began an intriguing two years inside the Department.

A complex personality, Barbara was fiery and formidable yet sometimes vulnerable. As a Departmental head, she was in full command; yet as an MP she was as meek and subservient to the Whips as the humblest Member. When her regional Whip, Jimmy Dunn, insisted that she stayed for votes in the early hours, no matter how exhausting her day had been, she stayed.

At the dispatch box in the House of Commons, she was fluent and passionate. Easily aroused, she would set about the opposition; to heckle her was to boost her adrenalin and provoke an even more rumbustious response. At her regular Monday morning Ministerial meetings, however, a more thoughtful, sensitive personality emerged. She sat at the head of a long, polished table in the Secretary of State's imposing room at the Department's headquarters at the Elephant and Castle, surrounded by her Ministers, adviser, personal assistant and me. Barbara mapped the agenda and made all the important decisions, yet she accorded full weight to the views of all those present. If agreement could not be reached, she instinctively knew when to overrule and when to give way gracefully.

At these complex meetings, Jack Straw, her political adviser, supplemented my lip-reading with voluminous notes. Fast, and often humorous, they were of tremendous help. Later, he was to win Barbara's Parliamentary seat at Blackburn when she retired from Westminster and went to the European Parliament. A barrister, he had the gift of quickly mastering complex briefs. Keen application allied to a lively wit made him a formidable debater and in due course he became a leading politician.

Barbara derived great benefit from having Brian Abel-Smith as a specialist adviser and Jack Straw as a political one. Untrammelled by Departmental protocol, and in touch with outside interests, they were able to give her fresh, alternative opinions.

(232)

At these regular meetings, we discussed the major policies of the Department, such as priorities in the NHS and social services, doctors' and nurses' salaries, pension schemes, pay-beds and many others. The contrast of styles between different Ministers was interesting, especially between Barbara and David Owen whose personalities were strikingly different. She was passionate and determined – though more diplomatic than her public image suggested – whereas he was detached. She laughed a lot; he smiled. The subtle interplay of these two was further complicated by their respective positions in the political spectrum; Barbara was on the left of the Labour Party, David on the right.

Although she was obviously boss, Barbara devolved considerable responsibility to David. He was authoritative, with a touch of natural arrogance, and although he always fought hard, he never pushed his views to the point of open conflict. The two respected each other and made a formidable pair.

The Monday meetings carried on through the lunch hour. I had heard that, in some Departments, lunch and wine were served. Whether or not that was the case, we could buy only unappetizing egg or ham sandwiches. Some of us took our own, Alf Morris taking bacon sandwiches and Jack Straw an apple and a piece of cheese. So the great affairs of state, and the fate of the nation's health services, were settled over these.

Barbara's capacity for hard work seemed limitless. I would saunter into her room after midnight to find her beavering away at her desk on which were piled three or four red boxes of documents.

'Let's have a drink,' I would suggest.

'Help yourself,' she would smile. 'I can't; I've got to finish these tonight', gesturing to the red boxes.

As she was also writing a daily diary at that time, it must have been a very late bedtime for her. Next day, she would still be the bright and energetic dynamo, driving the Department relentlessly.

No matter how busy she was, two things had a high priority. Visits by her husband Ted were very welcome, and she was obviously delighted to see him. Attention to her flaming red coiffure was also important, especially before a television appearance. Barbara was feminine and tough. I have occasionally speculated since her heyday what a riveting political drama it would have been if she and Margaret Thatcher had been of the same generation and directly opposed.

My close relationship with Barbara was of tremendous help to a number of campaigns which I held dear. She wrote in her *Diaries*: 'One by one I am trying to take his pet projects on board.' I tried my best to help her, keeping her informed of backbench opinion, discussing tactics and strategy and giving my views on the important issues. The job was far from easy. Contacting other backbenchers and seeking their views could be troublesome because of my deafness, and the most frustrating experience of all was when Barbara was speaking in the House or answering Parliamentary Questions. I had to sit behind her, and although I knew of her speeches beforehand, and had copies of the initial replies to Parliamentary Questions, it was a trial to be unable to lip-read her. But she was very understanding and more than made up for the frustration by her sensitivity and warmth towards me, something which continued after she went to the House of Lords.

One day in November 1974, as I was strolling through the Members' Lobby, Harold Wilson's PPS, Charles Morris, said Harold would like to see me. In his office behind the Speaker's chair, I found an amiable Prime Minister. 'I just thought you may like to know that I'm going to recommend that you should become a Privy Councillor,' he said. I was delighted by this totally unexpected honour. Membership of the Privy Council, a body which advises the Queen, would be especially valuable to me because the honour confers seniority in the House. If I were to become a Privy Councillor, I would be given preference in debates, and would no longer have to sit lip-reading for many hours. I thanked Wilson and after a few more words, conscious of the pressures on him, took my leave. I had no idea what the next step was to be and did not like to ask him. I would have asked Barbara Castle had I known at the time that she knew of this move. She recorded in her *Diaries* that Harold Wilson, having to appoint a Privy Councillor, said that 'he was left with only Roy Hattersley or Bill Rodgers, and he wasn't going to elevate either of them'. Hattersley was Minister of State at the Foreign Office and Rodgers Minister of State for Defence. Wilson's 'brilliant idea', she said, was to appoint me.

Brilliant or not, something – I have never discovered what – happened to change the plan. To my surprise I received a formal letter from Wilson a few weeks later saying that he had it in mind to recommend that I should be a Companion of Honour and asked if I would accept. I was mystified. Like many people I had no idea what most honours meant. So I borrowed a book from the library to find out. The CH was quite a distinction; the Order, restricted to sixty-five people, ranked higher than a knighthood. I could not find any comparison between the CH and the Privy Council. The press was no guide; when the Honours List is published, one newspaper puts the CH, if any are awarded, above the Privy Council while another gives precedence to the latter. That year, I became a Companion of Honour and Hattersley a Privy Councillor.

However, distinguished as it was, the CH gave me no precedence in Parliament. Nor was it generally understood. Despite its eminence, I received letters from people expressing disappointment with my award because they thought I should have got a knighthood. They knew as little as I had done.

One pleasant aspect of the CH was a twenty-minute personal audience with the Queen at Buckingham Palace. I went along with Pauline and Caroline, who was then eight years old. Caroline was allowed to explore a coach in the courtyard while Pauline and I were received informally by the Queen. Sensing that she was uncertain as to where she should sit to make lip-reading easiest for me, Pauline suggested that she should take one of the chairs near the windows with the light on her face. The Queen readily concurred. Relaxed, friendly and even humorous, she obviously appreciated the problems of total deafness. Throughout, as we chatted about my work and campaigns, she spoke clearly for me so there was little if any difficulty in following her. Her presentation of the exquisite medal at the end of our conversation was made without fuss but with casual and touching warmth.

My work as Barbara's PPS did not prevent me from being active in other spheres. Unlike many MPs in the 1970s, I always went to the annual party conference. Although I missed some of the noisy excitement because of deafness, I enjoyed them. Pauline always came and eased the strain of lip-reading with her notes. Despite the frequent disputes, there was still a great feeling of comradeship at conference. Many people felt they knew me personally, having seen me on television with my various campaigns, and I enjoyed a warm welcome.

Some constituencies sent the same delegate year after year, and the trade union representatives usually remained unchanged. So it was a bit like a holiday camp, greeting old friends and talking about issues of mutual interest. I felt at ease there and I always tried to speak. I was usually lucky enough to be called. At first I found it strange addressing thousands, in what was for me a silent conference hall, using a powerful microphone. Pauline would keep in my line of vision in case I was too quiet or too loud, but my old instincts worked well, and she never needed to signal.

I was pleased, but not hopeful, when in 1974 some colleagues suggested I should stand for the Labour Party's ruling body, the National Executive Committee. The seven constituency members were chosen by the constituency parties, whereas the rest of the NEC places were determined by the trade union vote. When the results were announced I was surprised and delighted to have got 205,000 votes; of those not elected, only Eric Heffer had more. At that time many constituency parties were predominantly left-wing, and I did not expect to be popular with them. The only right-winger elected in the constituency section in 1974 was Denis Healey, then Chancellor of the Exchequer.

The following year, 1975, Heffer was elected with 277,000 and I was the runner-up, ahead of Denis Healey, who lost his seat, Tony Crosland and Peter Shore, each of whom was a Cabinet Minister. When Barbara's *Diaries* were published some five years later, I was amused to note an acerbic comment in her entry for the day these results were declared. All her references to me as her PPS were favourable, even warm; but she must have reverted to left-wing tribalism that day. Commenting on the increased votes for victorious left-wing candidates, she said they were 'symptomatic, I suppose, of the party's mood of protest, though with typical illogic local parties put Jack Ashley, a well-known right-winger, in first place as runner-up, giving him 28,000 more votes than Denis [Healey]! Such are the quirks of democracy.' A quirk in her *Diaries* was that all her favourable mentions of me were noted in the index, but this one was omitted!

The next year, 1976, I was again runner-up. Soon after the election, Michael Foot became Deputy Leader to Jim Callaghan, thus becoming an ex-officio member. As runner-up, I automatically moved up and, to my great delight, became a member of the National Executive.

At the first meeting, in the historic conference room of Transport House, where the Labour leaders of the past had argued party policy, I found a remarkably relaxed and informal atmosphere. Was this really the place where the headlined party 'rows' took place? Sometimes it was like a family squabble. The informality was exemplified by Joan Lestor, when she was chairman. After an angry outburst by Eric Heffer against the Prime Minister, Jim Callaghan, she snapped, 'Oh, come off it, Eric. Shut up and let's get on with the business.' This was not the kind of ruling one got in the House of Commons but none the less effective for that; it was accepted without argument by Heffer. Most NEC members had been together in politics for years, and they had the kind of relationship that exists in a large and rowdy family, cantankerous at times but kept together by a basic bond.

It was agreed that Pauline could attend to help me with notes, and so began a period of fascinating meetings. I had no experience of the bitter divisions in the Labour Party during the days of Hugh Gaitskell and Nye Bevan, although they were obviously cataclysmic. In the 1970s, if the difference were not as bitter, they were certainly deep, and at the NEC they were clearly evident. As a result, members tended to be preoccupied with differences rather than the things they had in common.

Although there were many left-wingers on the NEC, their master of manoeuvre was Ian Mikardo. Some of the stories about Mikardo were legendary. In 1945, he dazzled a Labour conference with an electrifying speech in favour of nationalization. When he left the rostrum, Herbert Morrison said to him, 'Young man, that was a brilliant speech. But you do realize you have lost us the election?' Mikardo has been described as a man with a dark, faintly sinister face who could frighten more timid souls. The best-known remark about him was by Winston Churchill, who said, 'Mikardo is not as nice as he looks.'

At the NEC meetings, he spent much of the time reading the *Sporting Life* and seemed uninterested in the proceedings. After most people had spoken, however, he would intervene, analysing the most important points made, deftly attacking right-wingers, then shrewdly offering a 'compromise'. His compromises were probably what he had planned in the first place, but they were so cunningly presented that he appeared to be going out of his way to accommodate the other side. It was a political education to observe him.

At the next conference, rather to the surprise of the pundits, I was successful in the ballot and became an elected member. As Denis Healey later observed, he, Jim Callaghan and myself were the only three non-left-wingers to be elected in the constituency section between 1952 and 1987.

The debates, usually lively, sometimes angry, were always difficult for moderates, as the Left dominated the National Executive during my membership. They were also well organized, and I suspected that they worked at their tactics before the meetings, whereas the Right did not. The Left was then striving for constitutional reform, and one of the main objectives was to introduce reselection of MPs. Naturally, reselection did not commend itself to sitting MPs, but they were reluctant to speak against because most constituency parties favoured it. However, at a meeting of the Parliamentary Labour Party, I was critical, and a report of my comments appeared in the *Guardian*. The reaction was immediate. Scores of identically worded letters arrived from constituency Labour parties all over Britain supporting the principle and demanding to know why I was against it. They were clearly organized; whoever was behind the reselection campaign was working overtime.

Ironically, Ian Mikardo, one of the main supporters of reselection, was also attacked because he sought a genuine and sensible compromise, which left each constituency party to decide whether or not to activate the reselection procedure. The 'Mikardo compromise', as it came to be called, angered the Left, who took their revenge on their most outstanding tactician – and on me as well for my criticism at the PLP. At the next NEC elections in 1978, both Mikardo and I were defeated, to be replaced by Neil Kinnock and Dennis Skinner. After the election results had been announced at the party conference, I was due to respond from the platform to a motion on the death grant. It gave me the opportunity to quip about giving my own funeral oration.

It was expected that Neil Kinnock would win a seat on the NEC. When I congratulated him, he and his wife Glenys were exuberant. Although I was disappointed at losing, I was genuinely glad for him because I liked him and recognized him as a man of the future. His election to the NEC was a vital stepping stone to the eventual leadership of the party.

Dennis Skinner has made his own distinctive contribution in Parliament as well as on the NEC. An abrasive and earthy character, he is the living embodiment of the class war, confronting all Tories with hostility or suspicion. To a lesser extent, he mistrusts assorted opponents in the minority parties and treats right-wing MPs in his own party with disdain.

In his early years in Parliament, Skinner was himself treated with disdain by the Tories, who saw him as a rabble rouser who lacked respect for Parliamentary procedure and had more brawn than brains. He would have accepted the first criticism but soon disabused his opponents about his intelligence. He was shrewd, incisive and well informed. Although he had scant respect for Parliamentary procedure, he was a master of it. Successive Speakers were irritated and exasperated by his insolent, confident and often well-founded challenges to their authority.

Unflinching and dogmatic, he would never accept a 'pair' (an agreement that neither would vote) with political opponents, as nearly all other MPs did, in order to take a night off. I even found him unwilling to sign my Motions if a Tory was among the sponsors. As Chairman of the All-Party Disablement Group I often tabled Motions sharing sponsorship with MPs from other parties. Dennis would examine them and, the moment he spotted a Tory signature, scornfully reject them. Nevertheless he was generous about my work. On one much later occasion, in 1989, the Sunday *Observer* asked some MPs to choose the best backbench MP in their series 'The Experts' Expert'. Dennis was selected, but he himself chose me for what he called 'sheer persistence on important issues over a quarter of a century', and 'because he has been so effective over the years'. Coming from someone who acknowledged that we disagreed politically, it was a singular compliment.

From 1976 to 1978, when I was a member of the NEC, Jim Callaghan was Prime Minister and Party Leader, but he was not treated within the NEC with the kind of deference he received at 10 Downing Street and elsewhere. Constantly harried by the Left, often beleaguered, he displayed great strength and common sense. In practically every clash, I came down strongly on his side, because I shared his views and values.

On one occasion in the House, however, I lost my temper with Callaghan with embarrassing consequences. At Prime Minister's Question Time I asked him about unemployment; his response appeared to me to be a brief, curt dismissal. Angrily jumping to my feet on a point of order in a crowded House of Commons, I accused him of being 'arrogant'. He was the least arrogant person in the world. One of his greatest attributes was that despite holding the highest office he was never pompous. He remained unchanged, sensible, tough, fair and friendly. But because I was stung by his apparently dismissive rejection of my question, I threw this charge at him. Naturally the Tories opposite cheered, and I noticed Margaret Thatcher and Nigel Lawson nodding enthusiastically. Labour MPs sat silently observing this regrettable episode. They knew that for years I had supported him in the House, the NEC and elsewhere, and they were as taken aback as he was. I cooled down very quickly and knew that I had made a mistake by an unfair and unreasonable attack.

In retrospect, I can only hazard a guess as to why this happened. It may have been that to me the words, without hearing the tone of voice, seemed dismissive. I am sure, looking back, that they were not. Perhaps I was overstressed that day, or it may simply have been my determination never to be pushed around which, on this occasion, went too far. I wrote and apologized next day and received an undeservedly warm and generous letter from him saying he had not intended to upset me and was glad that I had written.

A major element of an MP's work is related to his constituency. Regular advice bureaux, a stream of letters from constituents and the local authorities, formal meetings and casual conversations all work together to create a strong, sensitive relationship. General issues can be taken up by any MP, but I was very conscious that only I, as Stoke South's MP, could take up local problems. So I was always anxious to be vigilant with constituency issues. One of the major issues in Stoke South was subsidence due to extensive coal-mining. I sometimes wondered how middle-class people in the suburbs of the south of England would feel if they had a dusty coal-mine across the road or backing on to their rear garden. The people of Stoke-on-Trent accepted the environmental blight of local mines with tolerance and good nature; perhaps because it was the livelihood of many, and they had no choice. But subsidence was different. They rightly felt that cracked walls and ceilings should be repaired by the Coal Board if mining could have been the cause. I agreed and fought many a subsidence battle on their behalf.

The law relating to subsidence is the opposite of innocent until proved guilty. It places the burden of proof for disclaiming responsibility for damage on the Coal Board, and I produced many detailed arguments on why the board should pay up. One of my party members, who happened to work for the local Coal Board, told me the management used to wince when they got 'yet another letter from that Jack Ashley'.

A variant of these troubles occurred in 1975 and 1976, when a series of earth tremors shook houses in the Trent Vale area of my constituency. In the first year alone, there were fifty tremors.

Walls cracked, flying china ducks flew from the walls, chimney pots fell, radiators rattled, and people ran panic-stricken into the streets. One man said: 'It was so bad I thought somebody had crashed into the house. I was nearly shaken off the settee and I thought the walls were going to cave in.' No one knew of the tremors in advance except a resident's dog which would dash for shelter under a settee just beforehand.

I visited the area to see the damage and talk to people. My arrival seemed to reassure them that as their representative was taking the reins all would be well. It did not turn out that way. As I was talking to them, another tremor occurred which jolted not only their houses but their faith. The local newspaper reported the comment of one woman, who said: 'I was leaning on the window-sill watching Mr Ashley. It was terrible. I can't stand much more of this.' I like to think she was referring to the tremor rather than my presence.

I found it difficult to believe that these events were natural phenomena. Suspecting a man-made cause, I called for compensation from the Coal Board, the most likely culprit, as well as a safety check on gas supplies. Without so much as a pause for breath, the Coal Board disclaimed responsibility. The Area Director wrote to me: 'it would be wrong at this stage to conclude that the alleged tremors are the result of current mining subsidence and that the Board should accept responsibility.'

There was no shortage of people who were certain of the cause of tremors. For water diviners it was heavy rainfall or an abundance of sunshine; for geologists and astronomers it was problems miles below and miles above the surface.

Reliable instant answers would have been welcome, but as they were not available there was no alternative to the slow grind of careful investigation. A working party was set up and an emergency relief fund established. Sophisticated seismology equipment, so sensitive it could record earth movements as far away as Turkey, was brought into the city.

The funding of this equipment, initially by the City Council and the Coal Board, became a source of dispute between the Secretary of

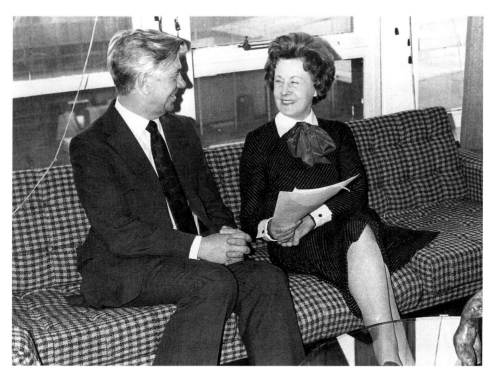

20. Parliamentary Private Secretary to Barbara Castle, Secretary of State for (Health and) Social Services, 1974.

21. With Neil Kinnock, at Stoke-on-Trent, 1986.

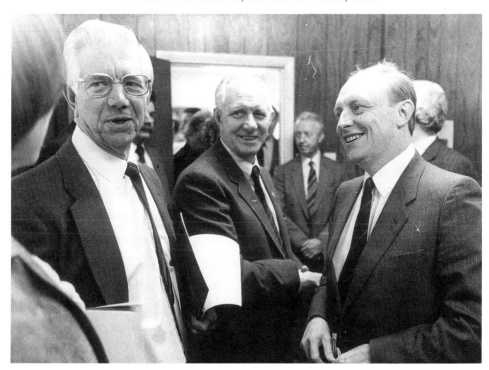

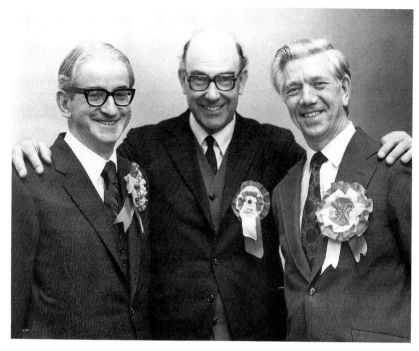

22. The three MPs of Stoke-on-Trent, having retained their seats in the 1970 election. Left, Bob Cant; centre, John Forrester.

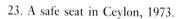

23. A safe seat in Ceylon, 1973.

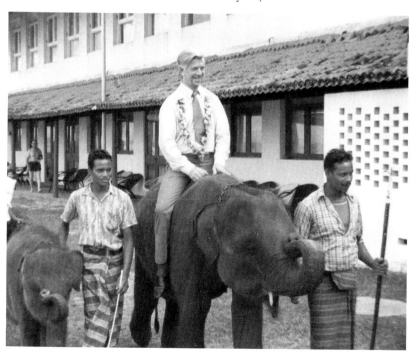

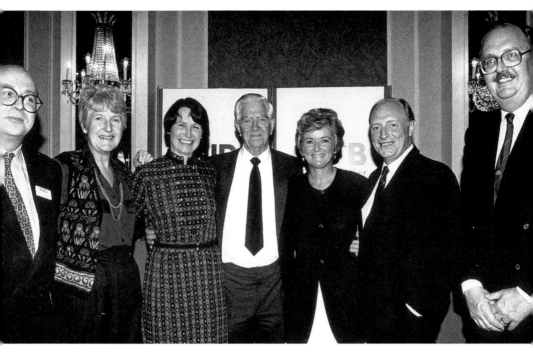

24. Celebrating twenty-five years in Parliament. Left to right: Stuart Etherington, Director of the RNID, Winifred Tumin, Chairman of the RNID, Pauline, Jack, Glenys and Neil Kinnock, and John Edmunds, General Secretary of the GMB Union.

25. Displaying caricatures from the House of Commons magazine. Left to right: Jack, Speaker George Thomas, Sir Keith Joseph and David Steel.

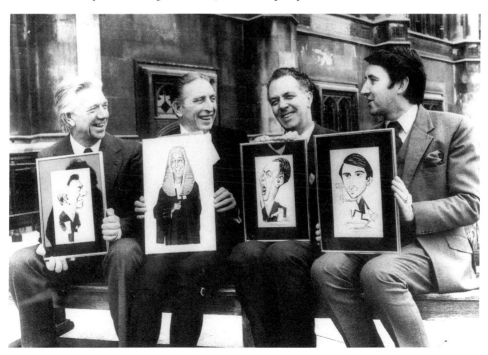

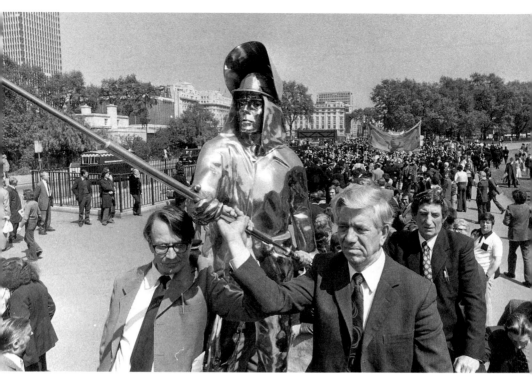

26. Marching with the steelworkers of Shelton in Hyde Park, 1975.

27. With former neighbours of Wellington Street, Widnes.

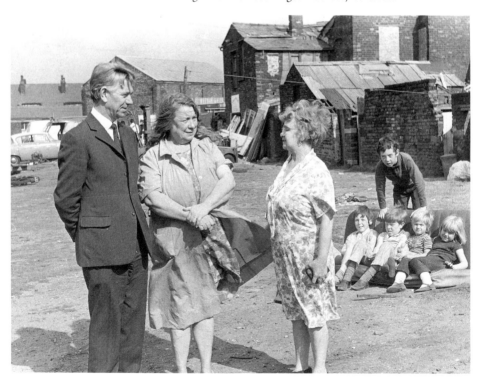

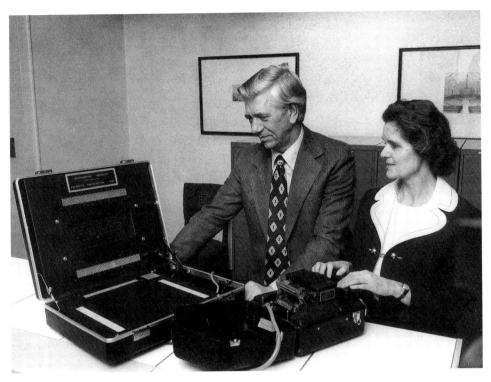

28. With Isla Beard, the Palantype operator.

29. The first official keyboard reading from the Palantype machine.

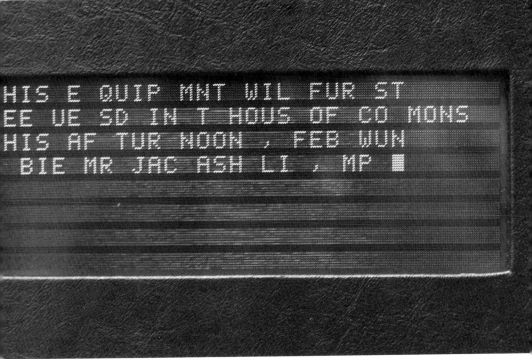

HIS E QUIP MNT WIL FUR ST
EE UE SD IN T HOUS OF CO MONS
HIS AF TUR NOON , FEB WUN
 BIE MR JAC ASH LI , MP

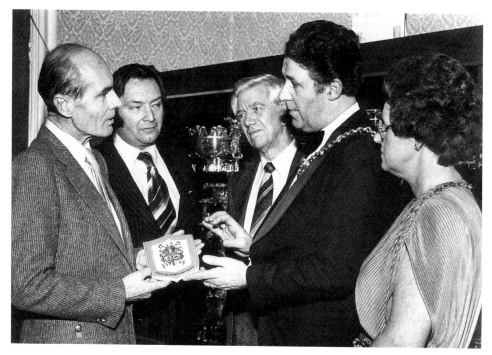

30. With Group Captain Leonard Cheshire (far left), receiving a city plaque from the Lord Mayor of Stoke-on-Trent, Jack's agent, John Wallis.

31. Protesting outside the House of Commons with a youngster on behalf of the Disablement Income Group, 14 November 1972.

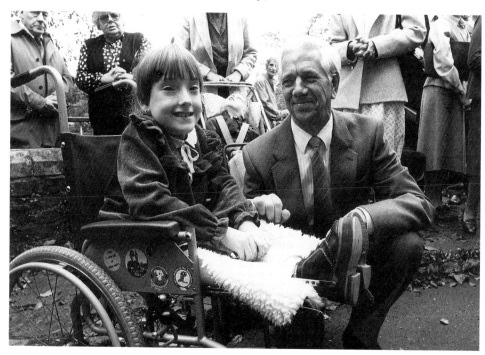

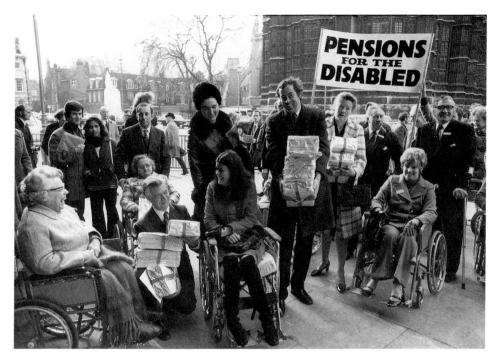

32. Jack receives a petition for a national disability income from disabled people outside the House of Commons, November 1972. Mary Greaves, Director of the Disablement Income Group, is on the extreme left.

33. Meeting Princess Diana at the Café Royal Young Deaf Achievers luncheon, 1989, with Mrs Gobel, wife of the British Telecom director (centre), and Pauline (right).

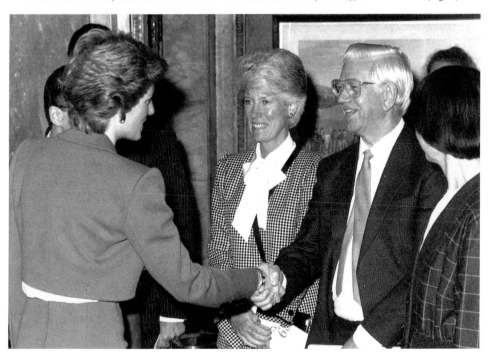

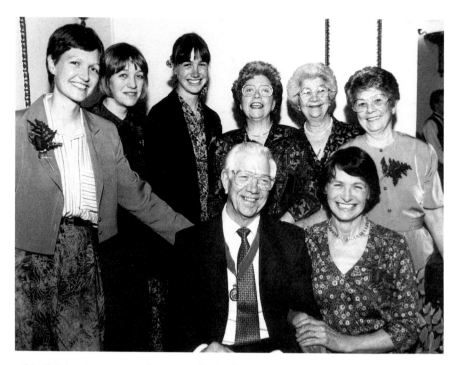

34. Celebrating twenty-five years in Parliament at Stoke Labour Party Dinner, with all the family. Left to right: Jane, Jackie, Caroline, Margaret, Mary and Helen. Pauline managed to persuade Jack to wear his Companion of Honour medal for the first and only time.

35. With grandson Harry, then aged two, London 1991.

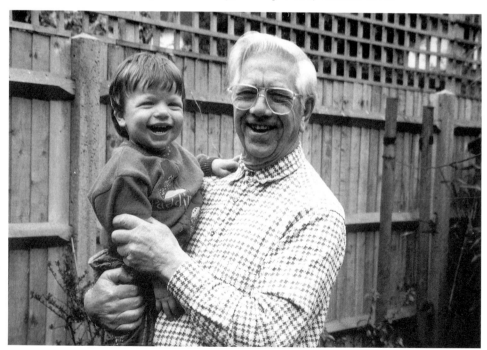

State for the Environment, Tony Crosland, and myself. We had become friends since meeting at the BBC when I was a television producer, and I had been to his home for dinner with him and his wife, Susan. One of the few first-class political theorists in the Parliamentary Labour Party, he seemed to be wryly amused at politics and politicians. His slight air of academic detachment did not, however, disguise deep commitment and great achievement. His early death soon after his appointment as Foreign Secretary was a tragic loss to the party and the country.

When I asked him to fund the equipment until the investigation was complete, he refused on the grounds that the Institute of Geological Sciences had advised him that it needed to withdraw equipment and staff to use elsewhere. Remarkably, he said: 'I am bound to accept this advice.' He was bound to do no such thing. As Secretary of State he was free to disregard advice from any quarter. Crosland had the responsibility, not shared by the Institute, to consider the social problems of those affected by the damage. I put these points to him, but apart from extending the period by a few months, he stood by the Institute's advice.

Soon afterwards, in April 1976, Peter Shore took over as Secretary of State for the Environment. I expected a battle with him. In an Adjournment debate, on 27 April 1976, I said that if the equipment did not stay as long as required 'I'm afraid that the Department and I are due for a long, hard, relentless grinding battle and there is no question whatever of me withdrawing.' To my surprise, and delight, Shore's Minister of State, Denis Howell, promised that both the equipment and advisers would stay in Stoke-on-Trent until the cause of the tremors was found, and that the Government would 'contribute effectively' to the cost. This was confirmed a week later by Peter Shore when I questioned him in the Commons.

So what was the cause of the tremors? There were two geological faults nearby and some NCB apologists pointed to these. However, mining had been carried on for two hundred years, and the underground was honeycombed with old workings which could collapse at any time. Aware of this, but unwilling to accept responsibility, one Coal Board official attributed the trouble to an 'Act of God'.

(243)

Residents responded that as the tremors only occurred when the pits were working, God must have been on a five-day week. They added that there were no tremors at weekends or during Wakes Weeks when the miners were on holiday.

Eventually the residents were proved right. The working party concluded that tremors were caused by mining, thus making non-sense of the Coal Board's repudiation of responsibility. Whereupon the board changed its mind, admitted responsibility and gave an assurance that mining in the relevant area would stop. Apart from some further argument about compensation to people living outside accepted subsidence zones, the board dealt sympathetically with claims and even contributed to the legal fees of people outside the zone. After two hectic years, tremors and their consequences were laid to rest.

The traditional industries of Stoke-on-Trent have long been pottery, coal-mining and steel. Shelton steelworks was small by modern standards, but with its long history it was important in the city. When it was announced in the early 1970s that 2,200 men were to lose their jobs because steel could be produced more cheaply at Scunthorpe, local people were outraged. The battle for Shelton began, led by Ted Smith, a fiery but thoughtful shop steward. Although Shelton was not in my constituency it was nearby and was of concern to the whole of Stoke-on-Trent. All the Stoke MPs took part in lively discussions, demonstrations and marches both in the city and in London. Even the local theatre participated, producing a play about the battle. Nevertheless, despite the magnificent campaign, the steelworks closed and the men lost their jobs. A symbol of the struggle, a steel cast of a steelworker, was prominently displayed throughout, and it now stands outside the museum, a reminder to all who took part in a losing but memorable fight.

Meanwhile, in the House of Commons, there were other subjects I wanted to press. Many people for whom I had campaigned had been in touch with lawyers at one time or another and they told me of their dissatisfaction with legal services. Inadequate solicitors or barristers, the rigid demarcation of function and the costs and delays all caused concern. In particular, people were dismayed by the lack of legal representation at tribunals, the informal courts which adjudicate on a wide range of benefits and entitlements of immense importance to people on low incomes.

I discovered in 1975 that poor people appearing before tribunals, except for specialized bodies like Mental Health Review Tribunals, were denied legal aid for representation. One hundred and thirty thousand people appeared before tribunals every year; they included old and disabled people, widows, war pensioners, redundant workers and immigrants, appealing about supplementary benefit, national insurance, pensions, redundancy, rent and tenancy agreements, and immigration. Without legal representation, most claimants could not contend with skilled and expert legal advocates used by Government Departments, employers and landlords. I wrote to the Lord Chancellor, Lord Elwyn Jones, somewhat stridently claiming this was 'outrageous' and accusing him of 'perpetuating injustice'.

I was to have many clashes with Elwyn Jones. Ever courteous, he must have been sorely tried by my many demands, especially when I telephoned him at home to press some point. On one occasion, I argued with him over the telephone, not knowing that he was in the middle of a birthday party. I learned later from one of his guests that, as he returned to the table, the normally serene Elwyn muttered, 'It was that bloody Jack Ashley.'

Not surprisingly, he was irritated by my constant pressure; sometimes he replied in kind. 'You have written in very forthright terms,' he responded, 'and I will try to reply equally directly.' He said that my case was based on the fallacy that if legal aid were made available for tribunals the imbalance between rich and poor would swiftly be corrected. 'I think this is much too superficial an approach.'

There was nothing superficial in my proposal that he should either allow poor individuals legal representation under the legal aid scheme or ban it for the organizations opposing them. That would be fairer than allowing the wealthy a legal advantage. He rejected this on the dubious grounds that if lawyers were withdrawn from tribunals it would be difficult to establish a satisfactory system in future. Legal aid, he said, would be extended to tribunals when the resources became available. My response was that, by depriving the poor of legal representation to match the legal advocates against them, 'we shackle the Davids and strengthen the Goliaths'.

A few weeks later, Elwyn Jones wrote saying he now fully accepted that in certain cases legal representation was needed before a tribunal. He added: 'I should very much like to be in a position to extend legal aid in the way you suggest.' But, he said, he was under pressure to make funds available for law centres – salaried lawyers working in the community – for example the Citizens' Advice Bureaux, and to raise the limits of the legal aid scheme. I appreciated his difficulties but was not satisfied.

Meanwhile, I presented a Bill in Parliament to change the system of allocating legal aid, aiming to take it from the control of the Law Society and place it under a new Legal Services Commission. The Law Society's prime function was protecting the legal profession's interests, whereas an independent commission could administer legal aid without any conflict of interest.

Shortly afterwards, I heard that an investigation by a Reader in Law at the London School of Economics, Michael Zander, had found that the cost to public funds of lawyers' fees for legal aid recipients in Crown Courts was some £24 million a year, but there was virtually no information about the way this money was made up or spent. Some members of the Bar Council were predictably offended by his findings and his call for an independent inquiry.

All these criticisms had a common thread: the inadequacy of the legal profession. So I began a campaign for a Royal Commission on the operations of the profession. On 6 January 1976, I wrote to the Prime Minister, Harold Wilson, asking him to set up such a commission. I suggested that it should investigate the legal profession's services, funding, monopoly rights of barristers, distinctions between them and solicitors, and unmet legal need. That call was reinforced by Parliamentary Questions and a Motion signed by over a hundred MPs.

Many lawyers, including the Lord Chancellor, were naturally opposed, but the *New Law Journal* supported the campaign: 'That it should be conceded, we have no doubt at all.' A leading article in *The Times*, while cautiously commenting that Royal Commissions ought not to be advocated lightly, concluded in favour of the proposal. Michael Zander was actively advocating it in articles and broadcasts, while less publicly, but of greater importance, Bernard Donoghue, head of the Prime Minister's policy unit, was pressing it at No. 10 Downing Street. He told me that Wilson was supportive.

On 12 February 1976, one month and six days after I had put the proposal forward, Wilson announced in the House that a Royal Commission on the Legal Profession was to be set up. Writing to me that day, he said he hoped I would agree that the terms of reference had fully met my wish to see a wide-ranging inquiry, because they effectively covered all the matters I and others had raised with him. So they had. It had been the shortest campaign I had known.

The next important question was the composition of the Royal Commission and its chairmanship. Bernard Donoghue proposed that the chairman should be either Adrian Cadbury, John Freeman, Peter Parker, Asa Briggs or Alec Cairncross, each of whom would have been a radical appointment. It appeared, however, that during the interregnum between Harold Wilson's and Jim Callaghan's Premiership, the Lord Chancellor's Department launched a shrewd counter-attack by nominating a conservative accountant, Sir Henry Benson, and he was chosen.

Although there were some excellent members, including Joe Haines, Press Secretary to Harold Wilson, Ralf Dahrendorf, Director of the London School of Economics, and Peter Oppenheimer, an Oxford don, the commission's eventual report was far from radical. Lacking dynamism, deferential to the legal profession and facing public indifference, it did not recommend sweeping change. The lawyers breathed easily again.

Ironically, thirteen years later, it was a reforming Tory Lord Chancellor, Lord Mackay, who introduced radical reforms. With his Legal Services Act 1990 solicitors were given new rights of audience and permitted to make conditional (no win no fee) agreements. But most important, and an echo from my campaign, was a 'Legal

Services Ombudsman' to oversee the handling of complaints against lawyers by their professional bodies. This was just the kind of impartial, investigative authority required.

When Jim Callaghan replaced Harold Wilson as Prime Minister in April 1976, he sacked Barbara Castle as Secretary of State for Social Services. David Ennals replaced her and invited me to be his PPS. I declined, mainly because I wanted more time and freedom to do what I knew best – campaign as a backbencher.

One of these campaigns concerned lenient sentences. Since my attempt to change the law on rape, I had been interested in sentencing policy because of the eccentric sentences of some judges. A sentence could be reconsidered on appeal if the convicted person felt it was excessive, and as judges sometimes erred by imposing excessively heavy punishment, this was reasonable. They could, however, also err by excessive leniency. One affected the individual, the other affected society. I felt that the one-way system of appeal against sentences was wrong, and both sides should have the right of appeal.

Another bizarre judgement induced me to press for appeals against lenient sentences. A guardsman, guilty of violent sexual assault, although gaoled for three years by the judge, was freed by the Court of Appeal, which said that a prison sentence would damage the man's career. I felt that men threw away their careers with their humanity when they embarked on crimes of sexual violence and they did not deserve special consideration. When the Court of Appeal stated that the man 'allowed his enthusiasm for sex to overcome his normal good behaviour', I retorted that the Great Train Robbers allowed their enthusiasm for money to overcome their normal good behaviour, but they were gaoled for thirty years.

I decided to go ahead with a Bill for appeals against lenient sentences. Although I wanted this to apply to all sentences, I confined it to sexual offences. I thought the prospects were better if I did this because some notoriously lenient judgements had recently been made. On 19 July 1977, the Bill I presented to the House gave the prosecution the right of appeal against lenient sentences for rape and other sexual offences. I argued that this right was already established in many other countries, and it was needed in Britain.

The Bill was opposed by a flamboyant Scottish lawyer, Nicholas Fairbairn, who claimed that in cases of rape there were so many variants and differences that criticism of the judge or judgement was dangerous. When a person had been brought to trial, found guilty of an offence and sentenced, that should be the end of the legal process. Disappointingly my Bill was lost by a vote of 114 against 52.

Some MPs opposed it because they feared double jeopardy. Others were influenced by Fairbairn's view that women can make false protestations of rape. I suspected that this argument had a disproportionate effect on them. Some months afterwards I brought in another Bill which gave the prosecution the right to appeal against the sentence for any crime. Presenting this on 14 February 1978, I quoted the case of a man given one year's gaol on a manslaughter charge after a policeman was killed. Such a case should be reviewed by the Court of Appeal; if there were mitigating circumstances to justify the lenient sentence, it would remain unchanged. Otherwise, it should be corrected.

Fairbairn again opposed the Bill. He reiterated the familiar arguments, adding that it would be 'improper' for a person to be unsure of his sentence until the prosecution had decided whether or not to appeal. Remarkably, only 30 MPs voted for my Bill and 293 against.

I was sure I was right, but given such an overwhelming vote against, there was no point in pursuing the issue. It was ironic that nine years later a Government Bill providing for the prosecution's right of appeal against lenient sentences was introduced by a Conservative Home Secretary, Douglas Hurd, and after a hiatus caused by the 1987 General Election, this was enacted in 1988. It was doubly ironic that this provision was embodied in the Criminal Justice Bill 1988 which resulted in a substantial reduction of civil liberties and I was consequently obliged to vote against the Bill as a whole. The compensating irony was that many Tory MPs who had indignantly opposed my original proposal trooped into the lobby to vote for it.

One of the interesting aspects of an MP's life is its diversity. During this period I campaigned for compensation for the relatives of those killed in the DC jumbo jet that crashed near Paris in 1975. With the US Ambassador I made the first ever transatlantic telephone call by a totally deaf person, typing the words carried over a telephone line, and opening up a new method of communication for deaf people. In what turned out to be a fruitless task, I also attempted to get compensation for deformed babies allegedly damaged because their mothers took hormone pregnancy tests.

I also spent much time trying to prevent the gas and electricity industries from using their monopoly power to cut off supplies to poor people who could not pay bills. I felt they should follow normal commercial procedures for unpaid bills, which were reminder letters followed by court action, if necessary, for repayment of debt. It was a vigorous campaign which did not succeed, although it did lead to the Government negotiating a code of practice with the fuel industries. This prevented disconnections of poor pensioners in winter, and gave £25 million to help people in difficulty with their fuel bills.

Similar marginal gains followed my efforts to secure the compulsory licensing of estate agents. At that time the 25,000 estate agents could choose from some ten different organizations to represent them or they could belong to none. Although I won no short-term gains, legislation was enacted in 1979, and extended in 1991, which limited the scope for dishonesty.

All these activities kept me busy, but I regretted missing visits abroad which many other MPs undertook. I had greatly enjoyed being on the delegation to Zambia before I lost my hearing.

When I became deaf no invitations to me were forthcoming, although many of my colleagues were travelling on Parliamentary delegations to various parts of the world. I mentioned this to the Chief Whip, Bob Mellish, who was friendly but non-committal. Within weeks, however, he told me that I was to go on a Parliamentary delegation to the Far East. Under the auspices of the Ministry of Defence, we visited military installations in the Far East and spoke to service personnel of all ranks.

The highlight of our tour was visiting Hong Kong, one of the last outposts of the old Empire. It was a glittering sight in the evening as our plane lowered itself into the bustling city, ablaze with light. The Governor, Sir Murray MacLehose, the military commanders and men in the garrisons all appeared confident, and so did the political and business leaders we met. At that time the reversion to Chinese autonomy seemed a small and distant shadow.

During my visit, a shipload of refugees lay just outside Hong Kong waters, refused entry by the authorities. That ship, and its unhappy passengers, became the centre of passionate controversy. Should it be allowed in, and the refugees be permitted to land? The visiting MPs were asked their opinion by Hong Kong journalists. I condemned the refusal of the authorities and urged them to permit entry on humanitarian grounds. I went to see the UN Commissioner for Refugees, who spoke in sympathetic but general terms, and afterwards I made more outspoken public comments. At a subsequent press conference, I faced some highly critical questions from hostile Hong Kong journalists.

All the Government officials I discussed it with were courteous and discreet although they too had undoubtedly had their fill of visiting MPs, dropping in for a few days, telling them how to run the colony and then returning to Britain unaffected by the proposed solution. On a subsequent visit to Hong Kong, some years later, I was chatting to the Governor, Sir David Wilson, and I told him of my earlier condemnation of the authorities but I could not remember the name of the boat. 'It was the *Huey Fong*,' he said. I congratulated him on his memory. He smiled. 'I was the civil servant in charge of immigration at that time.'

The *Huey Fong* was allowed into Hong Kong harbour on 19 January 1979, nearly a month after its arrival. In a letter he wrote to me ten years later, Sir David told me: 'The arrival of that ship presaged a massive flood of arrivals from Vietnam, mostly coming in small boats . . . from the beginning of 1979 to the present time some 150,000 people have arrived here from Vietnam.' My haranguing, therefore, may have played a minor part in the major problem of refugees which has bedevilled Hong Kong for so long.

Throughout these hectic years I did what I could to support and sustain the Labour Government. By 1979, however, it was enduring a difficult time and the fates seemed to be turning against it. With our perilous dependence on the Liberals in Parliament, we all knew that a crucial test was approaching. When it finally arrived, it was the end of an era.

15

Vaccine-Damaged Children

Helen, the second daughter of a Shipston-on-Stour housewife, Rosemary Fox, was born on 8 February 1962, a cheerful, robust baby. She was dubbed 'Hugh Gaitskell' because of a remote facial likeness and a tuft of hair on her forehead. For seven months she enjoyed excellent health and a happy, normal babyhood; but then, after a vaccination, her life was devastated. Severely brain-damaged, she suffers major convulsions, has neither talked nor learned anything since, and spends her time with building bricks and jigsaws.

The reason for this tragedy emerged six years later when Rosemary met an Oxford paediatrician who had researched vaccine damage. Helen was brain-damaged probably as a result of her polio injection. At first, Rosemary was relieved at a diagnosis she found believable and for a few years she was optimistic that Helen would be merely 'a bit slow'. Then in 1972, doctors advised that she would become worse over the years.

Fearing the long-term future, Rosemary, together with another mother, decided to find out how many other families were similarly affected. An article in the *Birmingham Post* resulted in twenty-eight letters, and these led to the founding of the Association of Parents of Vaccine Damaged Children.

Immunization has an honoured place in the long struggle against infectious disease. It has virtually eliminated smallpox and greatly reduced the prevalence of polio; and the numbers dying of measles, diphtheria and whooping-cough have declined drastically during this century. But so too has the number dying from scarlet fever for which there has been no vaccine.

In Victorian times, thousands of children died annually from infectious diseases. The great reduction in the death toll since those days has come from improved public health and individual living conditions. For example, deaths from whooping-cough fell from around 200 per million children per year at the beginning of the century to 6 per million in 1957, just before the vaccine was introduced for general use. Nevertheless the vaccine has been beneficial. Notifications of the disease fell from 85,000 in England and Wales in 1957 to 15,286 in 1990. The falls were welcome because whooping-cough, in addition to being distressing for both child and mother, can have long-term disabling effects.

Since vaccination began, the medical profession had been aware that, in rare cases, it can damage. Some doctors took care to screen out children thought to be at serious risk of an adverse reaction. In the 1970s, some experts believed that, of all vaccines, the whooping-cough vaccine was the least safe because, to make it effective, more of the active toxins had to be left in than with other widely used vaccines such as those for diphtheria and tetanus.

Rosemary Fox's Association included parents of children allegedly damaged by a variety of vaccines, and her own daughter was affected by the polio vaccine. Nevertheless, the whooping-cough vaccine became the focus of attention. Individual children benefit from vaccination because it helps them avoid the disease. Other children also benefit because, as the number of cases declines, so too does the risk of contact with an infected person. This so-called 'herd effect' was important with whooping-cough because, in the 1960s and 1970s, a child would be nearly one year old before completing their course of vaccination, and for a child of that age any serious risk of death from the disease had passed. So each child vaccinated reduced the prevalence of the disease as well as being protected themselves – and the first benefit was perhaps greater than the second.

In the early 1970s, other countries such as Germany and Japan acknowledged vaccine damage and compensated the children. But Britain refused to follow suit. So a campaign was launched by

Rosemary Fox, whom I first met on 26 September 1973. A quiet but determined woman, she moved me with the story of her experience; when she asked me to help her campaign, I readily agreed. At that time, the Conservative Government was still in office. I immediately wrote to Sir Keith Joseph, the Secretary of State for Social Services, asking for Government help. He left it to his Parliamentary Under-Secretary, Michael Alison, who replied with some head-patting comments.

Most adverse reactions, Alison said, were of a minor kind. I knew that already but I also knew there were some major reactions which destroyed the minds of children, and shattered the lives of their families. Regarding these Alison merely said he fully shared my concern. He did not, however, propose to do anything about them. His main point was that the protection afforded by vaccines outweighed 'occasional harmful reactions' and that vaccines were carefully controlled, monitored and improved. It was reassuring stuff for innocents but no help for the desperate families.

I challenged Alison's claim that only a 'very small' number suffered permanent damage. In an Adjournment debate on 31 January 1974, I asked him to say how small was 'very small'. Admitting under pressure that 'the majority' of adverse reactions were not reported, he dodged the question about specific numbers. But he admitted that about 170 reports of adverse reactions to vaccines were received each year. I knew that the medical profession acknowledged that doctors grossly under-reported damage caused by drugs. Estimates suggested that only one case in ten was reported. If the tenfold factor applied equally to vaccines, some 1,700 children might be suffering damage from adverse reactions every year.

As for compensation, Alison said it was neither appropriate nor feasible. Yet of course it was feasible – six other countries had schemes. Some of the many letters I was receiving showed how appropriate compensation would be for horrifyingly damaged children and anxious parents. One mother from Pembroke wrote:

At 13 Carolyn cannot walk, talk or help herself in any way. She is incontinent and has major epileptic fits which often result in pneumonia, although I have a supply of antibiotics and three suction units at home. Carolyn cannot even hold her head up and is of no mental age at all. She is tall and quite strong. We love her dearly and cherish and care for her 24 hours a day, but I feel dreadful that all this happened through an injection that should have prevented disease.

The mother of a boy born in Blackpool wrote similarly:

The same night he had the injection, he awoke screaming. He was rolling his eyes and jerking . . . ever since that day . . . he cannot help himself in any way, he cannot walk, talk, is still incontinent and has to be washed, dressed and fed. He has had the fits daily ever since the night of his injection; he can have as many as 12 a day. He has had to have three drugs three times a day for the last nine-and-a-half years, and has to continually wear a crash helmet to avoid injury to himself.

Incredibly it appeared that, at this time, some of the damage caused by the whooping-cough vaccine was unnecessary. Children had been vaccinated when there were contra-indications such as fever, a history of fits or serious reaction to the first vaccination making them vulnerable to damage. I quoted a study by Dr John Wilson, a paediatrician at Great Ormond Street Hospital, who found that no less than one-third of the children brain-damaged by vaccination should not have been vaccinated because of contra-indications.

The medical profession was aroused by the publicity, and its journals contained many claims and counter-claims on the value of the whooping-cough vaccine. But little interest was shown in the question of compensation for damage from this and other vaccines.

A year earlier, a Royal Commission had been set up under the chairmanship of Lord Pearson to consider civil liability and compensation for personal injury. Not only was the Government determined to wait for its report, but the Prime Minister, Edward Heath, said: 'No recommendation the commission may make could have any retrospective effect.' This statement upset the families in Rosemary's

Association. Their hopes had been raised by my Parliamentary activities only to be dashed by the Prime Minister's ruling. Despite this, they continued to campaign, accumulating case histories and adding to their membership.

I worked closely with them, but after the Labour victory in the February 1974 General Election Barbara Castle became Secretary of State for Health and Social Services and I became her Parliamentary Private Secretary; so I was unable to continue public campaigning. Other MPs nibbled at the subject, but none carried out a vigorous or sustained campaign. However, I kept in touch with Rosemary and arranged for Barbara to meet her. It was a formal meeting with two civil servants in attendance, but it was also friendly. I was disappointed that little substantial progress was made, although Rosemary subsequently told me that Barbara's personal advice to her was excellent. She said: 'There is no point in just saying you want compensation. Make your case, circulate it and then stick to the arguments you have made.' That is just what the Association did.

Because of my concern over the slow progress achieved, I warned at a Department of Health Ministerial meeting that I might resign as PPS if the claims were neglected. Barbara, who would normally have bridled at such a threat, diplomatically moved on to next business. I had to decide whether to leave in protest or continue helping on the wide range of major national issues in her Department. I was in two minds but I carried on, pressing the vaccine case whenever I could, although unable to raise it in the House. This was one of the factors which led me to refuse the invitation from David Ennals to be his PPS when in 1976 he succeeded Barbara Castle as Secretary of State.

With my new-found freedom, I began tabling a mass of Parliamentary Questions that Pauline had drafted. Ennals delegated the job of replying to his Under-Secretary for the Disabled, Alf Morris. In what the *New Scientist* called 'a dusty 400 word reply', he said that vaccination publicity was essentially a matter for individual doctors and health authorities, and – that old chestnut – it was a matter of 'clinical judgement' how much warning should be given to a patient. He adopted the Tory line when he said that he was unable to comment on the merits or procedures of particular compensation schemes, or on possible developments, in advance of the report of the Royal Commission.

Parents were distressed by Alf Morris's stonewalling response. I attended the Association's next annual meeting and was moved by the sadness and despair they expressed. Their children, healthy and happy before vaccination, had been transformed into pathetic babies, mindless, paralysed, deaf or blind. They agonized about when they could no longer care for the children. What would happen to them? Parents did not want them to go into institutional care, which was often of low quality. They were anxious to care for their children themselves in a loving home environment. The parents were seeking either a substantial lump sum in compensation, or a regular lifetime income adjusted for the degree of disability. They sought a scheme like those for servicemen or workers injured at the workplace. The damage done to their children was the result of no ordinary accident; it followed a specific Government-sponsored vaccination programme. They therefore sought specific Government financial help. Yet the Government was stubbornly refusing to provide it. Fortunately, Rosemary Fox was undaunted, continuing to plan, press and sustain all the other families. Her patient and courageous conduct heartened them all.

To outflank Ministers I asked the Ombudsman, Sir Idwal Pugh, to examine whether there had been official maladministration. He agreed to do so providing he was given specific individual or group complaints of alleged failures to warn of possible danger from whooping-cough vaccination. Rosemary provided these, and I told him of warnings given in the 1950s before mass vaccination was adopted. No sick child should be vaccinated, and if there was an untoward reaction to the first injection, there should be no more. The Medical Research Council trials of the vaccine in the early 1950s had excluded children considered to be at risk. But when local authorities were circulated in July 1957 with details of the procedure to be adopted for mass vaccination, there was no mention that some children could be at risk.

A further source of danger was that although the MRC trials

were conducted on children with an average age of well over one, the Department advised vaccination at three months and later at six months. One eminent virologist, Professor Dick, had pointedly asked: 'How did it come about that it was assumed that babies of only a few months of age would react in the same way as babies twice their weight?'

I asked the Ombudsman to investigate four cases which were typical of the many tragedies of vaccine damage. One child, with a family history of epilepsy, lost most mental and physical faculties after vaccination. Another, whose vaccinations were continued despite damage after the first injection, was retarded with no speech. Similarly, an adverse reaction was ignored with another child who became brain-damaged. In the fourth case the child, vaccinated four months after premature birth, suffered brain damage and constant convulsions.

Responding to pressure from me inside Parliament, and from Rosemary outside, on 8 February 1977, Ennals gave the House a lengthy explanation of the Government's position. Parents were reacting to the controversy by rejecting vaccination, and the big drop in take-up obviously alarmed him. Figures for diphtheria, tetanus and polio vaccination had fallen by 25 to 30 per cent in the last three years, and there had been an even steeper fall of nearly 60 per cent in whooping-cough vaccinations.

Reiterating his support for offering whooping-cough vaccine to babies, he claimed that the gains outweighed the risk. Vaccination caused about two cases of brain damage a year, whereas the disease of whooping-cough caused four.

Despite Ennals's admission of a brain-damage risk from the vaccine, he still refused to pay compensation to vaccine-damaged children, saying: 'I cannot consider the claims for vaccine-damaged children in isolation.' Repeating that he could not pre-empt the Pearson Royal Commission Report, he rejected my claim that an independent inquiry into the whooping-cough vaccine was necessary in view of the conflict among medical experts.

He was angrily attacked by MPs supporting me on all sides of the House. Tory MP Gerard Vaughan, later to be a Minister for Health himself, reminded him that six other European countries had compensation schemes. Labour MP Robin Corbett asked him to confirm that he and not the Royal Commission was running the Department.

I protested that a Government should not be prohibited from action by a Royal Commission. Harold Wilson had objected to the Tory Government using this device about thalidomide in 1972. At that time he told the then Prime Minister, Edward Heath, 'that the right of the Government to initiate legislation . . . will not be prejudiced by the setting up of a Royal Commission'.

I was concerned that the whole immunization programme could be damaged by the compensation dispute, but I was careful to say that I did not blame Ennals for that: 'he must do what he thinks is right. I must do what I think is right.' Soon after, however, stories began to appear in the press implying that Rosemary Fox and I were responsible for the reduced take-up of vaccines which was putting babies at risk. I felt sure that they were inspired by the Department to convey a message to me: 'Be quiet or be blamed.' I was furious.

I sought a confrontation with Ennals, and it took place a week later on 17 February 1977 in an unusually dramatic Adjournment debate. Because these debates take place late at night, a junior Minister usually replies; but on this occasion David Ennals, the Secretary of State, accepted the challenge. At 11.43 p.m. I began the attack. I told him that it was a story of 'Government incompetence, neglect and even deceit'. Healthy children whose lives had been 'shattered by blindness, deafness, paralysis or screaming convulsions' had been brushed aside. The risks of vaccination had been hidden from families, who had become tragic victims of crass official ineptitude, and as a result the crucial immunization programme was in jeopardy. Parents were resentful that a Government could advocate an immunization programme yet shirk its responsibility when things went wrong.

Naturally I repeated the crucial point that, while the community at large benefited through a high level of population immunity, it was the individual who bore the risk. As for Ennals's statement that only two children a year were damaged by whooping-cough vaccine, he was relying on the fact that only twenty-two cases of vaccine brain-damage were reported to the Committee on Safety of Medicines in the eleven years 1964–75. Yet the Department had admitted that most damage was not reported by doctors. In just one London children's hospital there had been more cases of alleged vaccine brain damage than were reported in eleven years to the CSM.

In a virulent attack I said that the Department was arrogant, dogmatic and intransigent. The only reason for Ennals's delaying action, I argued, was to ingratiate himself with the Treasury at the expense of helpless children – a shoddy bargain no self-respecting Secretary of State would touch with a barge-pole.

By now Ennals was looking grim, possibly wondering if he had been wise to come and sit through this. His reply was in kind, but with more restraint. I had accused him, he said, of being arrogant and dogmatic, but he had rarely heard a presentation of a case which was itself more arrogant and dogmatic than mine.

He insisted on awaiting the report of the Pearson Royal Commission and said there was no special obligation to pay vaccine-damaged children. One of his arguments was that the Department also recommended regular dental check-ups and treatment and there was always a small chance of serious damage from an anaesthetic. This flawed analogy revealed the weakness of his case, because children had dental treatment solely for their own benefit, whereas they were vaccinated in part for the social good.

Ennals admitted that not all vaccine damage had been reported, and, as he put it, 'the estimate of vaccine brain damage could be on the low side'. But he then accused me of creating serious dangers for children, whose health and lives might be put at risk, by insisting that I was right and the medical experts wrong.

At this I exploded. He knew quite well that I had not argued with any medical experts. Because I was not a doctor, I had scrupulously refrained from personally commenting on the vaccines. It was doctors from the universities of Manchester and Glasgow and London's Charing Cross Hospital who were critical. One of them wrote: 'Many, myself among them, regard the [whooping-cough] vaccine as

relatively ineffective and potentially harmful.' It was precisely because of this medical controversy that I had called for an independent
inquiry to try to resolve the conflict between doctors.

The last thing I would do would be to give a medical opinion.
Yet here was the Secretary of State for Social Services accusing me
in the House of Commons of insisting that I was right and medical
experts were wrong. I was beside myself with anger. He concluded
by proclaiming, 'to all parents throughout the country', that they
should not be misled by statements made by me, 'otherwise they
will put the safety of their children at risk'.

At thirteen minutes past midnight, with the Chamber silent as
Ennals collected his papers, I could not contain myself. I shouted:
'That was a shabby and squalid speech. The Minister should be
ashamed of himself. He didn't answer a single question that I put to
him. It was shocking.' On that bitter and angry note, David Ennals
strode out of the Chamber at one end, and I left from the other.

Throughout this emotional campaign, Pauline and I worked together, and I relied heavily on her research. Ennals had countless
doctors, scientists and civil servants to help him. The three of us,
Rosemary, Pauline and I, were a tiny group taking on a determined,
major Government Department. Despite support in Parliament, and
in the press, we seemed to be making very little progress. I was
beginning to receive abusive letters from the public. One doctor
accused me in a medical magazine of irresponsibility about the
deaths of unvaccinated babies. When I took legal advice and threatened a libel action, he apologized and paid me damages and the legal
costs, but the slur had been publicized. I was stung by the injustice
of these accusations.

As the Government was not budging, there was nothing for it but
to return again to the attack. Just over two weeks later, on 7 March
1977, I secured another Adjournment debate, this time at 2 a.m. In
my speech I accused Ennals himself of being directly responsible for
the damage to the immunization scheme because he had not responded to the widely supported call for compensation. By blaming
the campaigners, he was trying to shift responsibility and taking the
easy way out, and I was having none of it.

I pressed again for an independent inquiry into the whooping-cough vaccine and again I attacked Ennals's figures on vaccine damage. This time I gave a devastating quote from the Chairman of the Committee on Safety of Medicines, Sir Eric Scowen, who had confirmed that most vaccine damage was not reported: 'I don't know why the Secretary of State gave a figure [of two per year] for adverse effect of whooping-cough vaccine. I would not have given one. The data are not sufficiently reliable.'

The crux of Ennals's case was that the risk of brain damage from whooping-cough was greater than that from vaccination. He claimed that as many as four children a year were brain-damaged by the disease, but Pauline had discovered that this was based on one study which found two brain-damaged children among 8,000 who had had the disease. As there were some 16,000 cases of whooping-cough annually, the Department had simply doubled the two and claimed that the disease annually caused four children to be brain-damaged.

Unfortunately for Ennals, the detail of the research study showed that it was doubtful if one of the original cases had been due to whooping-cough – the child had recovered from it five weeks earlier – and, very important, both the children had recovered. His arguments rested on unsound figures, and I scathingly accused him of making a false statement in the House, abusing people who challenged him, hiding relevant facts in the dispute and defying Parliamentary opinion.

By now, the press was inflicting fearful damage on Ennals. Following a savage personal attack in the *Spectator*, the *Daily Mail* published a major article, 'The Blunders of David Ennals', subheaded 'Why he is the most disastrous Minister of Health in recent times'. No one had attacked Ennals more strongly than I, but I confined my criticism to his handling of the vaccine-damage issue. These articles, I felt, were vindictive. The *Daily Mail* was making political capital out of a non-party issue. Ennals was a scrupulous, sensitive man who I believed had made an error of judgement. By no stretch of the imagination was he the most disastrous Minister ever at the Department of Health; he had many fine achievements to his credit.

So, in the middle of my bitter wrangle with Ennals, I wrote to the

(263)

Daily Mail defending him and attacking their unjustified 'sweeping condemnation' of him. Ennals was no doubt bemused when the *Daily Mail* published my letter. The blows inflicted on him by the campaign, and the reduced take-up of vaccination, must have affected him. Apart from that, he was probably personally touched by the plight of the children. He began to indicate personal sympathy. When he met Rosemary and me, just before a rally of the parents, he seemed anxious to assure us that work was being done to help.

If he was accepting our case for paying compensation, the long and bitter battle was surely ending. But how could the Government surrender gracefully when it had irrevocably committed itself to awaiting the report of the Pearson Royal Commission, not due until near the end of the year, and maybe even later?

The answer came with an imaginative move. The Prime Minister, Jim Callaghan, wrote to the Chairman of the Royal Commission on 6 June 1977 and said that it would 'go far to relieve the anxieties and concern of myself and my colleagues, and to restore public confidence, if you were able to assure me that the Commission will be dealing specifically with the problem of vaccine damage and to give an indication of your thinking at this stage'.

Within three days Lord Pearson replied:

> The Royal Commission has indeed got very much in mind the problem of vaccine damage. We see it as a particular part of a very difficult field with which our Report will have to deal, but we have all reached the conclusion that some kind of financial assistance should be made available for very serious injury resulting from vaccination recommended by a public health authority.

This great news was followed by a statement to Parliament five days later. On 14 June, David Ennals announced that 'in the light of the conclusion which the Royal Commission has reached, the Government has decided to accept in principle that there should be a scheme of payments for the benefit of those who are seriously damaged as a result of vaccination, and that it will apply to existing, as well as new, cases'.

(264)

That was it. Payment was to be made and it was retrospective back to the founding of the National Health Service in 1948. It appeared that victory had been achieved, although I hoped, rather than assumed, that the payments would be generous. In his statement Ennals paid tribute to me and to Rosemary Fox and her colleagues in the Association for their efforts, restraint and concern. Pauline, having played no public part, was not mentioned, but she had made a significant contribution.

A few months later, in October 1977, the Ombudsman reported. He said the Department should have recognized earlier the desirability of alerting parents to possible reactions to whooping-cough vaccination. He noted that it was not until Rosemary's Association raised the issue in 1974 that the Department belatedly considered giving specific warnings to parents about these.

We had still to await the Royal Commission's report. The details of the scheme, including the criteria and amounts, could not be determined until this was published on 15 March 1978, some five months later.

Within two months of the report's publication, on 9 May, Ennals announced that the Government's payment scheme would provide £10,000, tax free, for those who had been severely damaged by vaccination since 1948. I was deeply disappointed. Ten thousand pounds abysmally failed to meet the lifelong needs of the children. I welcomed it as an interim measure but pointed out that it was only about three years' average earnings, and the children involved were irretrievably damaged for life. The Pearson Commission had recommended strict liability; this would mean that there would only have to be proof that a child was damaged by vaccination for him or her to receive a court award amounting in 1978 to about £115,000. I asked Ennals to introduce an adequate scheme.

Pleading for time, he gave an assurance that 'nothing I have said will pre-empt decisions which the Government still have to take on Pearson, and nothing . . . will prejudice the rights of those who will receive a lump sum payment from taking action in the future'. He was careful to say, however, that the payment was not compensation. The Government was intent on not admitting liability which would make it vulnerable to demands for realistic compensation.

As the Vaccine Damage Payments Bill passed its various stages in Parliament, I tried to amend it, particularly the provision that only those with 80 per cent damage or more would be paid. I felt strongly that all those damaged by vaccines should be paid proportionately to the damage suffered, as in the industrial injuries scheme. I also sought payment for those damaged before 1948. Ennals was adamant, however, and I was unable to extend the scope of the Bill.

The payments scheme, a step forward rather than a solution, was regarded by parents as an interim measure, though the Government had avoided saying this. The following year, in May 1979, Labour was swept from office and replaced by Margaret Thatcher's administration. Patrick Jenkin took over from David Ennals as Secretary of State, and Gerard Vaughan became Minister of Health. It soon became clear, however, that the new Government also was not prepared to pay adequate compensation. Patrick Jenkin ruled out any such scheme, claiming that it would mean cuts in other directions.

In Opposition, although both men had been sympathetic, neither had declared themselves unequivocally in favour of full compensation, although Vaughan had invited Rosemary Fox to discuss 'the pension idea'.

The families, indignant at Jenkin's attitude, had assumed that their previous support would be translated into legislative action. But the Ministers had taken care to avoid hostages to fortune, and they could not be pinned down. I maintained the pressure with repeated protests and scores of questions.

When Ennals was Secretary of State, he and his medical advisers had been embarrassed by his gaffe over the statistics about damage from the vaccine and the disease. Consequently the Committee on Vaccination and Immunization had commissioned a major investigation of all brain-damaged children hospitalized over a period of many months to assess the prevalence of brain damage from vaccination. The report of the National Childhood Encephalopathy Study, published in 1981, concluded that the evidence suggested that 'although the proof is not absolute, roughly one in 100,000 children who get the full course of whooping-cough vaccine may be damaged in some way'. But the committee believed that this was outweighed by the deaths and damage caused by the disease itself, although it provided no evidence of the extent of these.

With approximately 700,000 births a year, if all parents took the Government's advice and had their children vaccinated against whooping-cough, there would be some seven cases of severe brain damage every year. The number was small, but the individual tragedy was gigantic. If such small numbers were to be the future trend it was all the more reason for the Government to afford proper compensation. But it soon became clear that the case for proper compensation would continue to be rejected by the Government despite considerable media publicity and two Parliamentary lobbies by the families in 1983 and 1984.

In the early 1980s the parents, despairing of effective Parliamentary help, began to discuss legal action. Vaccine damage was soon plunged into a legal morass. The first case, brought on behalf of a sixteen-year-old, Johnnie Kinnear, collapsed because the negligence claim was not sustainable. Disappointed but not disheartened, the families made a further legal claim, and in 1982, the parents of Susan Loveday, an eleven-year-old girl, sued her doctor for damages when she suffered brain damage after whooping-cough vaccination. Hundreds of other claims depended on this case, which became a legal marathon, lasting till March 1988. The trial itself lasted four months. The court heard evidence from nineteen expert witnesses; and the judgement, read over two days, ran to 14 chapters, 6 appendices and over 100,000 words.

The case cost an estimated £1 million from the legal aid fund and an estimated £1.5 million in costs incurred by the pharmaceutical company, the Wellcome Foundation, which asked to be joint defendants with the former GP of the Lovedays, even though no negligence was alleged against the company.

The judge chose first to decide on the preliminary, but fundamental, question of whether the vaccine could be shown to cause damage. His judgement was a disaster for the families. Lord Justice Stuart-Smith held that 'it could not be shown on the balance of probabilities that pertussis [whooping-cough] vaccine could cause permanent brain damage in young children. It was possible that it did: the contrary cannot be proved.'

The families and I were incredulous. The judge's finding ran counter to beliefs long accepted in Britain; to an Act of Parliament; to the experience in courts in the USA where many whooping-cough vaccine victims had won damages; to the practice of six European countries with vaccine damage payments schemes; and to the actions of the Swedish health authorities, who had so little confidence in all whooping-cough vaccines then that they refused to have a Government-sponsored programme, despite a high level of whooping-cough. All these were being swept aside by one judge declaring that there was no proof that the whooping-cough vaccine caused damage. The most criticized vaccine of all was being given almost complete clearance. If the decision stood, the parents were worse off than if there had been no court action, as the judge's decision was bound to influence the Government's Vaccine Damage Payments Scheme.

The solicitors representing Susan Loveday wanted to appeal, but to get legal aid, they had to present a strong legal argument for doing so. The QCs concerned condemned Judge Stuart-Smith's decision as 'unsound'. They claimed he appeared 'to have thought of a number of reasons for disparaging or devaluing the evidence of the Plaintiff's clinician witnesses'. His attack on one of these witnesses, they said, was 'in many respects unfair and unwarranted'.

In the opinion of the QCs, 'the entire reasoning and conclusions of the Judge relating to the National Childhood Encephalopathy Study were misconceived and erroneous'. They quoted examples where he 'dismisses or disparages articles supportive of the Plaintiff's case yet uncritically accepts and relies on those which assist the Defendant's'.

Yet, despite their strong attack on the judgement, the QCs concluded that they could not recommend an appeal. This was because, although they believed the whooping-cough vaccine could cause damage, they did not think Susan Loveday was herself damaged by the vaccine, and accordingly her personal case would fail. The QCs' view blocked a legal-aid-funded appeal because, whatever the significance of the general 'causal' ruling – and it was very significant – legal aid can only be given to an individual who has a chance of success. The Loveday family had no resources for an appeal, and I was unable to find a philanthropist willing to help all the families with a challenge on causation. The Loveday case collapsed, and with it many people's hopes.

The Department of Health moved quickly and quietly. No vaccine damage payments were made for whooping-cough damage after the Loveday judgement. It was delivered on 29 March 1988, but the change of policy was only revealed in the spring of 1990 in response to Parliamentary Questions.

At a meeting with the Under-Secretary at the Department, and subsequently in letters, the position was clarified. Lord Henley told me that 'claims made solely on the basis of whooping-cough damage would, almost certainly fail'. But, he added, each case would be looked at on its merits, and payments would be made if appropriate. A few months later, I discovered that the Chairman of the Vaccine Damage Tribunals had earlier circulated copies of the Loveday judgement to all the tribunals. As these decide the claims, it was hardly surprising that all the whooping-cough applications were failing. I tried to persuade the new chairman to circulate counsels' opinion which gave the counter-arguments, but he refused.

The way out of the morass, I believed, was a judicial inquiry. It was absurd that the adversarial proceedings in a law court, where one side had the financial resources of a multi-million-pound pharmaceutical company, should determine whether or not whooping-cough vaccine could damage. But my request to Kenneth Clarke, the Secretary of State for Health, to set up such an inquiry was rejected on the specious grounds that other cases were being pursued in Scotland and in Ireland.

Pauline and I saw the effects of this long-drawn-out battle on the families when we attended another annual meeting of the Association of Parents of Vaccine Damaged Children in April 1990. By this time, the level of the one-off vaccine damage payment had been raised first to £20,000, and then to £30,000. But these changes kept pace only with inflation and they were not retrospective. There was still no proper compensation, and Rosemary Fox was faced by hundreds of anxious parents. The last time I had addressed them some ten years earlier, they were eager to fight, and I was warmly applauded. This time, even though they knew of the sustained efforts Pauline and I had made on their behalf, and they were warmly disposed to us, the reception was muted, and almost resigned. It saddened us, and as we left, we agreed that the fight must go on.

It did go on but only with difficulty. After the controversial Judge Stuart-Smith ruling, legal aid was withdrawn from all vaccine-damaged children. Only the determination of the co-ordinating solicitor, Jack Rabinowicz, led to it being restored for some fifty families by the autumn of 1991, and they continued with their legal fight.

It is difficult to quantify the effects of this campaign. The Vaccine Damage Payments Act was a welcome advance but no substitute for adequate compensation. The medical profession and the public were disabused of the myth that vaccines were a risk-free panacea. The element of risk, although small, became more widely recognized. So, too, was the danger of vaccinating children with contra-indications. This may well have saved scores of children from needless vaccine damage as doctors and nurses exercised more caution.

Despite all this, vaccine damage has not been eliminated. The official figures given to me for 1990 by the Minister for Health, Virginia Bottomley, were 748 reports of adverse reactions to vaccination, and disturbingly 199 of them were serious. Four children died, although the Minister claimed that only two deaths were due to vaccination.

The search for safer vaccines goes on, and perhaps the time will come when they are virtually completely safe. Meanwhile, until a British government meets its obligations, vaccine-damaged children remain the pathetic casualties of a state-sponsored immunization scheme.

16

Opposition Backbencher – the 1980s

I was not altogether sorry on the night of 28 March 1979 when the Labour Government was defeated in the Commons by one vote on a motion of confidence. Desperately needing a new mandate, the Government had been plagued for too long by its lack of a proper Parliamentary majority. Every important vote was a cliff-hanger. The Whips on both sides, like hyperactive sheepdogs, harried their flocks of MPs, allowing time off only for exceptional reasons. The strain affected everyone in this fraught Parliament.

Although, like other Labour MPs, I did not underestimate the difficulties, I looked forward to a General Election that would enable us to win a comfortable majority. The winter of 1978–9, the last one of the Labour Government, had been bleak as union after union went on strike against the Government's maximum 5 per cent pay policy. When the election came, the so-called 'winter of discontent' was trumpeted on the hustings by Tory candidates gleefully recalling that grave-diggers had refused to bury the dead, rubbish had accumulated in the streets, and cancer patients were turned away from hospitals. If their picture failed to match Dante's Inferno, it was not for want of effort. None of this, however, had much effect on the committed Labour voters of Stoke-on-Trent. The local campaign followed its traditional course of confident campaigning by the Labour Party and spirited, but slender, efforts by the Tories.

Nationally, I felt that we were the natural party of Government, even though this did not accord with history, and the Labour Government had recently suffered a rough passage in Parliament. I was unimpressed by the Tories, but perhaps I was victim of a syndrome which affects many MPs when their party is in power. Because opponents are unable to influence Government policy, let alone initiate it, they tend to be dismissed. I undoubtedly underrated Margaret Thatcher – although she was not then impressive as Leader of the Opposition – and probably some of her colleagues.

I was soon to find that, far from being the natural party of Government, we were to be relegated to opposition. With a swing of 5.1 per cent, giving them a majority of forty-three over all the other parties, the Tories took office. Margaret Thatcher became Prime Minister and made her cloying references to St Francis of Assisi, harmony, truth, faith and hope. Ahead lay her divisive, free market policies and eyeball-to-eyeball confrontations.

After elections, it is commonplace for leading MPs on the winning side to sit by their telephones awaiting a Prime Ministerial call to office. I never had that experience and knew that I never would after losing my hearing; but a few days after Margaret Thatcher was ensconced in Downing Street, I had a telephone call from Jim Callaghan, the man who had been Prime Minister up to a few days before.

'Jack,' he said, 'I'm going to recommend that you should be a Privy Councillor in the forthcoming Honours List.' Surprised at this totally unexpected honour, my thanks failed to convey my delight. I wondered if it might become a chimera, as it had done in Harold Wilson's time. But there were no slips, and my appointment was announced in the Honours List a few weeks later.

All Cabinet Ministers, and some Ministers of State, are Privy Councillors, but few backbench MPs are given the high honour. The Speaker, Bernard Weatherill, never forgot to acknowledge my new status and he invariably called me to speak as early as possible. As I no longer had to sit throughout lengthy debates which were so wearying with my deafness, it was a tremendous boon.

The 1979 election began a remarkable decade of British political history. The 'Iron Lady' and Thatcherism, the person and her creed, put an indelible stamp on the country and became famous or

(272)

notorious throughout the world. I doubt if many MPs then appreciated the extent to which dogmatism and dogma were to develop
over the years. It simply seemed to many, including me, that a
bright, tough woman was about to try her hand at reviving Britain.
The policies would naturally differ significantly from those of the
Labour Government, and we all waited and watched to see how the
new Prime Minister and her Government would develop.

Margaret Thatcher was always personally considerate towards me
in debate, looking directly at me and speaking clearly so that I could
follow. Even when I pressed her with hostile points, she still, while
replying in kind, showed the same consideration. At a reception she
held at 10 Downing Street for an anniversary of the Royal National
Institute for the Deaf, I saw the same genuine concern and thoughtful efforts to help deaf people. The helpful actions of the private
person were in sharp contrast to the harsh policies of the public politician.

She soon became a dominant Prime Minister. This was, of course,
due to many factors, but mainly a combination of high intelligence,
electoral success, recognition of a Prime Minister's authority and
strong determination. When she was riding high, none of her Cabinet
colleagues could argue with her. It was a matter of fidelity or
farewell. As her confidence in handling the Cabinet grew, so it did
in dealing with the House of Commons. Supreme confidence developed into oratorical stridency which became a fatal liability.

Her loudly proclaimed stand-on-your-own-two-feet philosophy
hit hard at the most vulnerable. Millions became unemployed as a
result of tough economic policies. The earnings-related supplement
to their unemployment benefit, valued by them and initiated by the
Labour Government, was abolished. They plunged from poverty to
penury.

Across the whole gamut of social policy, the Government imposed
burdens on the poor. Single social security payments for the simple
needs of the poorest, like bedding, heating or cooking, were replaced
by loans – but if it was felt that these could not be repaid they were
not granted. Child benefit was eroded by the simple device of
freezing it at a time of inflation. The link for old age pensions was

shifted from earnings to the lower one of cost of living. Cuts operated from birth to death as both the maternity grant and the death grant were buried. In terms of Europe's poverty league, Britain slid from second best in the 1970s to sixth out of twelve in the 1980s.

Thatcher's social and economic policies dramatically affected the people and industries in my constituency. By September 1980, the numbers of men and women unemployed in Stoke-on-Trent South had doubled to nearly 20,000. The next year they were marching for jobs but to no avail – in 1982, unemployment rose by a further 5,000. I attacked Margaret Thatcher in a Commons debate and asked her why, with moderate wages, technological advances and valuable exports, unemployment was so serious in the Potteries. In reply she blamed the world recession and – her familiar theme – the fact that 'people take more for themselves at the expense of jobs for others'. It was an absurd response about the low-paid workers of Stoke-on-Trent.

The city had long been concerned about the excessive reliance of the local economy on pottery, excellent though its products were. In Parliament, I constantly urged diversification of industry. Attracting new, modern industry to Stoke, never easy, was made more difficult by the honeycomb of underground tunnels, a legacy of coal-mining. Stabilizing these added to development costs.

The need for Government help to widen our industrial base became increasingly urgent as the Thatcher recession hit Stoke-on-Trent. It was the only large city without any form of designated status which would have qualified it for assistance from the Government or the European Community. Throughout the decade, from Keith Joseph in 1980 to Michael Heseltine in 1991, I went to Whitehall with deputations from the city seeking aid. All of them, at Ministries of Employment, Trade and Industry, and Environment, turned us down, apart from some help with land dereliction.

As is so often the case, one kind of deprivation led to another, and the low wages and high unemployment in Stoke-on-Trent were accompanied by inadequate infrastructure. An historically poor health record, insufficient health facilities, a housing shortage and congested roads depressed the quality of life. A particularly disturbing health summary published in 1989 showed that life expectancy in every ward in the city was below the national average; and in half of them, on average, children could not expect to live to collect their pensions at sixty-five.

The health provision was scandalous despite repeated demands for improvements by MPs and councillors. The Minister for Health and the Regional Health Authority must have been fed up with my frequent angry calls for more money and better facilities; but these were desperately needed. In the winter of 1985, local hospitals were on virtually continuous red alert – only emergency cases were admitted to hospital – but Ministers seemed undisturbed. Yet when just one red alert was declared in London the following year it was greeted with shock headlines and demands for immediate action.

The patience of people in Stoke-on-Trent, in the face of these difficulties, always amazed me. If anything, they should have gone to the barricades for improvements, but they tolerated them. A striking example was road congestion. The main road through my constituency, the A50, was blocked at most hours of the day; car and lorry drivers had to edge their way through, and occupants of terraced houses and shops had to suffer noise and fumes. Pauline delved into road traffic statistics and discovered that the A50 carried a higher percentage of heavy goods traffic than any other road in the West Midlands. Although I pressed the case for upgrading it and, better still, a proper bypass, it took many years for changes to be agreed, and they were not due to begin until 1992. Even then the constituency was left with a heavily congested multi-lane road slicing through it, and the bypass proposal was rejected by all Tory road Ministers.

I fought hard for my constituency on all local issues, many of which had national implications. But I was not at the forefront of the main political confrontations in Parliament and I regretted that. The compensation was that, not being a traditional politician chasing up the Ministerial ladder, I could fight issues of my choice.

A disturbing aspect of politics is learning the extent to which ordinary people are hurt by pompous bureaucrats, outdated customs, inadequate laws, domineering companies and heartless institutions, all of which hold power of one kind or another. The Thatcherite hands-off philosophy of the decade suited these perfectly and commensurately damaged the helpless. I pitched in to help where and when I could.

Some issues were straightforward Parliamentary ones such as trying, with MPs like Tam Dalyell, to prevent the tragedy of unnecessary death from kidney failure. People of all ages, but especially the old, were dying unnecessarily because no donated kidneys were available for transplant and there were no machines to treat them. Although this was not a problem that could be completely resolved, we persuaded the Government to give it a much higher priority.

One of my Parliamentary campaigns developed from a single constituency case. Unexpectedly, in 1981, a lorry driver from my constituency was released from prison where he was serving a life sentence for murder. An Appeal Court judge ruled that a forensic scientist, Dr Alan Clift, whose evidence had helped to convict him, 'had been discredited not only as a scientist but as a witness'. It subsequently emerged that Clift's forensic work had been involved in nearly 1,500 cases, but it took the Home Secretary, Leon Brittan, two years to refer just sixteen of them to the Court of Appeal.

For various reasons, including pleas of guilty, the Home Secretary deemed the other cases satisfactory despite acknowledged doubt about Clift's work. I failed to convince him to consider more cases, but the Clift saga jolted the authorities and public from the traditional belief that scientific evidence was infallible. As subsequent cases concerning Irish prisoners showed, forensic scientists can be as inaccurate and misleading as any other witnesses. Had I known at that time of the methods used by some police forces to get 'confessions', I would have been more relentless in demanding a review of cases involving Clift, regardless of whether defendants pleaded guilty or not.

There were two short but effective campaigns related to children. One was to persuade the Department of Health to copy the United States' example and ban the use of aspirin for children. It had been discovered that this could cause Reyes' syndrome, a rare but often fatal disease. Although it took some six years longer than the more vigilant US authorities, the Department did act in 1986, and I was glad to have contributed to this life-saving move.

The other brief campaign, largely outside Parliament, was to foster the use of a Hungarian technique known as 'conductive education' to help brain-damaged children and adults make more use of their limbs. In some cases it meant the difference between being unable to move and walking, albeit with great difficulty.

I met, and was impressed by, the main Hungarian practitioner, Madame Hari, and I worked closely with Andrew Sutton, the leading British expert. One of the main difficulties was to secure agreement between the conflicting views of the various authorities and charities involved. I chaired a crucial meeting which happily led to a consensus followed by the setting up of a conductive education centre in Britain. It subsequently played an important part in helping severely disabled children and adults.

It may seem churlish to complain about anyone supplying tins of baby milk free or at reduced prices. But when in 1981 I was approached by campaigners anxious about this practice in poor Third World countries, I readily agreed with them. The manufacturers were encouraging mothers to use powered baby milk by providing samples or making special offers. High-pressure salesmanship and blatant advertisements proclaimed its virtues. 'You, too, can have a happy, healthy child . . .' was the basic message – providing, of course, people bought their tins of powdered milk.

The effects were tragic. In poor countries the diluting water was often contaminated, and it was difficult to sterilize bottles. Poverty made many mothers give their children a weaker feed. Consequently, far from helping babies, the powdered milk was damaging and sometimes killing them.

The campaigners wanted all Governments to sign a World Health Organization code of practice which would restrict the activities of the manufacturers. I was pleased when Parliamentary pressure led to the British Government signing. This was a fine example of a small group of campaigners fighting powerful multinational manufacturers who were exploiting the weakness of Third World countries. In view of their lack of money and power, it was remarkable that the campaigners exerted so much influence.

A drug campaign in the early 1980s had echoes of thalidomide, although in this case it affected old people. It is a dream of many people suffering persistent pain that science should one day produce a magical cure. In March 1980, it seemed to sufferers of crippling and painful arthritis that this might have occurred. With a fanfare of trumpets, a United States pharmaceutical company, Eli Lilly, announced the discovery of a drug which could not only relieve the pain of arthritis but also modify the disease. Opren had arrived.

Opren was designed to move gently through the bloodstream so that it needed to be taken only once a day. But it was found to be moving too slowly for some old people. One tablet could take up to five days to be eliminated from the bloodstream, and this sometimes led to an accumulation of toxins.

Warnings by doctors from June 1981 led to an unprecedented number of reported reactions to the drug, including liver jaundice, kidney damage, bladder incontinence, stomach haemorrhages, eye sensitivity, detached finger- and toe-nails and excessive sensitivity to sunlight. Then, in August 1982, the Committee on Safety of Medicines suspended the Opren licence. Eli Lilly said later that month that it was withdrawing the drug. Overall, there were approximately 4,000 official reports of alleged adverse reactions including 76 deaths. Far from being a magical cure, Opren had been a human disaster.

Although its fatal effects on the liver and kidneys sparked the suspension, in the subsequent campaign for compensation, acute sensitivity to light (photosensitivity) received greatest attention. One patient described 'millions of pinhead blisters, and in forty-eight hours they all run together, crack open and it's like a gravel rash. They weep dreadfully and are very painful.' Some claimed to be prisoners in their own homes, unable to go out at all in sunlight because of the pain it caused.

Eli Lilly never denied that Opren caused photosensitivity but claimed that it had warned about this and it would be 'mild and transient'. The Minister for Health, Kenneth Clarke, complacently dismissed the tortured reactions of Opren sufferers as 'no more than the patient becoming lobstered'. His blithe suggestion that they could use sun-screens or simply stay out of the sunlight revealed deplorable ignorance.

Despite pressure from me and an Opren Action Group, as well as extensive media coverage, including two *Panorama* programmes on the marketing of Opren, Ministers refused to intervene, and the company did not budge. So a long and expensive legal battle began. Opren victims waited, many suffering acutely, as the lawyers and the medical experts prepared the legal case.

Five years later, in 1987, and only after the intervention of a financially strong pressure group, Citizens' Action, Eli Lilly made its first offers – without admitting liability – restricted to those it described as 'the deserving few'. These were the Opren victims who had suffered severe liver or kidney damage, or the relatives of those who had died. Richard Bailey, Lilly's UK Managing Director, said the company would not even consider compensation for the vast majority of victims because they suffered from photosensitivity about which the company had warned.

Nevertheless, by the end of 1987, sustained pressure from the Opren Action Group, Parliament, the media and Citizens' Action led the company to make an offer which did include photosensitivity victims. It was to go before Mr Justice Hirst, and Pauline and I went with Kathleen Grasham, Chairman of the Opren Action Group, to the High Court in the Strand in London.

As we sat waiting for proceedings to begin, my mind went back to my student days at a crowded debate at the Cambridge Union. During an opening speech of mine, when I was making a cheeky but oblique attack on one of the officers, I was challenged by the rather pompous Vice-President, resplendent in his evening dress. I gave him short shrift, to his great discomfiture and the delighted amusement of other students. Then, in the High Court as we stood at the command of the usher, in walked the former Vice-President, now Mr Justice Hirst, still resplendent, this time in crimson robes and wearing a judicial wig. Solemn, but not in the least pompous, his eyes caught mine, and there was a hint of a smile.

Mr Justice Hirst announced that claimants who accepted the offer would have to acknowledge Lilly's non-acceptance of liability, remain permanently silent about the amount of the award and under-take to abstain from further campaigns against the company in relation to Opren. He warned the majority of the 1,300 claimants who were legally aided that if they rejected the proposed offer there was a risk that their legal aid would not be continued. Lilly's concern for confidentiality ensured that the judge announced no figures. But it soon emerged that the total settlement was just over £2 million, an average of an abysmal £2,000 per person. These figures outraged the victims, particularly as the lawyers' fees were estimated to be £4 million.

In the next two months, I fought for a better settlement, using every Parliamentary weapon at my disposal. Pauline researched every aspect of the issue, but while the many letters to Ministers, petitions, Parliamentary Questions, Motions and debates secured media atten-tion, they had little effect. David Mason, the thalidomide parent, angered by the low level of payment after yet another drug disaster, inspired a spirited foray supported by the *Daily Mail*, but it was all to no avail.

Fear of the legal costs drove most Opren sufferers to accept the meagre offer. Yet they continued to write to me, and the letters movingly described their plight. A widow said about her husband:

> The drug caused his hair to fall out, his kidneys became infected, dried his toe-nails and finger-nails on both hands and feet, burst two toes on the left foot which never stopped discharging till his death . . . he couldn't even bear the weight of a sheet on his feet. It is only those of us who have witnessed the suffering from this drug who can tell of the agonies it produces on the human body.

Quoting from this letter in a final Adjournment debate held in March 1988, I fought desperately to save the faltering campaign and pressed again for a fair and honourable settlement by a trust fund. The junior Minister replying, Edwina Currie, refused a proper discus-sion. The debate ended with an angry attack from me on her Department of Health. I pressed for information on the Department's investigation into allegations that Lilly had failed to report drug damage, which by law it was bound to; but she refused to respond. It was my last fiery effort, because I knew that the political campaign had, after five years, run into the sands.

Why did the thalidomide campaign succeed so spectacularly while this one failed? An important factor was that the Opren parent company was located in the USA rather than in Britain and so its management were less amenable to pressures from the British Parliament. But the main difference was that Opren never caught the public imagination as thalidomide had done; public fervour was absent despite our efforts. People were sympathetic but not committed. They were moved and disturbed by limbless children but only marginally concerned by elderly people suffering severe internal injuries or skin ravaged by sunlight.

Both campaigns, however, had important lessons for the future. Thalidomide highlighted the need for greater drug safety, and many improvements resulted, while Opren strengthened the case for some form of no-fault compensation for medical accidents.

My relationship with Kenneth Clarke, never good, deteriorated further as a result of the Opren campaign. Assertive and bland, he disappointed thousands of Opren victims by his negative response. Of course I did not expect him to attack Eli Lilly, but he could have shown some concern about their behaviour. Instead, he went to great lengths to indicate that he had no complaint.

Despite political differences, I had good personal relationships with several leading Tories. John Major, in his brief spell as Minister for the Disabled, before moving to other posts and eventually becoming Prime Minister, was always personally friendly towards me. Norman Fowler, Cecil Parkinson and two very different Lord Chancellors, Lord Hailsham and Lord Mackay, were Tories with whom I was on good terms. The man, however, for whom I had the greatest affection on the Tory side was the calm and able Geoffrey Howe. Since Cambridge, when we had competed in the Union Society and opposed each other politically, we had maintained our friendship. Despite holding every high office of state up to Deputy Prime Minister, he was always warm and unassuming.

(281)

With Ted Heath, I had a friendly although not close relationship. When he was Prime Minister, he had always been considerate of my deafness. On one occasion a deputation from my union, the GMB, went to his room to discuss some industrial problem. As he was explaining the Government's view he glanced at me, paused a few moments, then adjusted a light on his desk so that it illuminated his face, which made lip-reading easier. It was a thoughtful gesture. Heath suffered much criticism from his Tory colleagues for his lone stand after losing the leadership to Margaret Thatcher, but I admired his courage and single-mindedness, even though it may have been self-destructive. However, he was above worrying about his image.

One of the great attractions of Parliament is the character and personalities of its 650 (since April 1992, 651) MPs. They include labourers and aristocrats, military men and pacifists, intellectuals and buffoons, idealists and cynics, self-publicists and the self-effacing. At one time, only a handful were well known to the public, but televising the House, which began in 1989, revealed far more public personalities. Some MPs and Peers had been vehemently opposed to televising the House because they feared it would change long-established procedures and reveal that the Chamber was often badly attended. Exhibitionists might hog the cameras.

The issue kept bubbling to the political surface during the 1980s. Whenever it did I was reminded of the debate in 1966, my first year in Parliament. I had listened incredulously to the Leader of the House, Richard Crossman, proposing a closed circuit experiment. I did not know Crossman well, but I never warmed to him, regarding him as an intellectual acrobat addicted to public displays. On this occasion, Crossman advocated television, then proceeded to argue the opposite case even more cogently. He emphasized worries about costs, the possible misuse of pictures and the selection of material. The effect of his speech was predictable. The motion was lost by just one vote – 130 for the experiment and 131 against – undoubtedly due to Crossman's asinine behaviour. Intent on showing himself to be master of the art of arguments, he lost the only argument that counted. His contradictory presentation resulted in the exclusion of television for many years. It is on such vain miscalculations by leading politicians that important decisions are sometimes made.

A few of us later made sporadic efforts to press the televising case with Bills. The most persistent was Austin Mitchell, and the most effective, Phillip Whitehead, a former friend and colleague from television and a distinguished MP. My own efforts were two Ten-Minute-Rule Bills, both of which were rejected. The first was opposed by John Stokes, a conventional, upright Tory, proud of all orthodox traditions. Joe Ashton, the earthy and articulate Labour MP for Bassetlaw, opposed my next Bill in December 1981. Joe's speech was a brilliant music-hall turn. Apart from one sensible comment that Parliament was about words, not moving pictures, he caricatured televised debates.

Parliament, Ashton said, would become a sort of *Match of the Day*, and television would be basically a *Candid Camera*. He created a Hollywood 'B movie' scenario of lunatics taking pot-shots from the gallery while MPs cowered on the green leather benches. Members enjoyed his act – and so would television viewers have done, had the cameras been there. I lost both the debate and the vote, 176 to 158. Nevertheless, I was sure the House would eventually change its mind.

The first indication of this came not in the Commons but in the Lords. They decided to televise their proceedings experimentally in 1984. From that moment, entry of cameras to the Commons was virtually guaranteed, the more so as the Lords' broadcasts were popular.

When the Commons eventually voted in June 1989 to allow the cameras in experimentally, none of the dire predictions were borne out. On the contrary, the presence of the cameras improved standards, because MPs were aware of the much larger audience watching them. Far more Parliamentary Questions were tabled by MPs, some of whom seemed to take on a new lease of life, not to mention a boost to their adrenalin. Some garrulous MPs became pithy, and even witty. The House became more of a political theatre in which MPs took care to avoid unbecoming behaviour and did their best to shine. Television did not cause a revolution but did induce a modest measure of reform. In so far as it brought the public closer to their representatives, it also give a minor boost to democracy.

Some laws, which would be rejected if introduced today, are accepted because of their antiquity, rather than their relevance. Yet changing them is always exceptionally difficult because change is usually expensive for the Government. One such ancient statute was Crown immunity from prosecution – something I was unaware of until 1983, when my union, the GMB, sought my help with their campaign for its abolition. Then I realized that it was creating two standards of health and safety.

Private employers observed health and safety and food hygiene legislation because they were prosecuted if they did not. But public institutions, like hospitals, defence establishments and prisons, protected from prosecution by Crown immunity, often had lower standards. For example, a 1977 survey published by the Institution of Environmental Health Officers found that food-handling areas in 60 per cent of the hospitals fell below the standards of Food Hygiene Regulations. Thirteen per cent of the hospitals would have been prosecuted but for Crown immunity.

Neither Parliament nor the public were aroused by these findings, nor by Crown immunity in general, until, in August 1984, nineteen people died and hundreds were made ill by food poisoning at the Stanley Royd Hospital in Wakefield. Contaminated beef, mouldy vegetables and liver with fluke had been lying around in the catering area. Staff food, different from that given to the patients, was of a higher quality and was specially prepared. The patients' kitchen area, infested with cockroaches, was inadequately separated from the toilets, and there were open and dirty drains. Food surfaces were cleaned with the same squeegee cloths used for cleaning the floor. Gully drains were unbearably foul smelling in hot weather.

These deadly conditions had existed despite recommendations for improvements made every year since 1977 by Environmental Health Officers. The Government's response was to appoint an inquiry.

Meanwhile, the GMB had prepared an impressive dossier, *The Case against Crown Immunity*. Claiming that the Stanley Royd tragedy had been wholly preventable, the union gave horrific examples of kitchen conditions in several London hospitals.

More kitchen hygiene cases emerged. In one hospital, it was reported that sparrows flew around the kitchen, dead cockroaches lay in the food store, and the slicing machines were coated with thick grease. In another, there was evidence of bird droppings in jelly, rice coated with bacteria and infestations of mice, ants and cockroaches. The General Manager of the Health Authority responsible was quoted as saying these conditions were 'absolutely disgraceful and indefensible'.

I discovered from Parliamentary Questions that about forty outbreaks of food poisoning were reported every year in NHS hospitals. One official blandly reported that the cockroaches found in stew some weeks earlier were sterile because they had been cooked. In sharp contrast, the organization representing pest control companies reported that vermin caused disease – polio, hepatitis, gastroenteritis and salmonella poisoning. Sickened by the detail and angered by the unnecessary threat to health, I introduced a Ten-Minute-Rule Bill, in June 1985, to remove immunity from all Crown institutions which infringed the Health and Safety at Work Act or Food Hygiene Regulations.

In the House of Commons, while I was speaking of the dangerous vermin and filth in hospitals, Kenneth Clarke sat smiling on the front bench. Possibly he was amused by comments made by one of his colleagues, but I assumed he was laughing at my speech. I lost my temper and asked what he had done about the nineteen people who lay dead because of negligence. Clarke stopped smiling. To present my Bill I had to walk past him to hand it to the Clerk of the Commons to read aloud. While he was reading, I berated Clarke, who sat nearby staring stonily ahead, as the Speaker called for order. Pauline told me later that my voice was so loud it could be heard clearly in the public gallery. From then on, Clarke was understandably even more icy than usual in his dealings with me.

He could not ignore mounting indignation about hospital hygiene.

But how could this be translated into legislative action? The answer was not long in coming. Richard Shepherd, an outstanding Tory backbench MP, was successful in the ballot for Private Members' Bills and he agreed to take on my Bill. Support flooded in from bodies such as the British Medical Association, the Association of Metropolitan Authorities, the Association of District Councils and many other organizations and individuals. To ignore one hospital disaster was one thing; to fly in the face of angry public opinion was another.

As the controversy raged in and out of Parliament, the report on the Stanley Royd disaster was published in 1986. It analysed and detailed the appallingly unhygienic conditions of the patients' kitchens which had led to the deadly food poisoning. Oddly enough, the report said the abolition of Crown immunity would have made no difference; but this view rested on the belief that local Environmental Health Officers would not have prosecuted even if they had had the power – a dubious hypothesis.

Shepherd wanted to pilot his Bill through the House. But on the day preceding its second reading, the Health Minister, Norman Fowler, announced that the Government was to introduce its own Bill to remove Crown immunity from health authorities.

The Government's reversal of policy on food hygiene was welcome, but it refused to remove Crown immunity from health and safety legislation protecting workers. Fortunately it was ambushed in the House of Lords by my old sparring partner, David Ennals, now elevated to the Upper Chamber. He pressed the point, and their Lordships voted in favour of his amendment to improve workers' safety. I was delighted. Crown immunity was not a quaint historic anachronism but a threat to people. Further changes will undoubtedly come, and it can only be a matter of time before this absurd relic is swept away completely.

One enjoyable facet of political life is its unpredictability. One can never be sure which of the masses of letters and telephone calls received every day will be routine, inconsequential or the first indication of something important. A journalist from the *Northern Echo* wrote to me in 1987 about the plight of 1,200 haemophiliacs infected by the Human Immunodeficiency Virus (HIV) through contaminated NHS blood transfusions. My immediate reaction was that the Government should accept responsibility and pay adequate compensation for this tragedy.

The Minister for Health, Tony Newton, quickly rejected my request for a no-fault medical accidents scheme with priority for haemophiliac AIDS victims. He claimed that compensation could only be awarded by the courts when negligence was proven. A few months later, the Haemophilia Society presented a briefing paper to MPs at a special meeting. The strength of their case and the support it gained from Conservative MPs induced a change of mind on the part of the Government. Within a week, Tony Newton announced a payment of £10 million to the Haemophilia Society for a special trust fund.

This looked suspiciously like a strategic withdrawal to me. The average *ex gratia* payment for each person would be only £8,000; the Government had made a concession which acted like a political poultice, drawing the sting from its supporters' criticism. The tactic was successful, and despite the efforts of the Haemophilia Society there were no significant political developments from 1987 to mid-1989.

However, during 1989, I received letters complaining that applicants were being means-tested. Some felt they had been unfairly rejected, others that the Government grant was inadequate. Lord Trafford, the Under-Secretary of State, defended the means test to me because, he said, 'the fund is not compensation'.

It was time, I felt, to take a tougher line. Haemophiliacs were dying, leaving distressed families in poverty. The consensual approach was not working. So I tabled a Motion condemning the Government for abdicating its responsibility, forcing the 1,200 haemophiliacs with HIV to fight in the courts, and calling for an immediate reversal of policy to give them generous compensation without acrimonious and exhausting legal action. Naturally, only Labour MPs signed. Within twenty-four hours another Motion appeared, sponsored by Tory MP Patrick Cormack and his colleagues. It congratulated the Government on its sensitive handling of the haemophiliacs and went on to claim 'every confidence' that the Government would act soon to resolve the difficulties, a confidence I did not share.

The *Sunday Times* meanwhile gave wide coverage to the campaign, supporting the demand for early Government payments. Legal action was obviously too slow a process for dying haemophiliacs. With the media pressure embarrassing the Government, a group of Tory MPs met Margaret Thatcher to discuss their problems. No doubt they were genuinely seeking help for the victims, but it would be naïve to assume that they did not warn the Prime Minister of the political damage that would result if the Government maintained its intransigence. The Government acted but it made a characteristically grudging and inadequate response – delivered with the sound of trumpets and applause from Tory MPs.

On 23 November 1989, in a written Parliamentary reply, rather than an oral statement on which he could be questioned, the Secretary of State, Kenneth Clarke, announced that the Government was adding an extra £24 million to the trust fund. This meant that each person could get an average of £20,000. It was an advance but still nothing like the £100,000 to £150,000 demanded by the Haemophilia Society. For actual compensation, Clarke reasserted, the victims had to fight in court.

At a subsequent meeting of MPs and haemophiliacs in the Commons, the extra money was welcomed, but it was agreed that we should continue to press the Government. I was moved by the passionate speech of an angry wide-eyed young man. Danny Morgan, a haemophiliac infected with AIDS by the contaminated blood transfusions, spoke of the reality. Ministers, he said, didn't realize the pain and anxiety, the terrible night sweats, the inability to insure for the families, the knowledge that they would die soon – all because of transfusions from the NHS. The chilling reality of his words was brought home to me again a year or so later when, in October 1990, I took part in a televised debate on the subject. One

(288)

of the speakers was Danny's widow, participating only because she felt an obligation to continue his fight.

The haemophiliacs themselves were very dissatisfied, and the court action continued. Approximately 1,200 were infected with HIV, and 960 of them or their relatives sued the Government for compensation. By 1990, 210 haemophiliacs had developed AIDS, and over 140 had died. It looked as if there would be a long legal battle. But then the *Sunday Times* revealed remarks made by Mr Justice Ognall to lawyers of his chambers. In a message with echoes of the thalidomide campaign, he said that the Government owed a moral as well as a legal duty to those in its care.

This dramatic intervention, seized upon by the media, together with splendid campaigning by the Haemophilia Society, pressure from MPs and growing public concern, would have been enough for most Ministers to settle. Clarke, however, was supported by the Prime Minister, Margaret Thatcher, and together they were adamant. Fortunately, Thatcher lost power and was replaced by John Major. Clarke was replaced by William Waldegrave.

MPs intensified their pressure. Significantly, the Tory backbenchers' committee – the 1922 Committee – moved to support the haemophiliacs.

Major then personally intervened. The dismissive formula, that it was a matter for the courts, was dropped. He spoke of a 'review'. Within weeks he announced agreement in principle between the Government and the haemophiliacs' lawyers. The Government was to provide an additional £42 million, which meant a total payment of £76 million. From this, £60,000 was allocated to those with families, and £23,000 for those who were unmarried. It was not as much as the haemophiliacs wanted, but much more than they were originally offered, and far better than a bitter and protracted legal wrangle in the courts.

As the Thatcher years passed, new and younger Labour politicians replaced the older ones. When Michael Foot retired from the leadership, the party decided to skip a generation and chose Neil Kinnock, for whom I had a warm regard and respect. Gradually he transformed morale and made Labour electable, which had seemed inconceivable in earlier years. His skill and courage were crucial to shedding outdated commitments, demolishing the extreme Left and initiating relevant new policies.

These were the prerequisites for electing a Labour Government. Achieving them without splitting the party reflected not only Neil Kinnock's determination but also his capacity to persuade. A gifted natural speaker, he could sway audiences with passionate oratory; but to me, his most appealing attributes were his intelligence, warmth and humour. Neil has a basic honesty and generosity which shine through in his dealings with people. Like his predecessors who were leaders of the party, he was attacked and sometimes vilified in the Tory press. Legitimate political criticism was one thing, personal vilification another. I admired the way he and Glenys stood up to what must have often been wounding attacks.

On the day I announced that I was standing down at the end of that Parliament, I was invited to the BBC studios to comment. When I arrived, Neil was being interviewed about my career. I watched on a monitor in the adjoining room and I was touched by his generous, eloquent comments.

Among other leading Labour politicians I was closest to Jack Cunningham and Jack Straw. I had known Cunningham's father in the GMB union in my early days and I watched the son enter Parliament as a raw recruit, gradually honing great natural political skills to become one of the most influential men in the party.

Jack Straw and I never lost the intimate sense of comradeship we established while working for Barbara Castle. The friendship and humour between us persisted as he rose from being a new back-bencher to Shadow Secretary of State. Of other younger Labour men, the most outstanding were Gordon Brown and Tony Blair. Each quickly soared high: Brown because of his outstanding capacity for research and fine debating skills, and Blair as a result of his natural political flair and presentation ability. Along with other gifted MPs like Robin Cook and Bryan Gould, these were some of the people who would lead the Labour Party in Parliament in the next decade and more. They brought to it the intelligence, verve and professionalism that were necessary for the challenge ahead. They helped to create the political climate that led to the downfall of Thatcherism, and qualified themselves to take on more far-reaching responsibilities of Government as and when the opportunities arose.

Naturally it was in the Labour Party that I had most of my friends. The person I worked most closely with on disablement, Alf Morris, had a similar working-class background to mine. For both of us, Ruskin College had been the ladder to a university education. Less extrovert than me but with a subtle mind and retentive memory, he was an effective politician with interests ranging from disability through science and technology to Parliamentary pensions. We both enjoyed tennis and snooker and often played together. Knowledgeable about all Westminster happenings, and with a gift for the apt comment, he was good company. For me there was the additional bonus that I could lip-read him without difficulty, although I sometimes pulled his leg about his Manchester accent. We travelled to many countries together when he was a Minister and afterwards, usually attending conferences on disablement.

Another good friend with the same working-class background, but this time with a Geordie accent, was Bob Brown, MP for Newcastle upon Tyne West. We shared the same sense of humour – when playing on a putting green with him it was no surprise to find my ball deeply indented in the turf after he had surreptitiously trodden on it. He had been a gas inspector, which was, I told him, a job which gave him impeccable credentials for sitting in the Commons.

I enjoyed a warm relationship with Merlyn Rees, a humane and experienced politician. He had excellent judgement and the capacity to put his finger on the central issue in discussions. Among my other friends were Lewis Carter Jones, a Welshman who couldn't open his mouth without telling an anecdote, and Bruce Grocott and Roland Boyes, both of whom shared many of my interests and views and took great trouble to help if I had any lip-reading difficulty.

Along with many others, people like this added immeasurably to my enjoyment of Parliament. I valued their companionship, the sense of fun, the conversations and shared interests. With them, life in the Commons was never dull or solemn.

During the Tory years, Pauline and I and our daughters became an extended family. As close and affectionate parents we had mixed feelings as the girls grew up and left home. Naturally we watched with great interest as they developed relationships and pursued their chosen careers.

Jackie was the first to leave, to read Philosophy, Politics and Economics (PPE) at St Anne's College, Oxford. A good and perceptive writer, she subsequently went on a *Daily Mirror* journalist training scheme and after a few months she became a news trainee with the BBC. A much coveted position, this gave her an excellent two-year grounding in all aspects of broadcasting journalism. After working on the BBC programme *Newsnight*, she transferred to ITN. I was particularly pleased when she began producing the House of Lords television programme and then became a political correspondent, because it meant that I would see much more of her at the House. That was the theory. In fact, we were each so busy in our respective spheres that our paths crossed only infrequently. But she became well known at Westminster, and I acquired the title 'Jackie's father'. She married Andrew Marr, a gifted Scottish journalist who at the age of thirty-two became political editor of the *Economist*.

Jane went to read Economics at King's College, Cambridge, and became President of King's Students' Union. During one student anti-apartheid protest, she clashed with the college authorities. Bernard Williams, the Provost, former husband of Shirley, was an old friend, and I had produced television programmes with Noel Annan, a former Provost. Jane aroused the ire of both, and it was with some amusement that I read an apoplectically angry letter from Annan denouncing Jane and supporting Williams. I admired Jane's idealism and determination. She later went to the University of Massachusetts at Amherst and to the London School of Economics for a Master's Degree in Economics.

One January, Pauline and I spent a happy few days with Jane in

Amherst, despite bitter cold weather. As the snow and ice were packed solidly outside her house I worked long and hard with a heavy spade cutting out space enough for the mail-van. Next morning we watched and waited expectantly, but after the briefest of pauses it rolled on. I had apparently cut space enough for a small British car rather than for one of the much larger American models. I had no option but to resume digging.

After gaining her Master's Degree, Jane worked for the Treasury, and then moved to the Labour Party's Research Department, where she had wide-ranging responsibility for economic matters. Both were excellent experience for her subsequent job as a producer for the BBC television programme *On the Record*.

Caroline went to Balliol College, Oxford, where she also read PPE. She, too, became active in student politics. As President of the Junior Common Room, she also clashed with her college authorities, but their response was less indignant than that of King's to Jane. She helped to persuade Balliol to remove its account from Barclays Bank, a move which helped encourage the bank to withdraw from South Africa.

Before going to university, Caroline spent five months in India, in a village just outside Bombay, living with the families and helping with the work. Later, during a college vacation, she went to China for six weeks, paying for the trip by first teaching English in Taiwan. As the Taiwanese demanded American tutors to teach English, Caroline, with her perfect English, had to pretend to be an American. She was caught out one day when she confused Flag Day with Independence Day in the USA! Her travels led on to a career in development work.

For a period of time nearly all the family worked at the House of Commons. In addition to Jackie and Andrew, who were based at Westminster, Jane had many meetings there when she was a Labour Party researcher and later as a television producer. She had married Martin Rosenbaum, a fine campaigner and journalist who frequently visited the Commons. Caroline, after obtaining a Master's Degree in Third World Development on a Fulbright Fellowship in the USA, became a researcher for Ann Clwyd, the Shadow Minister for

Overseas Development. Her partner, Richard Dewdney, had been with her at Oxford and was also a Fulbright scholar before getting a job in the House of Commons Library. As Pauline visited the House often, we naturally became known as the Ashley Mafia.

On 5 July 1989, Pauline and I became grandparents. We rejoiced when Jackie and Andrew had their son, Harry, who was to play an important part in our lives. As I pen these lines he is an energetic and humorous 2½-year-old. No doubt like all grandparents, we feel enriched by our grandson. We visit him often and play all kinds of games. I have resumed the habit I had when my daughters were children of telling stories, suitably embroidered, about my life in Widnes when I was a little boy. I have a fascinated, but already sceptical, listener.

Harry now has a sister, Isabel, who is now six months old. We already enjoy her company and look forward to her development. Equally exciting for us is that Jane and Martin have had their first baby. Ben is already taking an interest in life around him and will soon be a happy and involved participant. We are proud and delighted as our family grows.

17

Fighting the Forces

In March 1982, a crippled young man was wheeled by his parents into the room where I held my regular advice bureaux in Stoke-on-Trent. Martin Kettrick needed help with daunting problems undreamed of when, as a sixteen-year-old healthy adolescent, interested in hill climbing and vigorous sporting activities, he had joined the Marines.

Promoted to corporal unusually early, Kettrick was a success in the Marines until 16 November 1980, when his life changed dramatically. During a routine abseiling exercise in the Lake District, he stopped on a ledge to check why the rope had gone tight. The officer at the top shouted at him to 'Get on; get down!' Kettrick moved to continue his descent, but the rope had been cut, and he plunged 40 feet to the ground, landing on his back. With minimal medical help available, he was taken to hospital in the back of an Army Land Rover – a trip he would never forget. With a fractured skull, broken back, broken ribs and a punctured lung, his body registered every nightmare bump.

A month after he had been invalided out of the Marines, he came to see me. He was now a paraplegic, doubly incontinent and in continuous pain. He came not for sympathy but for justice.

While he was in the Marines, he had always taken for granted that if he were injured he would be well provided for. After the accident he assumed that the circumstances of his injuries would be taken into account, and he was certain that he had been the victim of negligence. The inquiry into his accident had led to a reprimand for the NCO who had cut the rope. But when he tried to sue for compensation, he was astounded to find that he was debarred. Like all service personnel, he had signed away this right on enlistment.

Section Ten of the Crown Proceedings Act 1947 specifically removed the right of service personnel to sue the Crown – meaning Government Departments and Institutions – or their colleagues, regardless of circumstances, and however blatant or serious the negligence. Every other public servant, like all civilians, had the right to sue for damages for personal injury. The 1947 Act had properly ended many of the traditional legal privileges enjoyed by the Crown. It had enabled civil proceedings to be taken against the Crown in the same circumstances as they could be against a private individual. The military, however, felt that the nature of the services was incompatible with the right to sue for personal injury in peace as well as in war. Section Ten of the Act provided for this exemption. It also removed the right, previously enjoyed by members of the forces, to sue their colleagues. As a result, forces personnel were denied any right to sue, leaving them with only official pensions for compensation in the event of disability. The level of their pensions was used to rebut criticisms when Section Ten was passed by Parliament. The Attorney-General at the time, Sir Hartley Shawcross, claimed that 'Pension entitlement . . . will in most cases – I will not say in every case – be as valuable for the soldier concerned as any lump sum for damages which he might recover.'

In 1947, just after a devastating world war, it was perhaps understandable that individual rights were not accorded the highest priority. But by 1983, most service personnel were engaged in routine duties, with only a few in anything like an active role. Section Ten was a monstrous deprivation of individual rights.

All that Kettrick got in 1982, when he left the Marines, was a lump sum of £6,822, a Ministry of Defence pension of £2,427 and a DHSS pension of £6,068, both pensions being inflation-proofed. Pauline worked on the figures and I spent the next couple of years haranguing the Ministry of Defence about the value of Kettrick's awards. The Parliamentary Under-Secretary, Jerry Wiggin, finally told me that the capitalized value was about £170,000 but that as some of the invalidity payments would have been payable to Kettrick had he been a civilian, the value of the payments attributable to his his service record was just £90,000. This fell far short of the £250,000 to £300,000 he could have expected from a successful court action. This would have paid Kettrick for loss of earnings, cost of care and specific requirements such as a suitably adapted home and additional heating, as well as for pain and suffering.

So much for the claim made by Shawcross in 1947. I was angry about the injustice, but my protests were rejected by the Ministry of Defence. Wiggin, admitted in a letter that, without Section Ten, Kettrick 'might have succeeded in a common law claim and obtained substantial damages more financially advantageous to him than his present benefits'. This was quite an understatement. I had discovered that an injured policeman or fireman would get pensions calculated on the same basis as for injured servicemen, but they could also sue. A court award, although allowing for their pensions, would be in addition to them and not a replacement.

A barrage of Parliamentary Questions resulted in little more than the information that Kettrick's disaster had led to a review of procedures and a requirement for instructors to check personally before ropes were cut. Although welcome, these were of no help to Kettrick. The only other advance was the establishment in October 1983 of an Inter-Departmental Inquiry into Section Ten.

I had no doubt that the law had to be changed, and it had to be retrospective to provide for Kettrick and others like him. The Ministry of Defence had other ideas. In response to my request for new legislation, Wiggin sent a magisterial letter rejecting it out of hand. Section Ten was 'essential' for the conduct of the armed forces, and in a series of letters and Parliamentary Answers he advanced four reasons. Allowing servicemen to sue for negligence would endanger discipline; it would create anomalies; the dividing lines between military action and other activities could not easily be defined; and servicemen might not be able to prove negligence.

I couldn't believe that these points were meant as serious

argument. In an Adjournment debate on 26 March 1985, I replied that discipline was irrelevant to legal redress; that an anomaly already existed because comparable public servants like police and fire-fighters could sue for negligence; that anyone in the services readily knew the dividing line between military and non-military activity; and that whether a serviceman could prove negligence or not was for the courts, not the military authorities, to decide.

A mother of a young apprentice in the Royal Navy, who had been killed, had heard of the circumstances of other horrific deaths. I quoted from a letter she sent me:

> Jonathan [her son] is dead. He sustained 60 per cent burns when a Seacat missile was fired by mistake. He was our son. He was just eighteen years old and he died before we could reach him. Steven was seventeen years old. He was thrown from an RAF truck, or was he? No one seems to know for certain. He was irreparably brain damaged anyway, and died within a few hours. Kevin took rather longer about it. When he was found floating face downwards in a vat of lethal cleaning fluid he was seventeen years old. When he finally died he was twenty-one years old and weighed less than four stone.

The Ministry of Defence was unmoved, but the media were quick to appreciate the weakness of the MoD case. The publicity they gave my Parliamentary efforts resulted in numerous tragic cases emerging, and I was inundated with sad and indignant letters.

The case of Snowy Clingham vividly illustrated the stark difference between the compensation for forces personnel and that for civilians obtained through the courts. A Naval Chief Petty Officer, Clingham was injured together with a dockyard worker when they were being lowered over the side of a ship in harbour. The apparatus broke and they plunged 40 feet on to a boat below. Clingham became a paraplegic with no control of his bowels or bladder. His naval pension was worth only a third of the capital sum the dockyard worker received in compensation because he, unlike Clingham, could sue.

(298)

Section Ten had also a curious side-effect. In some cases where the servicemen had been killed by alleged negligence, relatives were often unable to discover precisely what had happened. The services closed ranks, and without the scrutiny of a court case, there was no way of prising out information. The parents of Jonathan who had died of burns before they arrived at the hospital were upset by the clamlike secrecy of the military bureaucrats when pressed for scraps of information.

Many people wrote to me wanting to form an organization to press the Ministry of Defence. In response, I called a meeting at the House of Commons in February 1986. Kettrick and other severely disabled servicemen came, and so too did a number of widows and mothers of men who had been killed by alleged negligence. The most striking person was an ex-actress, the mother of Jonathan. Carol Mills, a sad, intelligent and determined woman, was soon to be elected chairman of the new group, which called itself STAG – the Section Ten Abolition Group.

From then on, the Ministry of Defence was badly buffeted. With Pauline's help I maintained a flow of Parliamentary Questions, letters and speeches inside the House, while Carol Mills captured media attention outside.

Soon afterwards, I took to the Ministry of Defence a deputation which included Carol Mills, Martin Kettrick, other disabled servicemen and Tory MP Winston Churchill. The Secretary of State, George Younger, accompanied by his senior advisers, appeared sympathetic as we explained the hardship, unfairness and injustice of Section Ten. He was particularly friendly with Churchill, who spoke strongly on our behalf. Although Younger made no specific commitment, we went away hopeful. Yet, as so often happened after discussions with Ministers, he wrote to me later rejecting our demands. He used the familiar stonewall defence of Section Ten, insisting that we should await the result of the review, which by this time had dragged on for almost three years.

STAG, now vociferous, reacted by arranging a rally in the town square of Woolwich, close to the Royal Arsenal and not far from the Royal Artillery barracks. The campaigners were joined by nuclear test veterans, also affected by Section Ten, who had long sought compensation for radiation injuries at tests in the Pacific in the 1950s. This rally was the first stage of a nationwide campaign to alert potential recruits to the rights they lost on signing on. A large poster was unveiled headed 'What They Don't Tell the Professionals' and it explained the potentially damaging effects of Section Ten on individuals. Carol Mills and I addressed the rally, and the media gave us good coverage.

On the third anniversary of the start of the Ministry of Defence review, I went to their headquarters in Whitehall with Carol and six widows of servicemen who had taken part in the nuclear tests. They were to present a petition of 5,000 signatures. The hapless recipient was the junior Minister, Roger Freeman, who, with microphones and television cameras hovering, had to listen politely to the views of angry and distraught widows before receiving the petition.

The campaign was undoubtedly winning widespread public support. To give further impetus, STAG extended their anti-recruitment activities and planned an application to the European Court. With the start of the new Parliamentary session in November 1986, I pressed for a full Parliamentary debate and tabled a Motion which was well supported by MPs on all sides. Suddenly, rumours began to circulate that the Ministry of Defence was weakening and even considering abolishing Section Ten. Either strong feelings on both sides of the House, or the effect of the campaign on recruitment, was shaking the Ministry. One or both together won the battle. On 8 December 1986, the Ministry of Defence surrendered.

All the Ministerial objections dogmatically reiterated over the years magically vanished. Service personnel disabled by negligence were to have the right to sue, and the Government said it would support a Private Member's Bill to achieve this. The campaigners were set to celebrate a famous victory. But George Younger soon quashed this by refusing to make the change retrospective. Kettrick and the other disabled ex-servicemen who had campaigned with me for so long were to get nothing. They were furious and frustrated.

In November 1986, Winston Churchill was successful in the Private Members' Ballot for Parliamentary time, and he took on the Bill to abolish Section Ten; but he made no provision for retro-spection. The hopes of Martin Kettrick and others hung on an Amendment which I introduced at committee stage to make the new provision retrospective. Would Churchill or any Tory support it?

I made a vigorous speech which Churchill praised. He was particu-larly supportive of the nuclear test veterans but he did not believe their prospects depended on a retrospective clause in his Bill. I knew then that my Amendment would fail; and so it did by 8 Tory votes to 5 Labour.

Ministers were claiming credit for the Bill, yet they had side-stepped responsibility for helping those to whom credit belonged. Carol Mills was scathing. She wrote to me: 'I am sorely tempted to remind some of those now attempting to take some of the credit for the proposed reform, just how dismissive and uninterested they were when their support and help was first asked for.'

I had no doubt that Churchill himself was genuinely anxious to help. His advocacy of other parts of the Bill had been impressive, and I could understand his fear that he might lose the Bill altogether if he supported me. Nevertheless, I would have preferred him to call the Minister's bluff.

Afterwards I put to him the compromise proposal of a trust fund to provide *ex gratia* payments for those disabled by negligence before the abolition of Section Ten. This at least would give some-thing to the excluded men, and, if accepted, we could then argue for a substantial payment. He agreed, and together we presented it to the junior Minister, Roger Freeman. This time, however, he would not be swayed.

As a last resort I wrote to Margaret Thatcher to ask if, in view of her well-known concern for service personnel, she would intervene. Her reply was firm; there would be no *ex gratia* payments to those previously disabled by negligence. Her objections were that such payments would be open-ended and would involve 'raking over' past actions, and that there was a lack of evidence.

Both Pauline and I felt that if progress was to be made it would come from attacking the Prime Minister's arguments, so we prepared carefully worded responses to meet her points. To avoid an open-ended commitment we proposed confining it to cases which had led to an official investigation and a conclusion of faulty behaviour, equipment or procedures. We also suggested that *ex gratia* payments be made only if there was adequate written evidence. The correspondence lasted from 30 March to 5 October 1988; but although we felt we had won the argument, it ended with her rejecting all our proposals.

I could see no justification for admitting the right to sue for negligence to one group of servicemen and denying it to others. Kettrick and the other men already disabled were bitter and aggrieved. They had trusted Parliament to give them a fair deal, particularly after the Government agreed to repeal Section Ten. I was angry and depressed at being unable to help them. These men, who loved the services yet were gravely injured in them and had campaigned for improvements, were entitled to a fairer deal.

In the course of the Section Ten campaign I became interested in the claims of nuclear test victims for compensation for radiation damage. In the early 1950s, 26,000 British servicemen had worked at the British nuclear test sites; 14,000 witnessed tests at the Monte Bello Islands off North-West Australia, at Maralinga and Emu in South Australia and at Christmas and Malden Islands in the Pacific. The first public signal that their radiation exposure might have caused damage was in 1983 when doctors at St Bartholomew's Hospital noticed that a number of cancer patients were nuclear test veterans. As a result of the ensuing publicity, 2,000 joined the Nuclear Tests Veterans' Association to fight for compensation.

The Association collected evidence that an unusually large number of men had leukaemia, multiple myelomas, cataracts, wart growths, stomach troubles and unusual forms of mental illness or infertility. As if that were not tragic enough, it was claimed that their children and grandchildren had a higher incidence of what were thought to be radiation-induced genetic disorders such as clubbed and webbed feet, menstrual disorders, lymph problems and physical deformities.

Official documents unearthed by the Association suggested that the veterans had a strong case. One read: 'Some degree of risk must be run by some people if we are to achieve the full purpose of the trial.' Another, a report from the Defence Research Policy Committee to the Chiefs of Staff, dated 20 May 1953 and marked 'Top Secret', stated: 'The Army must discover the detailed effects of various types of explosion on equipment stores and men with and without various forms of protection.'

This remarkable memorandum appeared to indicate that some men were not protected during the nuclear explosions. Yet the Ministry of Defence maintained that none of them had been adversely affected by radiation. Probing questions met with blunt refusals to answer, Ministers maintaining a denial of any damage to the men. But, realizing that the problem would not go away, they asked the National Radiological Protection Board to commission a comparative study to see if the nuclear tests had resulted in disproportionate mortality. Thereafter they refused substantive answers to questions until the NRPB study was published. And, although the study took place between 1982 and 1984, the publication of the results was delayed until January 1988.

The report identified a significantly higher evidence of leukaemias and multiple myelomas – two cancers which could be due to excessive radiation exposure. But it was disappointingly cautious about causation, acknowledging that there may have been small hazards of leukaemia and multiple myeloma but 'their existence is certainly not proven and further work is desirable'. The Ministry of Defence claimed that it fully vindicated its own view that the radiological protection measures adopted had been effective and the chance of anyone being damaged through participation was extremely small. It nevertheless agreed to ten years of further medical study. A softer line was taken by the Department of Social Security. Following the NRPB report, it agreed to give war pensions to men suffering from multiple myeloma and leukaemia, or their widows.

The report's findings were a blow to nuclear test veterans, but they were by no means conclusive. Veterans claimed that the evidence on which the report was based was taken from the National Cancer Register, which was opened only in 1974. The men who had died before then would be excluded. In addition, it was a study in mortality and therefore excluded living veterans. Submissions to the study closed in 1984, but as radiation damage took time to develop, a divergence in mortality rates could show up over time. Another vital omission was that the children and grandchildren of test veterans were excluded, so there was no consideration of genetic effects.

These were crucial points which at least merited careful scrutiny by the military authorities. Yet when, with the test veterans' support, I put them to Ministers, they simply refused to consider them. Proper precautions, they said, had been taken at the time, and that was that.

The Ministry of Defence left the veterans no option but to begin lengthy and expensive court proceedings. In the hope of short-circuiting legal action, I took another deputation to the Secretary of State for Defence, George Younger, to demand the establishment of a compensation fund. The deputation again included Winston Churchill; we were again given a courteous hearing – and turned down.

Meanwhile, test veterans in the USA had also been battling for compensation, but with more success. Their Defense Department decided to pay compensation to test veterans who developed any one of twenty specified cancers. In view of these awards, I felt it was inconceivable that the British Government could get away with rejecting all liability. Yet it did so; the Ministry of Defence maintained its stand. The injustice, and the sense of betrayal, rankled among the men. It remains to be seen whether the Ministry will maintain its battle against the men who served it loyally, and who are growing old and sick, or whether it chooses to somersault as it did with the right to sue for servicemen and servicewomen.

Because of my known interest in forces issues, I received letters from servicemen about all kinds of concerns. In the autumn of 1987, one or two of them mentioned bullying in the Army. At first I responded cautiously, because the line between tough discipline, vital in any army, and unnecessary bullying is not easy to draw. I became aware that there could be viciousness and intimidation when a series of courts martial revealed cases of horrifying brutality. The courts were told of 'humiliating and degrading' initiation rites suffered by recruits. Some soldiers pleaded guilty to brutality at these rites, which included enforced nakedness and buggery. A non-commissioned officer was found guilty of locking recruits in a cupboard and exposing them to CS gas. Other allegations were of young soldiers being kicked, punched, beaten and even burned.

Answers to Parliamentary Questions revealed that there had been 87 courts martial for assault in the last eight years, but in 1987 the Army had investigated only 75 allegations of bullying.

The publicity given to the courts martial and my subsequent questions led to a flood of letters. I had always taken a pride in our armed services, as indeed had many of the people who wrote to me, but I was appalled by the revelations in the letters. Most came from parents, grandparents, aunts and uncles who repeatedly said that their young men had eagerly entered the services only to become somehow different, shattered individuals. Servicemen feared reprisals if they complained about one corporal to another who might be his friend. Already apprehensive about scorn for telling tales, they were effectively silenced by warnings that any disclosure would break the Official Secrets Act. Many even hesitated to speak to their parents.

A sad letter came from a mother whose son in the Army Catering Corps used to come home on leave with burns on his wrist and bruising on his face. When questioned, he would say he had walked into a wall or burned himself on the cooker. One day, unable to take any more, he went absent without leave. Eighteen years later, that mother was still mourning her son, from whom she had not since heard.

Bullying appeared to be a long-standing phenomenon. An ex-serviceman wrote of how in 1969 he and others were made to bunny-hop around the barracks naked and with six inches of snow on the ground. He loved the Army, but the bullying forced him out.

Demanding action from the Ministry of Defence was difficult. Because of their fears, many letters from relatives were anonymously written, and others asked for the identities of the young men not to be revealed to the Ministry of Defence. Yet without identification, how could the allegations be investigated?

(305)

As the letters flooded in, Pauline scrutinized and tabulated the soldiers' allegations, relatives' complaints, general condemnation and public support. We decided to send a balanced dossier of the complaints to the Ministry of Defence, deleting identification except where there had been agreement to retain it. The allegations, ranging from the brutal to the degrading, included locking up, beating and starving a twenty-year-old soldier and depriving him of sleep for two weeks, leading to a mental breakdown, nine months in hospital and attempted suicide; dragging a young soldier from bed and repeatedly plunging him in and out of a bath of cold water until he nearly lost consciousness; forcible application with a scrubbing brush of boot polish, Brasso and toothpaste to the pubic area of a young soldier, resulting in blistering and swelling that needed medical treatment; burning young soldiers all over their bodies, including their genitals, with cigarette ends; binding a soldier's hands behind his back, tying his ankles, covering his head with a pillow and throwing him bodily downstairs; and beating up an Army cadet so badly that he could not walk and required eight weeks' hospital treatment. The Commanding Officer of the latter refused information to the parents on the grounds that they had signed over parental rights to the Army.

After sending the dossier, Pauline and I went to see the Under-Secretary of State, Roger Freeman, and the Adjutant-General of the Army, General Mostyn. Although they expressed concern, they were adamant that bullying and brutality were not a major problem, maintaining that such allegations were investigated. They spoke with the assured confidence of senior men in the Ministry of Defence, but I found the statement of an ex-warrant officer who wrote to me more believable. Complaining about the 'stupidity of the Tory statement that a soldier has only to complain', he said: 'I can assure you that a complaint against a "comrade" or superior can only bring oppression and misery to the complainer.' In any case, Freeman and Mostyn could not know how many cases there were – because in a Parliamentary Answer to me Freeman said that the information was 'not held centrally and could only be collected with disproportionate cost and effort'.

(306)

I suggested that they might have been given a laundered version of the truth. For example, a newspaper had carried reports of boys being paraded stark naked, and the Ministry of Defence had subsequently apologized, referring to it as an aberration. However, the mother of one of the boys involved wrote to say that far from being 'a one-off', it was a regular occurrence. The boy who 'spilled the beans' had been summarily dismissed; and everyone else had been warned about further disclosures. There were also even more horrendous activities, like marching boys naked through a river for over an hour in temperatures of minus six degrees.

The Ministry's complacency came under further attack when Parliamentary Answers revealed a high rate of wastage in the Army, with many deserting and others going absent without leave. At that time, 1985–6, 23.8 per cent of those who entered at sixteen, and 27.6 per cent of those who entered at seventeen, left the Army within six months. Although other factors would have been involved, it seemed likely that mistreatment was one cause.

The Ministry of Defence merely reacted to formal allegations, and that was too little and too late. I wanted it to probe the true extent of bullying and brutality, establish independent inspectors empowered to visit Army training centres or military establishments, give special training to junior officers and ban vicious medieval initiation rites.

I pressed these issues constantly at meetings with the Minister, in Parliamentary debates, on television and radio and in the press. As a result of the court cases and my campaigning, public concern was growing. Headlines included 'The Army Shame' and 'Crackdown on the Khaki Thugs'. An editorial in the *Independent* was headed: 'Inept reply to bullying charges'. An all-party deputation accompanied me to one of my meetings with the Minister and the Adjutant-General. Officials at the Ministry of Defence were beginning to look worried.

As more letters were sent to me I pressed the Ministry to order a full investigation. My suggestion for independent inspectors developed into a proposal for an Army Ombudsman which clearly horrified the Ministry. Among the anonymous letters I received was one which claimed that in one particular famous regiment there was a drinking initiation ceremony in which new young officers were stripped naked by the men and forced to drink cocktails of any available liquid, including urine. Another detailed, concerned letter alleged that a senior officer ran his Army unit by coercion and the imposition of unreasonable punishments on his men. These were said to include a fine of £500 for having an untidy room, a similar one for refusing to dismount from a bicycle and a fine of £150 for being late with mess bills. It was claimed that he had humiliated a corporal by forcing him to wear a badge embroidered with the words 'Numb-nuts' on his uniform after a parade-ground misdemeanour.

At the House of Commons, I spoke about my dossier of complaints including beating, starving, burning, stripping and tying up. I mentioned the regiment and named the senior officer in the Army unit in privileged Parliamentary Questions. That night and the following day, the dossier was a main item on all television and radio news bulletins and it got extensive press coverage the following morning. The focus was on my allegations about the regiment and the senior officer.

The Ministry of Defence reacted immediately with an investigation. Within a week it answered that it had found no evidence to substantiate the charges of initiation rites in the regiment, and it assured me that an eccentric was in the habit of making these charges. I accepted this and offered an immediate public apology to the regiment and its Commanding Officer.

With regard to allegations of unreasonable punishments, the Ministry of Defence confirmed that the heavy fines had been imposed for the untidy room, refusing to dismount from a bicycle and being late with mess bills. There was no mention of the 'Numb-nuts' charge, though this was later proved correct. The Ministry tried to justify these punishments by adding that in the first case the room was in an indescribably filthy and unhygienic condition; in the second, the officer was riding without lights and behaving in a disorderly manner in front of foreign visitors; and in the third, the serviceman was a persistent offender.

The Parliamentary Answer also said that the fines were well within the officer's power and entered correctly into disciplinary records. The evening paper headlined that the officer had been 'cleared' by the Ministry of Defence. The following day's press reports all took the same line; journalists uncritically reported the Ministry's view that the officer was acting within his powers.

So he was, but of course the real question was whether the fines were reasonable. Five hundred pounds, or eighteen days' pay, for a dirty room or failing to stop a bicycle and being disorderly, was the kind of punishment which would be laughed out of court if a judge imposed it. I felt that I was right, but the Ministry of Defence had won a public relations victory. Nevertheless, I regretted naming the unit's senior officer under Parliamentary privilege before I had the Parliamentary Reply and I apologized to him for that. As with my apology to the Commanding Officer of the regiment, I made it public, and wrote personally to each of them. The Commanding Officer of the regiment wrote of my 'generous gesture' in referring favourably to his regiment in the House when I apologized.

At a subsequent meeting with Roger Freeman and General Mostyn, the Minister said that the last six months had been very beneficial for the armed forces. General Mostyn said that after examining the evidence they were as disturbed as I was. Although he did not share my view of the extent of brutality, he conceded that there might be 'more under the water'; the problem was how to get it to the surface. He felt that it was not fear of reporting brutality to the authorities that prevented disclosure by soldiers, but fear of peers – if victims talked they were assaulted again. During his forty years in the Army, he said, no issue had been so thoroughly investigated at every command level.

The new proposals were extensive: the Army was to re-examine its responsibilities for man-management and foster a greater awareness among officers of their supervisory duties; junior and middle-level commanders were to be given more time to concentrate on leadership; welfare support to the chain of command was to be improved; administrative commitments were to be reorganized, guidance on man-management training to be revised and all harmful initiation ceremonies to be formally banned.

The cost of these changes was officially estimated at £2 million, and time and effort were to be devoted to their implementation. I was delighted. Despite the heat engendered between the Ministry of Defence and myself during the campaign, we ended up co-operating in our efforts to eradicate brutality.

Although the Minister, General Mostyn and I were now working together to implement the new procedures it would have been naïve to assume that everyone at the Ministry of Defence was pleased. At one of our sessions there, a beefy, red-faced senior officer simply sat and glared at me throughout the discussion.

Some time afterwards, I was invited to an Army Board dinner attended by the Chief of the General Staff, General Sir John Chapple, and his top generals. I went along to this very formal occasion wondering if I would be able to lip-read the generals, and what their attitude would be. During a discussion with General Sir John Chapple and the Quartermaster-General, Lt-General Sir Edward Jones, I asked for their frank opinion of my campaign. They both welcomed it. The Commander-in-Chief said that the reforms were very helpful. 'In any case,' he added, 'bullies will think twice about bullying because they know you will speak up about it in Parliament.'

18

Disability

When I was twelve years old I used to run weekend errands for a severely disabled woman who lived in an untidy flat near Wellington Street in Widnes. She had angular features and the sweetest smile and gave me a warm welcome whenever I entered her room – but I hated going there. I disliked her husband, a fat, irritable man who smoked a foul-smelling pipe and always seemed impatient for me to leave.

Not that I stayed long. On Saturday mornings I would take the written list from the woman on a sofa, the money and a shopping bag, and get her order. When I delivered her goods she thanked me profusely and gave me sixpence. That was why I went – for the money. I was glad of it but, even at that early age, I felt a trifle uneasy taking it.

So my attitude to her disability was casual indifference slightly tinged with pity. It characterized my generation's attitude to disabled people. In so far as we met any of them, and that was rare, we felt no real concern and left them to their own devices. No doubt their families helped, as they do today, but the public view was one of indifference bordering on neglect.

For many years, this woman was the only severely disabled person with whom I had any regular contact. Coincidentally, the next one also had angular features and the sweetest smile and always gave a warm welcome. There the resemblance ended. She had poise and charm but a will of iron and was determined to improve the lives of all disabled people.

A fragile and vivacious woman, Megan du Boisson was crippled by multiple sclerosis and confined to a wheelchair. I first met her in 1966, just after becoming an MP, and she was to have a great influence on me, capturing my imagination and stimulating my interest in disablement. Megan had a certain magic, a gaiety, even frivolity, which enlivened conversation with her. Yet she was also deeply serious, dedicated to a cause which she espoused passionately and intelligently. People listened to Megan du Boisson when she spoke on disability.

She was stirred to action because long-term chronic sickness and severe disability were then regarded as short-term illness indefinitely prolonged – and benefits were pitifully inadequate. Regardless of the severity of their disability, married women working at home for their families were excluded from social security benefits. Earning no income and supported by their husbands, disabled housewives were assumed to do no work for which financial compensation was required.

Incensed by this, Megan wrote a letter to the *Guardian* in 1965 calling for pensions for all disabled people including housewives. She also suggested setting up a Disablement Income Group to campaign for it. At a time when interest in disabled people was low, the effect of the letter was electric. Disabled people wrote to her expressing anger, frustration and despair. It was like a tidal wave of suffering, suddenly released, almost engulfing Megan with its passionate intensity.

The failure to tackle disability was a failure of democracy. Millions of disabled people were being ignored and their views disregarded. Disorganized, dispirited and sometimes desperate, they were often patronized. It was commonplace for people to address comments or questions to the person pushing a wheelchair regardless of the intelligence of the disabled person in the chair. Such an attitude was neatly mocked by the title of a BBC radio programme on disability: *Does He Take Sugar?*. Megan's initiative influenced the public and disabled people themselves because she articulated hidden feelings with a call that was to echo throughout the following decades – a fair deal for disabled people.

The Disablement Income Group (DIG) was set up in September 1965, and one of its early supporters was an unknown neurology registrar, David Owen. When he subsequently became an MP in 1966 he led the first delegation to present its case to the Minister for Health, Kenneth Robinson. Megan was pleased with his support but not above teasing him. When I suggested to her that we should try to get some working-class support for DIG she laughed and said affectionately, 'That's just what David [Owen] solemnly advised – with his middle-class voice as he tossed his hair back.'

It was through my association with Megan that I began to think seriously about disablement. I realized that the task was to translate the wind of change into political action. In the post-war era, disability was not mentioned in the manifestos of the main political parties, and there were no Commons debates on the subject between 1959 and 1964. The only time Parliament took an interest was to help disabled ex-servicemen to get jobs. The 1944 and 1952 Disabled Employment Acts, as their titles suggest, were aimed at encouraging the employment of disabled people. For the most part, it had been government by neglect, reflecting public indifference.

My first step was to initiate an Adjournment debate in October 1967, which gave me the opportunity of stating DIG's case in Parliament. My speech was sympathetically received by the Minister, Norman Pentland, but he made no specific commitment.

A few months after the Adjournment debate I lost my hearing completely and did not return to the Commons until the spring of 1968. It became clear to me then that some kind of Parliamentary organization was needed to stimulate political interest in disability and to establish co-operation between MPs and the voluntary organizations. In addition to a disability income, improvements were needed in many areas such as transport, employment, housing and education. I set about trying to organize a Parliamentary All-Party Disablement Group.

I approached John Astor, the Tory MP for Newbury, who had accompanied Megan on the deputation to the Minister for Health in 1966, and he readily agreed to help. One of the famous Astor family, he was a nephew of Nancy Astor, the first woman to sit as an MP.

There was about John a certain grandeur, a dignified bearing and disdain for publicity. With great sympathy and an understanding for disabled people, he tolerated some flamboyance from me and rarely if ever objected to any initiatives even when, as in the early 1970s, they were implicitly critical of the Tory Government. If I attempted to push the Group into outright condemnation of the Government he never said no; a clouding of his eyes was enough for me to beat a diplomatic retreat and soften the proposals – although this never impeded my own attacks from the Labour benches.

When the All-Party Disablement Group was officially formed, I was elected Chairman and John became Secretary. Thus began many years of intense activity in Parliament. We held regular fortnightly meetings with disabled groups, and many informal ones with their officials or disabled people themselves. Having learned of the problems, we asked Parliamentary Questions, spoke in debates and took deputations to Ministers. We gave disabled people access to the corridors of power.

The Group played a prominent role in the Chronically Sick and Disabled Persons Bill, which substantially helped to restore my confidence in the House after losing my hearing. Ideas for the Bill and active participation were required from MPs of all parties and so too was harmony. Had there been the usual party political acrimony, the Bill could not have been enacted before the General Election in June 1970. Members of the Group took part in briefing sessions, helping to get an agreed backbench line to put to Ministers and officials. This was particularly important as the Secretary of State, Dick Crossman, showed a marked lack of enthusiasm for the Bill, so much so that when its sponsor, Alf Morris, went to discuss it with him, Crossman suggested that he should drop disability in favour of organ transplants. But faced with united all-party support, Crossman could hardly oppose it outright. The role of the Group was crucial.

Outside Parliament, Megan's Disablement Income Group was growing in strength and having a big impact on public opinion. On Saturday 10 May 1969, the fourth Annual General Meeting of DIG was held, at which Megan was to report progress and plans for the following year were to be formulated. On her way to the meeting,

(314)

she was killed in a car crash. Her husband, Bill, who was with her, lost a wonderful wife, and disabled people lost a charismatic champion. In one newspaper she was described as 'a saint' with creative imagination and likened to Florence Nightingale for her pioneering work. In a mere four years, as the Chairman of DIG, Denis Saunders said, 'She captured the hearts and minds of all who heard her.'

Despite the blow, DIG continued its work. Mary Greaves, an ex-civil servant, who was also disabled, succeeded Megan. Possessing different qualities, she was a warm, thoughtful, knowledgeable person who ably built on the foundations laid by Megan. The most important social security improvements for disabled people during her term of office were an Attendance Allowance, which enabled severely disabled people to pay for personal care, and a long-term invalidity benefit.

Although these were small beginnings, they encouraged DIG to redouble its efforts. One of the highlights of 1972 was a DIG petition for a national disability income signed by a staggering 258,404 people. When I presented it formally to the House of Commons, a relay of attendants were required to carry the impressive pile into the Chamber.

I was sorry when John Astor left the House in 1974 and saddened when he died some years later. His work for disabled people, although little known, had been outstanding. He was replaced as Secretary of the All-Party Disablement Group by John Hannam, an able and considerate Conservative MP with sound judgement. Despite being an executive member of the Tory 1922 Committee, their powerful backbench group, he was often outspoken in his criticism of Government policies on disablement, albeit in much more discreet and diplomatic language than mine. As with John Astor, he and I found little difficulty in maintaining an all-party stance while sustaining our own individual vigorous party political activity.

The Group kept some 150 MPs and Peers in touch with disability issues through the circulation of its minutes, but it was generally a score or less of committed people who attended the meetings. Those who joined the Group tended to stay with it, partly because they often had a personal interest in disability. Dafydd Wigley, a lively

Welsh MP who was the Plaid Cymru leader, fought disablement issues with conviction and passion. He spoke not for publicity but out of feeling because his two sons had died of a rare hereditary disease. He and I were once invited to Hungary to visit a disablement centre. But the 1987 election was in the offing and Dafydd decided he could not risk being away because, had he gone, the Parliamentary Plaid Cymru group, with just two MPs, would have been halved. I saw his point, and we put off the visit.

Lewis Carter-Jones specialized in technology for disability. He was a director of Possum, a firm which developed technical devices to help disabled people to control their environment. One of the Group's researchers made an apt comment about Lewis, saying that, on Select Committees, 'If he disagreed with what witnesses were saying, he would question them with a degree of amazement in his voice, akin to a caveman seeing an aeroplane for the first time. By the end of the discussion he normally had the witnesses questioning facts they had previously been sure of.'

David Price was a Tory MP whose disabled wife was in a wheel-chair. Understandably he was particularly interested in access issues. Although he was less fiery than the two Welsh MPs, he was no less effective.

Other MPs who were stalwart members of the Group but with no close personal links with disability included Alf Morris, Peter Thurnham, Tom Clarke and Bob Wareing. These all had a natural interest in the subject and some had steered their own Private Members' Bills on disability through Parliament. Alf Morris, in particular, focused strongly on disability throughout his Parliamentary career. No MP was more knowledgeable and none achieved more genuine help for disabled people.

The Group was well supported by members of the House of Lords. Some of them – Sue Masham, Davinia Darcy de Knayth, Felicity Lane Fox and Martin Ingleby – were known as the wheel-chair brigade. They made a formidable group and, together with Denis Carter, Beatrice Kinloss, Barbara Loydon and others, were able to ambush the Government in the Lords on several famous occasions, although regrettably the Government sometimes reversed

their successes when the Bill returned to the Commons. Nevertheless, particularly in the Thatcher years, they were able to achieve
more than the Commons MPs. The Lords could be astute tacticians.
Once, when one of them was moving a disability Amendment,
another, a Tory, took five new Conservative Peers for a drink at the
crucial voting time so they would not vote against it.

The Group was fortunate in having remarkably able and caring
people as research assistants. The most outstanding was its first,
Peter Mitchell. No one was more knowledgeable about disability or
quicker at spotting the place in a Government Bill to propose an
Amendment favourable to disabled people. Five women subsequently held the position; despite youth and, in some cases, only
slight experience, they, like Peter, rapidly and accurately absorbed
information and presented its essence to busy MPs. Their excellent
briefs were carefully angled to the temperament and politics of the
MP to receive it, although one researcher later admitted to her
chagrin that I never stuck to my script and would deliver my own
personal broadsides. I suspect, however, that they were sometimes
more frustrated by the all-party nature of the Group, which needed
a fair measure of diplomacy. Not that MPs were mealy-mouthed.
Particularly on the floor of the House, they would add to their briefs
and make hard-hitting attacks on the Government. The MPs were
given the credit, but it was the researchers who seized opportunities
and provided the ammunition to maintain the momentum of the
disability lobby.

The pressure in Parliament for the rights of disabled people was
gradually becoming irresistible. Not only MPs but political leaders
began to take note of the campaigns. It was a major step forward
when in 1974 the new Prime Minister, Harold Wilson, created a
new post of Minister for the Disabled. Alf Morris was given the job
and although he was attached to the Department of Health, he
liaised with all other Departments on matters affecting disabled
people. A capable and knowledgeable Minister, with the necessary
good eye for publicity, he had established himself by piloting the
Chronically Sick and Disabled Persons Act.

When the Labour Government took office in 1974, everyone

realized that stringent measures would be necessary to get the economy right. Morris was therefore caught in the crossfire of pressure from the Treasury to avoid spending commitments and pressure from our Group and disabled people for extensive and expensive reform. Despite the difficulties, he instituted many changes to help disabled people, some of which were of direct benefit to disabled housewives. In 1977, recognized at last, they were given a non-contributory invalidity pension. This had been introduced two years earlier for those with insufficient national insurance contributions. Congenitally disabled people who were never able to work were thus brought in from the cold, and the later extension of this benefit to married women gave DIG great satisfaction. Other important advances introduced while Morris was Minister were the Invalid Care Allowance, for those unable to work because they cared for a severely disabled person, and the Mobility Allowance, for those who could not walk.

The Parliamentary Group was deeply involved in the legislation bringing about these changes. The sharp end of disability is often cash not pain. Disability means extra costs yet it reduces if not eliminates the ability to pay for them. So, over the years, every benefit change was scrupulously monitored by the Group's researcher and MPs.

There were many successes as well as disappointments, but one particularly welcome advance was the granting of Mobility Allowance to deaf–blind and to mentally handicapped people in 1989. It seemed so obvious to members of the Group that the ability to put one foot in front of the other does not give effective mobility if, say, a mentally handicapped child runs in all directions at random. The mother of such a child cannot get from A to B by walking or using public transport, and she deserves the Mobility Allowance as much as the mother whose child is immobile. But it was only after many deputations that Ministers and their officials accepted our case.

The world of disability is like a turbulent sea. New thoughts, ideas and beliefs are constantly rising to the surface, being tested and then carried on either an outward or inward tide. The Group was the channel through which the new sustainable ideas were funnelled into Parliament and legislation. For example, it used to be assumed that the physically immobile or brain-damaged child should be tucked away in a special school, and a helplessly disabled adult should be tended, albeit often somewhat inadequately, in an institution. Disabled people themselves demolished these ideas. The Group conveyed the new thinking to Parliament, and new legislation emerged for both young and old. The 1981 Education Act provided for all handicapped children to be educated with their peers in normal schools, but with special appropriate individual provision. Adults so disabled as to be virtually paralysed were enabled to live in their own homes with their own selected form of care paid for by the new Independent Living Fund, for whose preservation MPs fought hard.

One of the Group's researchers once commented to me that it was the task of Sisyphus to organize MPs on disablement. I had to turn to the dictionary to find that Sisyphus was a Greek condemned to push a stone up a hill and begin again when it rolled down, an image which aptly reflected the work of the Group. No sooner was one disability issue dealt with than another took its place. Over the years, all aspects of disabled life were addressed, from perinatal mortality and antenatal care for babies to income and access for those of working age, and then to the major concern of old age – 'community care'.

We used every Parliamentary device to push the disability cause. It was sustained pressure, but much depended on the resistance of the relevant Minister, and in particular of the Minister for the Disabled.

None of the Tory Ministers who succeeded Morris, following the election of Margaret Thatcher in 1979, made any great impact. Even the one who later became Prime Minister, John Major, failed to make any significant advance. I was impressed by his obvious interest and willingness to listen, but his short tenure from October 1986 to June 1987 was marked more by hope than by achievement. Yet I recognized his talent. After he first addressed the Group, at a time when he was just a junior Minister, I told the Group's research assistant that I thought he would be the next Leader of the Conservative Party. As she said later, if only we had put money on that!

Many of the disabled people were exceptionally interesting person-alities, and I learned a great deal from them. One of the most outstanding was Peter Large, a civil servant who got polio in 1973 when he was thirty years old. He was confined to a wheelchair, his legs useless and his arms weak, but his mind was one of the keenest I have known. On all aspects of disablement he spoke with know-ledge, clarity and authority.

It was through Peter, and his wife Susy, that I began to appreciate fully that flights of steps, kerbs and narrow doorways – all taken for granted by able-bodied people – created major barriers for him and others like him. The lack of personal mobility was emphasized whenever he took a car journey; Susy would hoist and manoeuvre him into the car with specially adapted lifting gear. Getting in and out, which most of us never think about, was for them a slow, cumbersome and wearying process; though it was carried out with great dignity, the burden on them both was obvious.

Susy made her own contribution on disability and she could be scathing about mindless bureaucracy or Ministerial ineptitude. She obtained a first-class honours degree with the Open University, and, with her vigour and intellect, would certainly have been a powerful disability activist had she not suffered kidney failure. Tragically, after two unsuccessful transplants, she died in 1982.

The majority of disabled people feel that lack of access is a form of discrimination, and one experience at Westminster illustrated this. Access in the rambling, beautiful but old building has always been a problem despite some improvements like ramps and places for wheelchairs. There was no difficulty, however, when the crippled Deng Pufang, head of China's national disablement organization and the son of China's leader, Deng Xiaoping, arrived for a meeting. I alerted the police to carry him up a flight of stairs at the end of Westminster Hall to the room. But, surrounded by his entourage and embassy officials, he was lifted without difficulty, still smiling and chatting, before the police could help.

I therefore assumed that there would be no difficulty when Rachel Hurst, a well-known disability activist in a wheelchair, was to attend a meeting I had arranged with some foreign visitors. Because it was to be filmed for a television programme, I booked one of the few rooms, off Westminster Hall, in which cameras are permitted. It was down just five steps. Rachel thought the room was inaccessible, but I assured her that as Deng Pufang had been carried up twenty steps without difficulty, she could be carried down five. I knew the police would be willing to help. However, because of her desire for independence, she had a powered wheelchair with a lead battery; and it was so heavy that four policemen were unable to lift it. Her concern was justified and, as a result of my miscalculation, she was excluded from the meeting.

I subsequently asked the Services Committee if, under these special circumstances, they would permit television cameras into the committee rooms which were accessible to wheelchairs, but they refused. Only official meetings in the committee rooms could be filmed – a quite unnecessary piece of discrimination against disabled people.

Denying access to any buildings or rooms causes great frustration to disabled people, but the denial of jobs causes distress and suffering because it leads to poverty. Yet little is done to help. The 1944 Employment Act was supposed to tackle the problem by providing that all firms with over twenty employees should not be allowed to take on more able-bodied workers unless they employed a quota of 3 per cent disabled. Excellent in theory, it was a cardboard crutch because the Department of Employment showered exemption permits like confetti on thousands of firms, allowing them to evade their quota. I could see neither sense nor fairness in this and I continuously pressed successive Governments to copy French and German practice and enforce the legislation, tighten the permit system and impose levies on evading firms. The Group was very supportive, but this was not a battle we won. Instead, all sorts of advisory schemes, aimed at persuasion rather than prosecution, were put to the rogue firms – those with neither the quota nor a permit – but they were often brushed aside.

What I really wanted to do, however, was to tackle discrimination against disabled people, which extends over a very wide field. In education, transport, holiday accommodation and the provision of goods and services, it was rampant. To study this, a group of experts, under the chairmanship of Peter Large, was appointed by Alf Morris in January 1979. Their report, published in February 1982, provided just the ammunition needed.

The report said that discrimination was just as extensive in relation to disablement as to race or sex, and quoted examples which were bizarre or absurd. In one case a draughtsman with an artificial leg was offered a job which was withdrawn when his disability was discovered. In another, a holiday camp refused to accommodate disabled people in summer, claiming that it was because of the hills in the area; but it offered to accept them in the spring or autumn.

I was more annoyed than surprised by the Tory Government's response to the report when it was published. Ministers clearly intended to take no action on the recommendations for new legislation, and they were supported by some Tory members of the All-Party Disablement Group. I strongly favoured action and within days I drew up the first Bill to outlaw discrimination on the grounds of disability. It provided for a commission, with powers to conciliate and to take appropriate action when necessary. Presenting it, I emphasized that I was only concerned with unjustified discrimination. Like the committee, I was not demanding blind bus drivers or deaf piano tuners, nor seeking action if safety hazards were created, or where costs would be disproportionate to benefits.

With no allotted Parliamentary time, my Bill had no chance of being enacted but it highlighted the issue to MPs. I was pleased when Donald Stewart, Leader of the Scottish National Party, who was successful in the ballot for Private Members' Bills, took it up and I waited expectantly but warily for the second reading debate.

Ministerial misgivings were expressed, gently at first but with increasing stridency. The then Minister for the Disabled, Hugh Rossi, had said earlier that he would reserve judgement on legislation but he would need good evidence of significant breaches of human rights. Just before the important second reading debate on 11 February 1983, more Tory MPs began to walk the familiar political tightrope of expressing reservations while claiming to support the principle.

Storm signals were flying two minutes after Donald Stewart ended his opening speech in the debate. Jill Knight, an influential senior Tory backbench MP, was quick to complain about the words 'unjustifiable discrimination'. 'How', she demanded, 'are we to judge what is justifiable and what is unjustifiable?' I knew immediately that her speech was not going to be supportive. She welcomed the idea behind the Bill but called for its rejection on the ground that it was impracticable. When Hugh Rossi warned that the House would be ill advised to embark on this legislation, there was no doubt we were sunk. Most Tories withheld support, and it failed to get its second reading by twenty-three votes.

A major chance for improving the lives of disabled people occurred in 1986 when the Labour MP Tom Clarke, a pleasant, quietly spoken Scot, was successful in the ballot for Private Members' Bills and chose disability. His Bill began as a modest measure to improve the rights of disabled people, but at the planning meetings voluntary organizations, local authorities and the All-Party Disablement Group worked together to construct a radically reforming Bill. Its proposals included the right to appoint a representative to act on their behalf, the right to a voice in the assessment of their needs and an improvement in the co-ordination of services for them.

The Minister for Health, Barney Hayhoe, spoke of 'a useful, if modest, development' and, more menacingly, of his 'sceptical neutrality'. But, after an adroit exercise in political tactics, Tom Clarke saw his Bill enacted in July 1986 – victory appeared to be complete. Ministers thought otherwise, however. They refused to implement some of the important clauses.

When it became obvious that the Government had no intention of budging, a mass lobby was proposed. The plan was to get disabled people in wheelchairs into Westminster Hall and blind and deaf people in the Central Lobby. At first it seemed as if the ambitious exercise was to be a disaster. House officials said Westminster Hall could not be used; the police said no special parking facilities would be available; and there was no press interest.

Our Group wrote to all MPs informing them of the lobby and inviting them to attend. After much effort, everything suddenly began to work. Westminster Hall was made available, the police allowed special parking, and even National Car Parks gave free spaces in their car park close to the House of Commons.

The day itself, 8 April 1987, was a triumph. Westminster Hall and the Central Lobby were packed with disabled people. MPs came to the lobby – over 200 of them – and so too did the spokesmen of the political parties, including Neil Kinnock.

The quick appropriation of a blackboard and a police loudspeaker meant that at times Westminster Hall looked like a cross between a betting shop and a fairground. While I tried to get order using the loudspeaker, House officials were sanguine enough; but when Brian Rix got hold of it and began a long, passionate speech, they became worried. Apparently only MPs can speak in Westminster Hall. I managed to persuade Rix to keep his speech brief, and all was well in the end. It was a memorable day. The Government eventually implemented more parts of the Act, though not to the extent that we wanted.

Although the lobby did not achieve all its objectives, it was of great significance. Previously, disabled people had not themselves lobbied on any scale. They mainly left action to the officials of the voluntary organizations. Now despite the difficulties of travel, over a thousand had come in wheelchairs with guides or helpers to Westminster. They had shown that they could represent themselves effectively. A feature of the lobby was that for the first time hundreds of deaf people came with their interpreters, proving that they too were capable of highly organized protest.

This mass demonstration reflected a profound change in attitude regardless of the type of disability. Recognizing the need to fight, disabled people had founded their own organizations, run by rather than for them. It was a tenuous beginning of a disablement rights movement comparable with those for racial and sexual equality. A few disabled people adopted extreme positions, condemning all able-bodied people, just as some feminists would have no truck with any men, but most were moderate and reasonable.

It is right in principle that disabled people should speak for themselves, and they know better than anyone what the problems

(324)

are. Their first-hand experience enables them to convey the nature of the disability and the consequence of unnecessary man-made obstacles.

Bert Massie, a man crippled by polio as a baby, exemplified to me how this works in practice. After a poor childhood in Liverpool, he had to overcome immense difficulties before getting a university degree, because the local colleges were inaccessible to his wheelchair. His intellect, and his anger about neglect of disabled people, led him to work for the Royal Association for Disability and Rehabilitation. In 1991, he became its Director, the first disabled person to lead a major disability charity.

Massie was a member of a deputation I took to see Lord Ferrers, Minister of State at the Home Office, to discuss the Orange Badge scheme for disabled drivers which gives them special parking rights. The abuse of this badge by able-bodied people was damaging the scheme, leading some local authorities to withdraw from it. But Massie was certain that the solution was to make it an offence to display the badge when the disabled person was not in the car. We knew that the Home Office was strongly opposed to this, but Massie argued it forcefully, using his own experience, with the MPs playing a supporting role.

Soon afterwards, Lord Ferrers told me that he had accepted the proposal. It is rare to persuade a Department to change its mind, and the All-Party Disablement Group got the credit. The reality was that Bert had won a fine victory.

Another person who won impressive victories was Group Captain Leonard Cheshire VC OM, who later became a Peer. A quietly spoken, gentle man, but with a will of iron, he is regarded with devotion by many disabled people, and his achievement in establishing a chain of Cheshire Homes for them across the world has been striking. We have been good friends for many years, and I have noticed that one of his characteristics is to give rather than receive.

I saw this most clearly in Beijing when he discussed with the Chinese authorities the establishment of the first Cheshire Home in China. They were none too enthusiastic at first, possibly chary of Western interference in their domestic affairs. Perhaps they were

(325)

expecting money and were no doubt disconcerted to find that Cheshire Homes all over the world are supported by local donations. But Cheshire gently emphasized his wish to help disabled people in China, and gradually one could see the change in attitude which ended in total agreement and acceptance of his idea.

In 1981, the International Year of Disabled People, when a group in Stoke-on-Trent, which included some disabled ex-airmen, heard that I knew him, they excitedly asked me to persuade him to attend a meeting they were organizing. I was reluctant to press him because I knew how exceptionally busy he was at home and abroad. But I asked him if he would be free, and characteristically he said he would make time free. In Stoke-on-Trent he spoke very quietly from the platform but held hundreds of people spellbound as he related his experiences across the world.

Many disabled people dislike the term 'the disabled' because it presumes that they are a homogeneous mass of humanity. Instead they prefer to emphasize that they are individuals who have a disability, and they consequently use the term 'disabled people'. One person who felt very deeply about this was Lord Snowdon, who has worked with disabled people for many years. He organized an award scheme in 1981 financed initially by royalties from his photographs of the Royal Family, which provides help with the further education or training of young disabled people. I served as a trustee for a long time and knew how passionately he felt.

Nicholas Scott was 'Minister for the Disabled' in 1990 when Tony Snowdon protested about his title. Why couldn't a Minister in this particularly sensitive position drop the term 'the disabled' from his title and be called Minister for Disabled People? This valid request, of singular importance to many who are disabled, was accepted by the Government, and Nicholas Scott thereupon became 'Minister for Disabled People'.

Throughout my years of campaigning on disability, I found that when disabled people were mentioned in the House, MPs tended to nod approvingly. Well disposed, they were anxious to express support, rarely attempted to make political capital, but equally rarely did they press for extra resources. Despite substantial differences between the main parties, debates lacked the venom and point scoring which often characterized clashes on basic political issues. Because of this, disablement was often seen as a political side-show.

The official Office of Population Censuses and Surveys study of 1988 found that there were some 6 million people with varying degrees of disability in Britain. Most able-bodied people assume that disability will happen only to others, and they are therefore often indifferent. At any one time, the vast majority of people are not disabled. Nevertheless over time very few will avoid being affected by disability either personally or through their families. Attitudes will change as this is perceived, and as the numbers of disabled people increase because of greater longevity. Already, on average, people spend more time caring for dependent elderly relatives than looking after children. As middle-aged people come to appreciate that they face years of caring, then being cared for themselves, so disability will gain recognition as an important social issue.

Although some 18 million members of families affected by disability are potential campaigners for change, the greatest impetus is likely to come from disabled people themselves. This has been the pattern in the United States, which has led the way. Spurred on by disabled Vietnam war veterans, the protests and lobbying have achieved substantial gains, and mobilized massive support. In the USA, emphasis has shifted from 'cures' advocated by non-disabled people to 'rights' demanded by those who are disabled.

The American campaign was triggered by a four-year-long refusal of the US Government to implement existing but limited anti-discrimination legislation. A deadline for its enactment was given by disabled people, and when this passed without implementation, thousands from all over the USA converged on the regional offices of the Department of Health. The most successful and effective sit-in was in San Francisco, where disabled people stayed in offices for a 25-day siege. It became a media story, an embarrassment for the Government and a symbol of disabled people's determination. The result was victory and implementation of the legislation.

A vital lesson had been learned, summed up succinctly by one of the leaders, Judy Heumann, who said: 'No matter what anybody tells you, being quiet and passive ain't the way to go.' The Americans built on this progress, demanding more and stronger legislation. In July 1990, President George Bush signed the Americans with Disabilities Act, legislation as wide ranging as the 1964 Civil Rights Act. The culmination of more than twenty years' effort, it outlawed discrimination against disabled people and effectively ended their status as second-class citizens. It protected them against discrimination in transport, employment, public accommodation, hotels, restaurants, shops, telecommunications and services provided by state and local governments. While the USA was leading the world in rejecting this discrimination, Britain, under Conservative rule in the 1980s, was lagging far behind.

Throughout the world, even in developing countries, the 1981 Year of the Disabled stirred concern about the plight and the rights of those who are disabled. It led to action such as the United Nations Decade of Disabled Persons 1983–1992, and its World Programme of Action. The task is enormous, because, according to the UN, at least one person in ten is disabled, and some 25 per cent of most populations are adversely affected by disability within the family.

There could be dramatic gains at relatively little cost. At a United Nations conference in September 1991, it was stated that in the next decade at least 30 million people could be saved from disability through preventive action. If basic surgery were available, over 40 million disabled people in developing countries could have their sight, movement or hearing restored. Mental retardation, affecting 16 million children every generation, caused by iodine deficiency, could be prevented by distributing iodine capsules at an annual cost of 5p per individual. Fifteen million children disabled every year by diseases could be saved by new and combined antigens in vaccines. A million children are born each year with brain damage caused by birth asphyxia – lack of oxygen in the first twenty minutes of life. This could be prevented by a simple resuscitation gadget which a village midwife could use. Already a start has been made on tackling some of these problems. In 1990, 1.2 million cataract operations were performed in India at a unit cost of about £8. Just imagine: a person's sight for £8!

Unless there is general recognition of their difficulties, disabled people will remain in the shadows of the world. Their anxious, and sometimes desperate, striving for independence should be accepted, and the need for assistance from society and government recognized and met whenever possible. Adequate resources are the key. Only then will disabled people escape poverty and patronage, and begin the long, slow climb to fulfilling their own rich potential.

19

Deaf World

Total or profound deafness destroys normal communication, robs people of their confidence and imprisons them in a cocoon of silence. A man can be blind but not isolated, lose his limbs but retain his confidence – but the chilling consequence of loss of hearing is alienation and insecurity. Cut off from the hearing community, a deafened person is deprived not only of communication but often of the will to bridge the chasm to the rest of mankind.

The great Helen Keller, after a lifetime of being both deaf and blind, had no doubt that the problems of deafness are deeper and more complex than those of blindness. Speaking from harsh personal experience, she said: 'I have found deafness to be a much greater handicap than blindness.'

A disturbing truth lies at the heart of her observations. Blindness evokes sympathy, while deafness provokes irritation. Since losing my hearing I have noted the contrasting public attitude to the blind and the deaf. People automatically guide and help a blind person. All too often, having done so, they seem to feel, consciously or unconsciously, that they have done their good deed for the day. The Boy Scout and Girl Guide ethic lives on in most people, but is rarely manifest in their dealings with those profoundly or totally deaf. Yet the burden of deafness is uniquely amenable to sharing; even a slight effort to speak clearly by a hearing person can reduce the difficulties of one who is deaf. Such effort is not, however, always welcome to hearing people.

The instinctive assumption is that a failure of communication is due to stupidity. How can a person, visibly apparently normal, fail to understand? A totally deaf person's reliance on the flicker of silent lips is difficult to comprehend, and the absence of visual evidence makes it doubly so.

No one is at fault, yet between totally deaf and hearing people lies an invisible barrier. A meeting between them may appear normal, but appearance disguises reality. The conversational experience of each is strikingly different. For the one who is deaf, every word he or she tries to follow is a potential pitfall because just one word misunderstood can obscure or distort meaning. There is little difference in the lip movement for such opposite phrases as 'I can do that' or 'I can't do that'.

The difficulties only become apparent to those who can hear when the deaf person's lip-reading fails. Up to that point, it seems to be an ordinary conversation. Then the hearing person suddenly realizes that he or she is unwittingly being drawn into a web of misunderstanding. He or she has to decide whether to continue or break off what has become a disturbing relationship. Any impatience or irritation, noted by the deaf person, leads to anxiety and frustration. Thus friendly or constructive dialogue can be destroyed.

Despite the difficulties, fluent communication between profoundly deaf and hearing people is possible. Nevertheless, hearing people find it easier to speak to each other than to a deaf person and, just as water naturally runs downhill, they gravitate towards each other. Over the years I have watched a conversational pattern develop. My discussion with a hearing person would progress reasonably well until another joined us. Then I would gradually be squeezed out as they began to talk one to the other. No unpleasantness was involved, but it was natural for them to react to each other's comments rather than break the flow to explain things to me. I had then to decide whether to stay out and be content with fragments, or intervene to keep the conversation within my range of understanding. This meant interrupting, and asking for sentences to be repeated, something I dislike doing. With Pauline present I could always rely on her to give me the gist of a conversation, but her presence was not an unmixed blessing. People would often turn away from me and speak to her instead.

'Forgetting' the deaf person absolves those with hearing from speaking more slowly or explaining what is happening. Although I understood the reasons for this, I always found it difficult to accept. On one occasion, just outside Parliament, to the astonishment of two MPs, I gave vent to my feelings. I was walking down Whitehall from the Commons to attend a meeting, accompanied by two friends, Fred Peart and Bob Brown. Peart, a cheerful extrovert, was Leader of the House of Commons. Brown, a down-to-earth Geordie, was Minister for the Army. They chatted and laughed together as the three of us walked from the Members' Lobby, through the House and New Palace Yard and part of the way down Whitehall. Naturally, as I could not understand the conversation, I felt isolated; then I became increasingly resentful and angry at being excluded. As we approached the meeting place I could contain myself no longer. I stopped and blasted my anger at them in extremely colourful terms.

Both were taken aback at the vehemence of this attack; they stood silent as I delivered it, then I stalked off. They were perfectly entitled to chat to each other. Yet I felt insulted because of my deafness. As they were friendly and tolerant men, they never held this against me, and we later resumed our friendship. But the episode must have damaged it in the short term. This was one of the many sad consequences of deafness and my attitude towards people reacting to it. Without my deafness, of course, we would all have been laughing and chatting together.

An even more upsetting experience occurred when I went to discuss some mining problems with the chairman of the local Coal Board in Stoke-on-Trent. For meetings like this, when I could not be certain whether I could lip-read those present, I would normally ask Pauline to accompany me to make notes and, if she couldn't, I would ask for a secretary. Sometimes a fellow MP would help out. When they were MPs John Forrester and Bob Cant, the MPs for the other Stoke seats, had been very considerate. On this occasion, Pauline was unable to go, and the only other MP attending was less familiar with the problems of deafness. I asked him if he would help with some notes of the discussion. He agreed but, when the meeting began, after writing a few sentences he embarked on an hour-long two-way discussion with the Coal Board official. I was totally excluded. I understood that he was anxious to explain his own views and hear those of the Coal Board; but nevertheless the meeting left me angry and depressed. Such experiences, though, were rare. With goodwill and some prior organization, I generally had little difficulty with meetings.

In the early days I worried about my friendships. If I had to rely on interpretation of one sort or another, would they become strained and stilted? In the event, I lost none of my friends when I became deaf, but it was not until I was deaf that I knew who my friends were. I quickly recognized the signs of subtly changed relationships. The middle distance acquired a new fascination for some as they passed. Others would become aware of a sense of time, even urgency, for other appointments. People who had formerly been friendly passed by frowning as if preoccupied with solemn innermost thoughts. The contrast with former enthusiasm and warmth was saddening.

At first, I felt as if I were living in a twilight world, with deafness a badge of shame. Rejection was the more traumatic for being sudden. Yet I came to realize that the loss of some relationships can be as useful to a man as shedding fat is to an athlete. Ultimately we rely on the love of our families and the affection of our true friends.

People's reactions were remarkably varied. Not long after I became deaf, I was invited to join the BBC's General Advisory Council. Outside Broadcasting House, I met my old colleague Huw Wheldon, who was then Managing Director of Television. After the mutual greetings he peered at me keenly and asked, 'Jack, how can I help?' Typical of Wheldon: he was frank, warm and practical.

Some of my less extrovert friends were embarrassed. They felt for me, yet did not like to ask how to help as Wheldon had done. They needed encouragement and had to be persuaded, chivvied even, into believing that a discussion was possible. Part of the reward was the pleasure the other person got from breaking through the deafness barrier, and reaffirming our friendship. Similarly with acquaintances

(333)

who were puzzled by deafness, I would explain the difficulties and how they could be tackled by slower, clearer speech. Usually the response was helpful.

In Parliament, some people tried patronizing me, albeit in an oblique manner. If anyone tried to be patronizing I always pricked it immediately, sometimes perhaps too aggressively, but the attitude needed to be challenged. People are tempted, I noticed, to behave dominantly in the presence of a person with little or no hearing, particularly if that person's confidence is low. Confidence damaged by the uncertainty induced by deafness is further undermined by condescending attitudes.

There is no simple solution, and little point in urging a timid person to act like a lion. But deaf people sometimes permit the public to judge them more by their deafness than by their personality.

A curious reaction to deafness was that after I lost my hearing some MPs would defer to me in the Commons rather as Victorian men did to ladies. For example, when two of us reached the narrow exit of the Division Lobby, a common occurrence as they are usually crowded, colleagues would often, regardless of their age, beckon me to precede them. Not wanting to offend them, I usually accepted; then I realized that although it was done with goodwill, usually with a smile, they were treating me abnormally. I was no longer one of them but a courageous invalid. Kind though they were, I began to insist on them preceding me.

In the early days I was particularly appreciative of help from the public because I was then extremely sensitive about my deafness. Previously simple tasks such as asking the price of goods, or directions in a strange place, or information about train times suddenly became difficult. If I, with my extrovert approach and refusal to be patronized, found it so worrying, what must it be like for a shy person to lose their hearing?

It was not long before I realized that most people did not know how to deal with total deafness. If I could not follow, I had to explain my deafness and the need for lip-reading, and ask people to speak more clearly. This happened frequently at first, and if I still could not understand, I had to proffer pencil and paper. Some people were irritated, others embarrassed. The majority were astonished, not knowing how to respond, but a surprisingly large minority automatically said, 'I'm sorry', then spoke more clearly. I could soon tell how people were going to behave. They betrayed their feelings with a sudden change of expression, a flicker of eyelids or a glint in their eyes; a few smiled and took the problem in their stride. I learned to react accordingly.

When I am recognized, people are exceptionally courteous and pleasant despite the difficulties, but if I am not, the reactions are the same as towards other deaf people, ranging from kindness to irritation. The frustration, and occasional contempt, shown by some of the public when confronted with deafness can cause great distress. I have occasionally faced fierce irritation in shops or at ticket counters, understandable perhaps with a queue of impatient people behind. On one unhappy occasion, my request for a railway ticket was answered by a query from the counter clerk which I could not lip-read. As he repeated it, I concentrated hard, but again I could not follow. Explaining that I was deaf, I asked him to repeat it slowly; he raised his eyes to the heavens and shouted the information. Still unable to follow the flickering lips, disguised by a moustache, and conscious that all those behind would be watching and hearing, as well as waiting for their turn, I asked him to write it down, which merely resulted in further bawling.

My patience snapped. 'Look,' I said. 'All I want is a bloody ticket. There's the money; just get it!' Such drama for such trivialities! Yet deaf people cannot help being occasionally caught up in such episodes.

I have often been amazed by the insensitivity of some people to the implications of deafness. In noisy environments such as a party with loud music or an office with a pneumatic drill outside, hearing people grimace at me and shout: 'You are lucky to be deaf.'

I learned from such comments that most human beings are infinitely more conscious of their own difficulties than those of others. This was borne out when I found that problems in communicating with me were readily overcome when someone needed my help or advice. An example was a former MP who for years had made no effort to speak to me clearly, or indeed at all, in Parliament. Suffering defeat in the General Election, she wanted to apply for my seat after I decided to retire and approached me for information. Her speech was strikingly clear.

I often wish my lip-reading was better, but only a few totally deaf people are very skilled at this. They are usually very gifted people who lost their hearing as children but after acquiring language. Malleable young brains are capable of adapting to this new form of communication and, with experience, develop an impressive command of a near-impossible art.

The vast majority of good lip-readers, however, are not totally deaf. Time and again, I have been told of someone who was far better than me – a truly incredible lip-reader – only to find that he or she had some hearing, buttressed by a powerful hearing aid. No wonder such people are good; they are communicating with both ears and eyes. When I first left the Liverpool ear, nose and throat hospital and had a whisper of hearing, many people commented on the excellence of my lip-reading. But to lip-read well with no hearing at all is staggeringly difficult.

At normal speed there is little clear movement of the lips, and the invisibility of many consonants and vowels poses formidable problems for lip-readers. Even some of the consonants most visible on the lips are indistinguishable from each other. For example, 'p', 'b' and 'm' all look alike, adding to the confusion. These are basic difficulties, quite apart from bushy moustaches, straggly beards and strong accents.

In some books on lip-reading, I have read that a slight puff of the lips with the letter 'p' helps to distinguish it from 'b' and 'm'. This is perhaps slightly discernible when a teacher illustrates it with exaggerated lip movements, but for normal speech 'p', 'b' and 'm' can only be distinguished by context. Equally illusory is the idea that lip-reading is an adequate substitute for hearing. Yet it is a vital crutch which, in the case of totally deafened people, becomes a lifeline. Tenuous and unreliable as it is, it has nevertheless enabled me to survive in Parliament for over twenty years.

(336)

Lip-reading helps with straightforward communication, but tone and inflexion provide vital information which most people absorb immediately and take for granted. I used to pride myself on being able to assess people accurately as soon as I met them. But deprived of sound, I have had to rely on observation and instinct. Natural politicians – not by any means all MPs – have sensitive antennae which enable them to sense an atmosphere. Mine had always served me well and became even more important when I lost my hearing. I got clues to reactions, moods and personality from a slight turn of head, a shift of gaze, extra blinking or speed of body movement.

Useful as these can be, however, they are not infallible. The concentration and energy required for sustained lip-reading detracted from my capacity to observe, and I sometimes got the wrong impression. In rare cases I have thought that a person, perhaps tired or preoccupied, was indifferent to the point of hostility, until a gesture or comment indicated that this was not the case.

Loss of independence, and the need for some help from others, is an inevitable consequence of total deafness. I became sensitive, perhaps hypersensitive, if assistance was given indiscreetly. For example, the Whips, the business managers of Parliament, occasionally came to me as I sat in the Chamber, to explain changes in the order of debate or with messages from the Speaker about when I might be called to speak. A few in particular ostentatiously gesticulated and pointed as if communicating with a moron.

Some people who were kind could not resist displaying it. On one important Parliamentary occasion, I asked a friendly Tory MP to signal to me if my voice became too loud. As it happened, no signal was required. But a few days later a political gossip columnist reported how MPs, including this one, were kindly helping me with signals. I resented the exaggerated story and never again asked that MP for help.

Despite daily pitfalls, I usually managed to avoid major errors in the House, but on one occasion I made a spectacular one. A group of Labour MPs had been trying to persuade the Chancellor of the Exchequer, Tony Barber, to concede extra cash to disabled people. His officials told us just before the debate that although he was

sympathetic he intended to reject our request. Accordingly, I prepared a hostile speech. When Barber addressed the House, no colleagues were near me to make notes and I had great difficulty in
following him. I felt relieved that I knew what he would be saying.

When he finished, the Speaker called me first, and I strongly
attacked his meanness and lack of humanity to disabled people. Immediately I could sense shock on both sides; a Labour colleague rushed
up with a note to say that Barber had changed his mind and accepted
our proposal. Naturally embarrassed, I promptly apologized for the
misunderstanding and sat down. Next day I looked in Hansard, the
official verbatim report of proceedings, to check my unfortunate
tirade against the Chancellor. It was not included. Probably for the
first time in the history of Parliament since proceedings were
recorded, a speech was deliberately omitted. It emerged later that
the Speaker, together with MPs on both sides, had agreed on the
omission, although some Labour Whips had to be persuaded.

The possibilities of this kind of gaffe, and the strain of lip-reading
and relying on occasional notes from colleagues, meant that something had to be done. Pauline suggested that as Hansard reporters
took shorthand notes in the press gallery, we should find out whether
a camera could record these on a screen for me. This would entail
the agreement of the House authorities, provision of a camera,
acceptance by Hansard reporters and mastery of shorthand by me.
These were a lot of provisos, but I set about investigating them.

The BBC kindly agreed to provide a camera for a trial session, a
first step which unfortunately came to nothing. I found that all
shorthand writers have their own idiosyncrasies, and Hansard reporters explained that it would be impracticable for me to acquire
sufficient expertise to understand all of them, much less at speed
and under pressure.

Then we heard that Alan Newell, a scientist at Southampton
University, was developing a device for deaf people which enabled
them to give or receive messages. This turned out to be merely a
brooch worn on the lapel that displayed a few words. It would be
fine for things like 'hello' and 'goodbye', but hardly a solution to my
problems of following detailed speeches in the House.

(338)

Pauline and I, our hopes rising and falling, continued with our inquiries and learned of Palantype, a mechanical shorthand device which enabled an operator to type at the speed of normal speech. The operator pressed various combinations of special keys according to the phonetic sounds she heard. A pattern of dots, meaningful to the operator, emerged on a paper roll and was transcribed by her into properly typed English. If the operator could 'read' the pattern of dots, Pauline thought that a computer could do so and produce phonetic English for me to read on a monitor. Then we heard that scientists at the National Physical Laboratory had found that it was too complex and costly to translate Palantype into perfectly spelt English; but, when we visited them, they suggested that we should approach a few small electronics firms to see if they could produce a system adequate for my needs.

Any workable system could transform my life in Parliament and be a great advance for deaf people – but I had no money for experiments and no authority from the House to pursue them. Nevertheless, two small electronics firms were interested. In mid-1974, six years after I lost my hearing, they set to work.

It was time to approach the House of Commons authorities. I wrote explaining the possibilities and asking for their agreement. The Services Committee quashed the idea in diplomatic language, saying that the equipment would be too large and too expensive to develop; in any case, it could not be seriously considered until it was seen working.

One electronics firm subsequently withdrew, but the other, owned by an enterprising and innovative man named Postlethwaite, continued. In addition Alan Newell, the scientist from Southampton University, decided he too would like to explore the use of Palantype. I told both Postlethwaite and Newell that the cost of the trial equipment must be low, and the size of my monitor small. In addition, neither I nor Parliament could pay for development costs. Nevertheless both went ahead.

It was an exciting but tense period. As the technical experts made progress, I set to work to win acceptance of the project at Westminster. The Government Chief Whip, Bob Mellish, the Minister for

Disablement, Alf Morris, and the Leader of the House, Edward Short, were all helpful. Mellish wrote to the Services Committee, saying: 'I am sure cost ought not to be a consideration, for I believe that the whole House would want to do everything possible to enable Jack Ashley to give of his very wonderful best.' This was excessively generous but helpful to my cause; and, in addition, he wrote to the Prime Minister asking him to help in any way he could.

Behind the scenes at 10 Downing Street I had another fine ally. Bernard Donoghue, a great and trusted friend, was the senior policy adviser to the Prime Minister. Although I did not know at the time how he influenced opinion, he wrote in his book *Prime Minister*: 'Perhaps the greatest satisfaction I enjoyed in Downing Street was in helping to provide Palantype equipment in the Chamber to enable Jack, who is totally deaf, to follow the proceedings.'

Once Southampton University and Postlethwaite had developed their systems I invited the members of the Services Committee to view them at the House, where Pauline and I, together with the operators and scientists, waited expectantly. The MPs strolled warily into the room, wanting to be clear about what they were being asked to permit in the hallowed Chamber of the House. Would it disfigure the august benches? Would it distract from Parliamentary business? How costly was it going to be and, above all, would it work?

I had worked desperately to understand the oddly abbreviated phonetic language that appeared on the screen. It still looked like gobbledegook, and I was by no means certain that I could comprehend it at this vital testing time. Translating such abbreviations as 'cheim', 'dwic', 'hoyfr', 'mfr', 'reg', 'syrcs', 'sti' and 'op fyuts' at the speed of normal speech was not easy. It was not blindingly obvious which words they represented; for example, the translations of the above symbols were: 'chairman', 'difficulty', 'however', 'manufacture', 'regulation', 'circumstances', 'society' and 'obvious'.

Thankfully two of the committee's earlier requirements were met: the cost was less than £5,000, and the visual display unit was only 9 inches by 9 inches. But would it work? The chairman, Tory MP Robert Cooke, tall, languid but sharp, stood in front of me and asked questions. As the operator typed her coded messages I carefully watched the small visual display unit before answering. The conversation was halting, but seemed to be going reasonably well. Cooke was reflective, and I guessed that he was wondering if I was supplementing information from the screen by lip-reading him. I was right – and so was he.

He walked behind me, and as the rest of the committee watched, the operator began to tap out his next question, which came up on the small screen. I stared intently at it and half-calculated and half-guessed that it was: 'Just suppose for a moment that I was the Foreign Secretary, what would be your reaction to me now?' My mind raced as I decoded this message while the committee awaited my response. At that time, Labour was in power, and when I replied, 'To suppose that you were Foreign Secretary would be to face disaster, because you are a Tory MP', the laughter changed the atmosphere. I was exhilarated. For the first time in eight years I had communicated directly with a person I could not see. He asked more questions, and other committee members did so as well. Then, commenting favourably on the equipment, they left to consider their verdict. It turned out to be full acceptance, and of the two they chose the Southampton University version.

That day, 19 May 1976, marked the victorious end of a two-year battle for me to 'hear' via Palantype. I first used it on 1 February the following year. It was a turning point in my life as a deaf MP; proceedings in the House were now far more accessible to me. My main operator, Isla Beard, used the equipment with great skill, making the text as comprehensive and clear as possible in subsequent years as she had done in the test for the committee.

I chose to sit at the end of the third row in the Chamber, a vantage point giving me a view of Members on both sides to comple-ment the words on my screen. Two sockets were fixed under my seat on the Government side to provide electricity for my equipment. I became the only MP with a permanent seat. After the defeat of the Labour Government in 1979, I discovered that two sockets were waiting for me across the Chamber under a seat on the Opposition benches.

No speech is faster than repartee in the House of Commons; but

Isla, sitting high up in the press gallery listening to proceedings and tapping them out on her keyboard, kept me well in touch over the years. The system was subsequently taken up by the Research Development Council and then by Possum Controls. The script became vastly more comprehensible, and in later years it was practically perfect English. Deaf organizations and some individuals have found it tremendously helpful; its one limitation is the shortage and high cost of skilled operators.

There is not enough help for most deaf people, but remarkably, in the face of monumental difficulties, many do surmount the obstacles. Often they do much more than that, flourishing despite adversity, calling upon untapped reserves to overcome their disability and go on to greater accomplishments. The triumph of the human spirit against deafness is a marvel; how else can we explain the success of deaf poets, mountaineers, actors, musicians, engineers and athletes? Ostensibly trapped in a silent world, they escape by virtue of their spirit, determination and resilience.

Although those losing their hearing are always aware of what they have lost, people born deaf face daunting difficulties. The natural ease with which hearing children develop speech and language contrasts starkly with the obstacles facing those born profoundly deaf. Without hearing a word, they have to acquire language as a vehicle for thought and a means of communication. Only then can they learn to adapt to a hearing environment and find an appropriate niche in a world for which nature has left them ill adapted.

Sometimes, with the devoted help of parents and professionals, the results are excellent. Powerful conventional hearing aids, and radio aids, backed by teachers and parents, give some very deaf children excellent language and lip-reading ability; they obtain good jobs and have a secure place in society. In other cases the deaf child becomes a poorly communicating, ill-educated young adult.

The most impressive profoundly deaf child whom I have met, relying virtually entirely on lip-reading, was Wendy Craig. She was the daughter of two Canadians, who helped to organize the Alexander Graham Bell Convention in Toronto, which I attended in 1982. Despite having to concentrate intently on using her tiny remnant of hearing, she was a balanced, happy, communicating six-year-old. The dedicated efforts of her parents and teachers were fully rewarded. But Wendy was not typical. Unless they receive intensive support, some profoundly deaf children cannot benefit from hearing aids and, if they do not use sign language, they can become educationally and socially deprived. For many years the extent of this deprivation was not appreciated. Instead, speaking and lip-reading success was emphasized.

Parents of deaf children usually accepted the views of professionals. But, in 1977, a study by the British psychologist Dr Conrad showed that the average profoundly deaf child left his or her special school at sixteen years of age with the reading age of eight, a very limited vocabulary and speech which was often difficult to understand. Studying all profoundly deaf children rather than focusing on the exceptional ones showed that a vast gulf existed between deaf and hearing children in general – and some of the deaf children were virtually living in a communication vacuum.

How can these standards be raised? A historic conflict between advocates of lip-reading and those favouring the use of sign language has bedevilled deaf children's education for over two hundred years. The so-called oralism and manualism controversy still continues, although with less bitterness. The obvious answer is to provide the appropriate method for each child. But this is easier said than done, because a child's natural oral skills can only be assessed after the crucial early learning years. Parents often have to take vital decisions in the dark.

Ironically, deaf children who can communicate and who have a good education face another hurdle – discrimination. I have come across many examples since I lost my hearing, one of the most striking being that of Matthew James. A profoundly deaf 22-year-old graduate with an upper-second degree in biological sciences, he had won his university's Dean's Commendation for Excellence. I met him when he won the Deaf Achiever of the Year award, and again the following year when he was an adjudicator. On the second occasion he sat between me and the Princess of Wales, who was presenting the award. With both of us, he communicated without

(343)

difficulty. Friendly, intelligent and brimming with initiative, he was the kind of young graduate companies would normally rush to employ. Yet he had no job despite many applications. It was an absurd waste of talent, and unjustified discrimination.

As he specialized in ecology, I asked Chris Patten, Secretary of State for the Environment, if he knew of any vacancies or if he could assist this exceptionally talented young man to find a job in that field. Patten's response was generous and comprehensive, outlining not only possible opportunities in his own Department but also those in the wider area of ecology. I kept in touch with Matthew, and six months later he told me that of the eighteen establishments he had applied to, only six had offered interviews. A mere two had offered jobs, but not the ones he applied for, and they were well below his competence. In desperation he took one of the inappropriate jobs because he needed the money.

In striking contrast to those prejudiced against deaf people, Princess Diana did all she could to help. Her warmth and clarity of speech, as well as her moral support, gave great encouragement to all those at the Deaf Achievers lunch. As Patron of the British Deaf Association, she learned to sign, and this was but one of the many ways she helped deaf people in general and young deaf people in particular. Her royal example meant a great deal.

The vast majority of hearing-impaired people are neither profoundly nor totally deaf, and for them a hearing aid gives access to the hearing world. My mother's life was transformed when she started to use one. Instead of retiring when visitors came to the house, she joined in all the conversation and became an active participant in many pensioners' activities. The change came in the early 1970s when I bought her an ear-level aid. At the time, the NHS aid was an old-fashioned body-worn aid, efficient enough but cumbersome and unwieldy. It had to be fastened to clothing and connected to the ear-mould by a long wire cord. Private hearing aid firms manufactured small aids fitting neatly behind the ear, but some of their advertisements were designed to make deaf people feel uncomfortable about 'unsightly' hearing aids – a contributory factor to deaf people feeling ashamed of their disability.

I felt it was deplorable that the Government should refuse to provide modern ear-level aids to the 2 million people moderately and severely deaf who could benefit. Many of them could not afford up to £100 for a private aid; yet because of the potentially large numbers required, the Government could purchase ear-level aids for a capital cost of only £8 each and distribute them for a further £8.

In 1973, I began to press the Secretary of State for Health, Sir Keith Joseph, to provide all deaf people with ear-level aids. Pauline had noticed the junior Minister's fudged replies to my constant demands; he was 'actively considering', 'seriously considering', 'expediting the study', 'looking into it', 'still looking into it' and 'had not yet completed the study'. In the House one day I catalogued these pathetic variations on a negative theme and, as the whole House dissolved into laughter, I suggested that he should 'change his line of patter or work the trick'. Soon afterwards, Sir Keith Joseph announced that all deaf people were to receive a behind-the-ear aid free of charge.

In the longer term, of course, preventing and treating deafness by furthering fundamental research are even more important than improved hearing aids. With most conditions, doctors can at least explain what has happened even if they cannot reverse the damage. But when I lost my hearing, I found there was much medical ignorance about deafness, and doctors could do neither. This was because I suffered from the most intractable form of hearing loss, sensorineural or nerve deafness. Once this occurs, through noise, drugs, illness or other unknown factors, doctors are helpless – unable either to alleviate or to explain it, except in the most general terms.

Disturbed by the medical ignorance, I tried in October 1968 to get support for an international seminar of experts to advance knowledge. The CIBA Foundation has a high academic reputation for scientific research, and I asked the Director, Dr Gordon Wolstenholme, if they would organize and fund an international seminar on nerve deafness. In a friendly but disappointing response, he regretfully refused because CIBA was over-committed. I thanked him, said I would look elsewhere and asked if CIBA's meeting rooms could be hired. Soon afterwards he wrote to say that they had

(345)

changed their minds and intended to set up the seminar. It was a fine gesture leading to an important event, attended by experts from Europe, the Middle East and the USA. No simple solutions were forthcoming, but the exchange of ideas and the meeting of minds were valuable steps forward in furthering fundamental research.

My next opportunity to encourage research came in March 1974, when I became Parliamentary Private Secretary to Barbara Castle. I asked her about establishing an Institute of Hearing Research, which, together with a hard-of-hearing MP, Laurie Pavitt, I had tried unsuccessfully to promote during the passage of the Chronically Sick and Disabled Persons Act in 1970. The most we were able to achieve was a clause imposing a requirement on the Secretary of State to 'collate and present evidence to the Medical Research Council on the need for an Institute for Hearing Research'. As the MRC was opposed to an institute, that clause did not get us very far.

Barbara was willing to help and raised the matter with her civil servants. She found that most were unenthusiastic, and the powerful MRC was still firmly opposed. Although Barbara was undeterred by that, she was not convinced of the need for an institute. So she called a special meeting to hear both sides. I spoke of the inadequacy of research into deafness. Fragmented and sometimes duplicated, it had no co-ordinating body, no dynamism and minimal funding. Closely co-ordinated multi-disciplinary work was required to include specialists in clinical otology, audiology, physiology and sociology. Lacking that unified approach, deafness as a research subject was languishing in a backwater.

The opposing civil servants claimed that co-operation did exist between various research centres, and that such an institute would centralize control, leading to rigidity. But their strongest argument was that it would be costly. This case, persuasive to most Ministers, must have been attractive to Barbara, who was under great financial pressure.

After both sides had argued the case, and answered questions from Barbara, we awaited her decision. She was reflective, weighing the pros and cons. Then she said quietly but firmly that an institute should be set up. Once she had made up her mind, she brooked no opposition from civil servants or the Medical Research Council.

Her published *Diaries* record that, on 7 July 1975, she wrote of a long-planned meeting to be held with Sir John Gray of the MRC:

> It was originally arranged with the idea of my making it clear that I intended to go ahead with the Institute of Hearing Research on the lines Jack Ashley has rightly been fighting for and that, if the MRC stuck to its opposition, DHSS would go ahead immediately and finance a chair of hearing research at a university. In the event, the MRC has climbed down and agreed to make £500,000 available for a new building to conduct and coordinate multi-disciplinary research . . . So once again we politicians have been right and our officials wrong . . . Of course, officials opposed us all the way.

Barbara and I both believed that the Institute would greatly benefit deaf people, and so it has proved. Under Professor Mark Haggard, with headquarters in Nottingham and clinical out-stations in Southampton and Glasgow, the Institute is in the world's front rank of research centres. In 1989, the Medical Research Council reported that referees were enthusiastic about the research, which was of high scientific merit.

Pauline had developed a keen interest in hearing research following her appointment as a Governor of London's Ear, Nose and Throat Hospital in Gray's Inn Road, and subsequently chairman of its associated postgraduate medical school. From her work there she realized that, despite the excellence of the research, its development was curtailed and frustrated by a serious shortage of funds. Research into most disabilities got well over half its funding from charitable sources, but deafness had no charity devoted solely to research. With help initially from the specialists at the Gray's Inn Road centre, she established the Hearing Research Trust in 1985.

It soon won the support of authoritative people, together with royal backing from the Duke of York, who became its Patron. Professor Haggard became its Chief Scientific Adviser. I was made

(347)

President, but the real head of it, the driving force, was Pauline. Devoting immense energy and determination, she established the Trust as an influential and important means of stimulating and funding research.

An early aim was to provide answers to the many unresolved questions regarding sensorineural deafness. The cochlea, the crucial inner ear, is tiny and inaccessible, which is why its complex mechanism has been a mystery for so long. Sophisticated computers, powerful microscopes and space-age materials were at last enabling scientists to discover how it worked and why it sometimes failed. The Trust supported the research of a network of scientists across Britain, all investigating the cochlea. Before long it was asked to help with many other problems such as the early detection of deafness in babies, genetic deafness, cochlear implants and ways of improving hearing aids and ear-moulds. Money for the Trust did not flood in – deaf charities face the same indifference as deaf people – but with hard work it came in a reasonably steady stream. Five years elapsed before the Trust raised its first million, but I am sure that before long Pauline will achieve her ambition of raising at least £1 million annually for research into deafness.

One of the most promising developments in the 1970s and 1980s was the cochlear implant. In a healthy ear, sound waves travel through the outer and middle ear and are picked up by the inner ear – the cochlea. Here, with incredible sensitivity and accuracy, they are transformed by the cochlear hair cells into nerve impulses which travel to the brain. Damaged hair cells cannot be restored, and when damage is severe even the most powerful hearing aid is useless. A cochlear implant bypasses the hair cells and directly stimulates the auditory nerves, enabling the brain to understand sound.

The early implants were valuable supplements to lip-reading, while the sophisticated ones developed later give greater understanding of speech, even enabling some exceptional patients to follow simple messages on the telephone. A further benefit is that most people so deaf as to require an implant cannot hear their own voice and an implant enables them to do so, thereby improving their voice modulation. By 1989, over 5,000 deaf people had received cochlear implants in other countries of the world, most of them successfully. Many British surgeons had been sceptical, but there was one determined pioneer – Graham Fraser, at University College London. Supported largely by the Royal National Institute for the Deaf and the Jules Thorne Charitable Trust, he set up a special unit and between 1982 and 1990 gave cochlear implants to over fifty deafened people. He knew, however, that NHS funding was essential if cochlear implantation was to be routinely offered to those of the 100 people losing their hearing annually who could benefit from it.

This seemed a fine but unobtainable objective. Local District Health Authorities were short of funds, and cochlear implants apparently did not fulfil the criteria for central funding. To break this bureaucratic impasse, I took a deputation to see David Mellor, Minister of State at the Department of Health, in March 1989. It included Fraser and a woman patient who had been fitted with an implant. Mellor listened carefully as we put the case for £3 million to fund a comprehensive programme. Then he turned to the woman, Christine Harding, whose life had regained some semblance of normality, and quizzed her. We all sat silently as she watched him and listened to him intently; she understood and answered his questions. It was a moving occasion, and I knew that Mellor had been impressed. Although he could make no immediate commitment, I got a clear impression that he wanted to provide the money. He had to argue the case with the Treasury, but before long it was agreed that £3 million was to be provided by the Department over four years to fund up to six NHS centres – a major advance for deaf people in Britain. The surgeon, Fraser, and the politician, Mellor, had ensured that deafened people in Britain would no longer be deprived of cochlear implants.

Given more research and development, many profoundly deaf people and perhaps even children born deaf will greatly benefit from implants. Although it seems improbable that they will ever restore perfect hearing, electronics and the science of sound are advancing so rapidly that in the middle or near the end of the twenty-first century there could be no more totally deaf people – just some who are hard of hearing.

The cochlear implant also relieves tinnitus in some people, and
one day it may be used specifically for that purpose. Tinnitus is one
of the most bizarre conditions ever to afflict people. With a name
derived from the Latin *tinnire*, to ring, it has no known origins and
no cure. One researcher has said that tinnitus is as much a mystery
and a problem for the specialist medical practitioner as it is for the
patient. It can involve roaring, hissing, buzzing, thundering, whis-
tling and shrieking, and sometimes a combination of these. Some of
the noises in this bedlam are constant, others pulsatory. All of them
vary in pitch and intensity.

I have had to endure this searing cacophony almost daily since
that dreadful time in hospital in Liverpool just after losing my
hearing. Every morning since then, instead of my former instant,
alert anticipation of the day, I am first aware on awakening of the
intensity, pitch and type of tinnitus, and then I try to adjust to it.
On rare occasions when it is unbearable, with a jet engine noise
screaming full pitch inside my head, and combining with other
roaring noises, I take sleeping pills and try to go back to sleep. Most
days when the tinnitus is severe, I simply get up and immerse
myself in my work. Occasionally, it is less intense and more bearable.
There are even good days when there is only a roar or hiss in the
background. For me, tinnitus is as disturbing an affliction as total
deafness; and if, by some magic wand, I was to be offered an
overnight cure for just one of them, I am not sure which I would
choose.

Unfortunately only those affected and a handful of experts appreciate the intensity of tinnitus suffering. Jack Vernon, an American
expert, has said that after severe and intractable pain and severe and
intractable vertigo the worst thing is 'severe and intractable tinnitus,
for nothing robs man of the quality of life in the manner which
tinnitus does'.

Jonathan Hazell, a British consultant, says that

Many sufferers experience multiple noises apparently spread
throughout the head. These may change in pitch and intensity
and may equal in volume the loudest sounds in our environ-

ment. It is not surprising that the most stalwart citizen may disintegrate after years of such diabolical torture, and indeed suicides do occur. What is perhaps more surprising is how many sufferers manage to adapt and adjust to their tinnitus.

Some sufferers fear that they are going mad, unable to understand these apparently crazy noises in their head. Some feel isolated, unable to explain this unique form of suffering. Others feel bitter that they get so little understanding and sympathy. The overwhelming response to occasional media publicity showed that many people wanted an organization that those afflicted could belong to, seek advice from and discuss common problems and press for research with.

Clearly something needed to be done. In November 1979, I booked a large room in the House of Commons for a meeting. It was attended by hundreds of tinnitus sufferers, RNID representatives and Jonathan Hazell, the tinnitus consultant. That day we set up the British Tinnitus Association, and it has since been of great assistance to many people. With branches all over the country, it maintains an informative newsletter and keeps sufferers in touch with each other. They no longer have to suffer alone, and research into the condition is being intensified and extended.

As there is no cure, help is necessarily of limited value. Yet some progress has been made by experts including counselling, relaxation and drug therapy. The most beneficial form of treatment appears to be 'maskers', a method of feeding sound of the same frequency as the tinnitus into the ear. With careful selection, the device produces a band of noise of the appropriate frequency, content and intensity to mask the noise of the tinnitus. Much credit for persuading the medical profession to take tinnitus seriously belongs to the RNID, with its long-standing support for Hazell and his tinnitus clinic at University College London.

The RNID, an old-established organization, had an elderly feel when I first came into contact with it. After speaking at the Edinburgh conference in 1968, just after losing my hearing, my relationship with it was restricted to keeping in touch with its officers and speaking at occasional meetings.

However, in 1986, with new leaders and a more demanding membership, it became more thrusting and effective. Its Chief Executive, Mike Whitlam, gathered together a team of professional directors, clarified its image and adopted a higher profile. The Institute, he insisted, should become modern and dynamic. He was supported by an energetic, intelligent Chairman, Winifred Tumim, the mother of two deaf daughters. They put in hand plans to improve the organization and initiate campaigns to improve community services, employment opportunities and communications in technical and medical services.

I served for a while on its General Management Committee and then, in October 1987, I was elected President. As the RNID's first deaf President, I became far more involved in its activities and in particular with its campaigning in Parliament. One of our most successful joint campaigns, together with the Deaf Broadcasting Council, was for an increase in subtitled television programmes. In 1989, the subtitles on BBC's Ceefax and ITV's Oracle were teasing deaf people rather than easing their frustrations: a mere two hours per channel per day gave but a glimpse of their value. For the rest of the time, television, being two-dimensional, was almost impossible to follow because of the difficulty of lip-reading. The most important medium of communication was largely inaccessible to some 300,000 severely deaf people who found it extremely difficult to follow speech on television.

In 1990, a Broadcasting Bill was presented to Parliament to establish a franchise for Channel 3 and the new Channel 5. A provision of the Bill required that there should be at least a 10 per cent increase in the average number of hours subtitled compared with the year before the new franchise took effect. This meant a statutory requirement for just another twelve minutes per channel per day – a pathetic improvement.

When I raised the point in the debate on the Bill, the Minister handling it, David Mellor, now at the Home Office, interjected to assure me that the Independent Television Commission (ITC) would set an increasing target in subsequent years. I explained that the words already in the Bill – 'a greater increase' – could be interpreted to mean one as little as 0.1 per cent by reluctant ITC executives, particularly if they were pushed by TV moguls concerned about the extra costs.

Mellor again seemed sympathetic. When I met him in the corridor later he said he would do what he could to help. True to his word, at the committee stage he said he had changed the proposal so that with the new franchise 50 per cent of all ITV programmes would have to be subtitled by 1998, and the ITC would be exhorted to build on that.

This decisive change of Government policy was heart-warming to those of us who had campaigned on subtitling. It meant that deaf people would share in and enjoy much more of the rich variety of entertainment and information provided by television. Personally I derive great pleasure from subtitled plays and films, and find subtitled news and current affairs programmes invaluable.

Unlike most other disabilities, deafness has several distinct groups of sufferers. The vast majority of Britain's 7 million deaf people have lost some hearing over time, and many of them can escape the full force of deafness by using a hearing aid. Others lose so much hearing that they have no escape route, but there are only some 5,000 deafened people with virtually no hearing. They do, however, have language, and the written word remains available. Those born totally or profoundly deaf, some 50,000, form another distinct group. Their language difficulties and limited education usually meant a restricted and paternalistic way of life which at one time was passively accepted. This began to change in the 1980s when the National Union of the Deaf, led by a young and vigorous deaf man, Paddy Ladd, campaigned for recognition of their own distinctive culture, especially the use of sign language.

They were influenced by the activities of deaf people in the United States, particularly at Gallaudet University in Washington, DC. The world's only liberal arts university for deaf students, it has provided high academic qualifications for many intelligent deaf people. Signing is the basic form of communication at Gallaudet; all the classes are conducted using signs, finger-spelling and the spoken word simultaneously. People who can hear are the odd ones out. On our first visit in 1977, Pauline and I found that deaf students and staff conversed with impressive fluency, unselfconsciously using sign language as their natural means of communication. Even those members of staff who had hearing signed as they talked together, partly from habit but also to include deaf colleagues. The atmosphere was happy, relaxed and brisk as some 1,500 young deaf people enriched their minds and social life in this unique institution of learning.

On that first visit we had a strange feeling of being in a different world. Our guide introduced us to various deaf students who smilingly addressed us in rapid sign language. I had to explain that I was unable to sign, so the students spoke slowly for me so that I could lip-read. They were patient and good humoured, but I felt I was disabled whereas they were not.

In 1977, Gallaudet honoured me with an Honorary Degree. During the ceremony in Washington's Roman Catholic Cathedral, the graduates were animated as they received their degrees. Pauline was particularly struck by the strange, silent liveliness of the great cathedral. Outside in the sunshine, hundreds of students and their families gaily celebrated their educational achievements. On that day, deafness was both natural and irrelevant to them, although they were soon to enter a new and perhaps alien world where, despite their qualifications, they would certainly find their disability a burden. Yet at Gallaudet, they had been given not only an education but confidence and faith in themselves, so lacking in many deaf people. They were fortunate.

The extent of their confidence could be judged by a demonstration in March 1988 which gripped the attention of the US media and changed the course of Gallaudet University. Although it had had only four Presidents since its Congressional charter in 1964, and one, Ed Merrill, served with distinction for fourteen years, there were two between 1983 and 1988. When the last of these resigned for a business appointment after a relatively short time, the students felt it was time for radical change; for them that meant a deaf President. Another hearing President, they argued, would be as unacceptable and paternalistic as it would be to have a white President of a nearby predominantly black college.

At a large rally on the campus they pressed their demand, but the Board of Trustees rejected it. Despite having two deaf applicants out of three on the final short list, they chose the hearing person. The board argued that Elizabeth Zinser had better administrative experience than the other two candidates. She was the one with hearing. None of this impressed the students; they blocked the entrances to the university, closing it completely, marched to the Capitol a mile away, and later to the White House. They had a persuasive argument: 'The blacks already have their black college Presidents, the women have female ones, and we want a deaf one.' Their silent, firm campaign, given vast media coverage, caught the imagination of the USA and won widespread public support there and abroad.

They got their deaf President. After Ms Zinser resigned, without having been allowed to set foot in the university, Dr King Jordan, a warm and intelligent deafened man, was appointed President. The students of Gallaudet had proved that they had the character, will and confidence to determine the leadership of their university. By their campaign, they won not only the battle but respect from the public.

Such remarkable victories for the rights of deaf people are rare in any country. This disability does not lend itself to drama, still less to victories. So often deaf people are defeated by the limitations and frustrations imposed by deafness. To be deaf in a hearing world is to be an alien. It is victory enough for some deaf people to be accepted as part of a community. Yet, as Gallaudet University has shown, deafness need not anchor people. Deaf people, even the totally deaf, can cope. Public respect can be won. Deafness, a disability which can devastate, nevertheless poses a challenge which can be met and conquered.

20

Looking Back

It is relatively rare for a person's life to be divided into two fundamentally different parts as mine has been. Until I was forty-five, I felt that life, for all its vicissitudes, was a joy. Any disappointment, frustration, anger or regret was superseded by a *joie de vivre*, extrovert eagerness and lively optimism that were never dimmed for long. I had a voracious appetite for living.

The sudden, devastating onset of total deafness and acute tinnitus changed all that. Not to the extent of making me morose or pessimistic; nor did I lose my love of life. The change was more subtle than that. I was forced into a different mould. Deafness became not merely a facet of my life but a profound and dominant influence. Like a shaken kaleidoscope, my life pattern was suddenly redrawn, leading me to adopt a new perspective.

Although my sense of humour remained unchanged, repartee and banter, which marked many of my relationships, became difficult. The loss of this lubricant, and the need to concentrate intently on lip-reading, made me appear more solemn than I felt. Gradually I began to seek normality. Total deafness, however, is an abnormality, and maintaining a balance between realistic acceptance and dogged defiance required dexterity.

Acceptance of a profound disability can bring peace of mind. Yet it can also induce passivity. This is alien to my nature and upbringing. Acceptance was not a genuine option for me, but my capacity to fight back was drastically diminished, at least in the beginning. A

(356)

blow to the morale can be as devastating as one to the body. Total deafness is no insignificant matter, and I faced the wreck of my hopes, as well as the loss of my hearing.

I felt this nowhere more devastatingly than at a conference of my trade union in the Isle of Man, just months after deciding to attempt to retrieve my political career. Determined, with the matchless help of Pauline, I had struggled through the formal sessions. But during a party at the end of conference, as I watched everyone laughing and joking and dancing, including Pauline, I began tumbling towards depression. For the first time in my life, I was with people but not of them. Physically a part of that occasion, I felt totally apart, no longer having a rapport with those to whom I had an affinity. In addition to the wreck of my political career, I was witnessing the collapse of valued relationships.

I was angry with the burden of deafness, the loss of a vital faculty, the disdain of the public and the indifference of some friends. None of this made for tranquillity but it helped fire my resolution and boost my adrenalin.

The main deprivation of deafness is not, as many imagine, the loss of music and birdsong, sad though that is, but the severing of easy communication. It is the end of radio, the emptiness of television, the difficulty of small-talk, the absence of conversational nuances and the lack of company which mark the mind. Deafness separates humans from humankind

No one can reasonably expect the public to understand total deafness. I am sometimes bewildered by it myself. But with the right kind of help, a person deprived of all hearing can still get by. What matters is the support he gets, the attitude of people and, above all, his own determination. These are the means of escaping from the apparently inescapable, and rejoining society. Blessed with a marvellous wife and family, I got by better than most.

In truth two families were supporting me. In Epsom, Pauline gave all she had to give, and our daughters were a constant source of encouragement. In addition, in Widnes, Mam and my sisters could not have been more helpful. Mam had watched my early development with a mixture of apprehension and pride. She worried at first that I was so outspoken in public, yet delighted that, despite the poverty, I became the youngest councillor and trade union leader in Widnes. It must have been the zenith of her aspirations when I was elected to Parliament, although I suspect she then raised them further and assumed I would become a Minister.

Mam gave me more than encouragement. Her example, shy courage and quiet resolution affected me. Unknowingly, in those early years, I was absorbing her spirit of gentle defiance, and if my own attitude to adversity lacked gentleness, it at least embodied defiance. I can only imagine how she felt when I lost my hearing and said I was resigning. All her hopes and ideals for me were shattered overnight. She saw me overcome the initial problems of being a deaf MP, and I am thankful for that; but I shall always be sorry that she did not live to see my major campaigns or the rest of my career in Parliament.

My twenty-five years in Parliament were a mixture of sadness and achievement. I was never reconciled to the deafness which prevented me from savouring the great Parliamentary occasions, especially in the years before I got Palantype. I also missed the minor dramas, irreverent asides, witty interjections and spontaneous laughter at unexpected quips. I was part of it but out of it.

Fortunately, the House of Commons is a unique arena, able to accommodate diverse individuals. MPs are guided into roles by their experience, inclination or luck. Each makes a choice and decides what to be – Ministerial aspirant, loyal party supporter, rebel martyr, constituency specialist, headline catcher, political blunderbuss, Parliamentary rapier, champion of the needy, friend of the greedy, conscience of the party, scourge of the Government, left-wing radical, right-wing die-hard or all things to all men.

I accepted that many of these roles were not for me. Deafness had removed the most desired one – Ministerial aspirant. But I might have tripped before getting office even had I retained my hearing, or handled a post badly had I got one. The loss of opportunity, however, is something I shall always regret – although not in any deeply disturbing way, because life has been too busy for such brooding.

Every politician wants to further the cause he or she believes in, and Ministerial office is a major way of achieving that. But it can be a fickle one; Ministers are often less powerful than they seem. They can be shunted into uncongenial posts and be vulnerable to the constraints of the Treasury and the whims of a Prime Minister. Their jobs are worth having, but not worth pining for. One way to negate an MP's opportunities is to hanker after office. Without office there is more time to pursue important human issues. Deafness meant an enforced exchange of opportunities for me.

Despite my deafness I was able to be more than a spectator in Parliament, voicing my beliefs, fighting my corner and making a constructive contribution. For all its dramatic impact on my life, deafness did not prevent me from participating in the House of Commons, that great theatre of remarkable and unremarkable talents. In no other place would I have simultaneously experienced friendship, hostility, humour, boredom, loyalty and intrigue – sometimes all in the same day. The House of Commons is a perpetual drama. Six hundred and fifty Members play their roles, yet, by some unerring instinct, the House seems able to evaluate each one accurately.

At Westminster, I learned of the ordinariness of great men and women. Gifted statesmen and outstanding politicians discarded their greatness in the tea room, smoking room or committee. Only the most obsequious MPs treated them differently, yet talent was recognized and respected.

Entering Parliament in 1966 was the stuff of my dreams. I felt a sizzling exuberance, an uplift of the spirit and a glowing excitement I had not known before. Sensing the history pervading Westminster, I wondered how the leading lights compared with giants of the past. Did we have a Disraeli, a Churchill or a Bevan? At that stage in my career it was impossible to tell. Orators like Michael Foot and Enoch Powell were always a delight to hear. Harold Wilson, then in his heyday, mastered the House and dominated the Opposition. Personalities like Ted Heath, Willie Whitelaw, George Brown, Tony Crosland and Roy Jenkins added their own distinctive colour. They were the leading players on an exciting stage, and I looked forward to working in the political cast.

(359)

From then on I saw leaders and Ministers come and go. Most were aware of the transience of fame. But for those who believed their own propaganda, or became infected by the trappings of office, there was always the banana skin of a reshuffle, or the catapult of a disastrous General Election. The most effective antidote to pomposity is loss of power. Few sights equalled the incredulity and dismay of the over-mighty when they were transformed overnight from Government to Opposition.

The set-piece party battles, important in the struggle for power, rarely lived long in the mind. Often they were anticlimactic, however distinguished some speeches were. It was individual contributions which left a mark, and everyone has their own treasured memories.

Mine include the amiable Geoffrey Howe wielding a civilized political dagger to assassinate his Prime Minister, Margaret Thatcher; Roland Boyes passionately advocating euthanasia after the agonizing death of his mother; and Margaret Thatcher rendering her political swan-song.

The House has been variously described as living history, a fun factory, the nation's greatest debating chamber and a workshop. It can be all of these things, but above all it is a democratic forum. Governments don't decide policy in the House but they explain it there, and are sometimes forced to change it.

In a troubled world, the House of Commons is an enduring beacon. Some people scoff at its ancient traditions and archaic procedures, its rhetorical careerists and occasional eccentrics. Yet the House is indispensable to our freedom. For twenty-six years I participated, espoused causes, represented individuals, questioned Ministers and supported my party. From eager young backbencher to retiring old Member, I always regarded it as a remarkable privilege. I experienced pleasure and anger, enthusiasm and frustration, a sense of accomplishment and a sense of failure – all in the company of people I miss. For me, the sight of Big Ben and the House, symbols of those people, years and events, always bring a twinkle to the eye and a catch to the throat.

Index